Drug Hepatotoxicity

Editor

VINOD K. RUSTGI

CLINICS IN
LIVER DISEASE

www.liver.theclinics.com

Consulting Editor
NORMAN GITLIN

February 2017 • Volume 21 • Number 1

ELSEVIER

1600 John F. Kennedy Boulevard • Suite 1800 • Philadelphia, Pennsylvania, 19103-2899

http://www.theclinics.com

CLINICS IN LIVER DISEASE Volume 21, Number 1
February 2017 ISSN 1089-3261, ISBN-13: 978-0-323-49652-0

Editor: Kerry Holland
Developmental Editor: Meredith Clinton

Clinics in Liver Disease (ISSN 1089-3261) is published quarterly by Elsevier Inc., 360 Park Avenue South, New York, NY 10010-1710. Months of issue are February, May, August, and November. Business and Editorial Offices: 1600 John F. Kennedy Blvd., Ste. 1800, Philadelphia, PA 19103-2899. Customer Service Office: 3251 Riverport Lane, Maryland Heights, MO 63043. Periodicals postage paid at New York, NY and additional mailing offices. Subscription prices are $281.00 per year (U.S. individuals), $100.00 per year (U.S. student/resident), $476.00 per year (U.S. institutions), $403.00 per year (international individuals), $200.00 per year (international student/resident), $590.00 per year (international instituitions), $347.00 per year (Canadian individuals), $200.00 per year (Canadian student/resident), and $590.00 per year (Canadian institutions). Foreign air speed delivery is included in all *Clinics* subscription prices. All prices are subject to change without notice. **POSTMASTER:** Send address changes to *Clinics in Liver Disease*, Elsevier Health Sciences Division, Subscription Customer Service, 3251 Riverport Lane, Maryland Heights, MO 63043. **Customer Service: Telephone: 1-800-654-2452 (U.S. and Canada); 314-447-8871 (outside U.S. and Canada). Fax: 314-447-8029. E-mail: journalscustomer service-usa@elsevier.com (for print support); journalsonlinesupport-usa@elsevier.com (for online support).**

Reprints. For copies of 100 or more of articles in this publication, please contact the Commercial Reprints Department, Elsevier Inc., 360 Park Avenue South, New York, NY 10010-1710. Tel.: 212-633-3874; Fax: 212-633-3820; E-mail: reprints@elsevier.com.

Clinics in Liver Disease is covered in *MEDLINE/PubMed (Index Medicus)*, Science Citation Index Expanded, Journal Citation Reports/Science Edition, and Current Contents/Clinical Medicine.

Contributors

CONSULTING EDITOR

NORMAN GITLIN, MD, FRCP (LONDON), FRCPE (EDINBURGH), FAASLD, FACP, FACG
Formerly, Professor of Medicine, Chief of Hepatology, Emory University; Currently, Consultant, Atlanta Gastroenterology Associates, Atlanta, Georgia

EDITOR

VINOD K. RUSTGI, MD, MBA
Clinical Chief of Gastroenterology/Director of Hepatology; Professor of Medicine, Robert Wood Johnson School of Medicine; Professor of Epidemiology, Robert Wood Johnson School of Public Health, New Brunswick, New Jersey

AUTHORS

JAWAD AHMAD, MD, FRCP, FAASLD
Professor of Medicine, Division of Liver Diseases, Icahn School of Medicine at Mount Sinai, New York, New York

OMAR ABDULHAMEED ALMAZROO, MSc, CCTS
Department of Pharmaceutical Sciences, University of Pittsburgh School of Pharmacy, Pittsburgh, Pennsylvania

CHALERMRAT BUNCHORNTAVAKUL, MD
Division of Gastroenterology and Hepatology, Department of Medicine, University of Pennsylvania, Philadelphia, Pennsylvania; Assistant Professor, Division of Gastroenterology and Hepatology, Department of Medicine, Rajavithi Hospital, College of Medicine, Rangsit University, Bangkok, Thailand

NAGA P. CHALASANI, MD, FACG
David W. Crabb Professor and Director, Division of Gastroenterology and Hepatology, Department of Medicine, Indiana University School of Medicine, Indianapolis, Indiana

YNTO S. DE BOER, MD
Liver Diseases Branch, National Institute of Diabetes and Digestive and Kidney Diseases, National Institutes of Health, Bethesda, Maryland; Department of Gastroenterology and Hepatology, VU University Medical Center, Amsterdam, The Netherlands

MICHAEL A. DUNN, MD
Division of Gastroenterology, Hepatology and Nutrition, Center for Liver Diseases, University of Pittsburgh, Pittsburgh, Pennsylvania

ALISON JAZWINSKI FAUST, MD, MHS
Assistant Professor, Department of Medicine, Division of Gastroenterology, Hepatology and Nutrition, University of Pittsburgh Medical Center, University of Pittsburgh School of Medicine, Pittsburgh, Pennsylvania

SWAYTHA GANESH, MD
Thomas Starzl Transplantation Institute, University of Pittsburgh, Pittsburgh, Pennsylvania

HUMBERTO C. GONZALEZ, MD
Department of Transplant Surgery/Center of Advanced Liver Disease, Methodist University Hospital, University of Tennessee Health Science Center, Memphis, Tennessee

ZACHARY D. GOODMAN, MD, PhD
Director, Liver Pathology Research and Consultation, Center for Liver Diseases, Inova Fairfax Hospital, Falls Church, Virginia

STUART C. GORDON, MD
Division of Gastroenterology and Hepatology, Henry Ford Health System, Detroit, Michigan

ALBERT GOUGH, PhD
Research Associate Professor, Department of Computational and Systems Biology, University of Pittsburgh Drug Discovery Institute, Pittsburgh, Pennsylvania

SHAHID HABIB, MD
Staff Physician, Department of Medicine, Southern Arizona Veterans Affairs Health Care System, Tucson, Arizona

ABHINAV HUMAR, MD
Thomas Starzl Transplantation Institute, University of Pittsburgh, Pittsburgh, Pennsylvania

CARLO J. IASELLA, PharmD
Department of Pharmacy and Therapeutics, University of Pittsburgh School of Pharmacy, Pittsburgh, Pennsylvania

SYED-MOHAMMED JAFRI, MD
Division of Gastroenterology and Hepatology, Henry Ford Health System, Detroit, Michigan

HEATHER J. JOHNSON, PharmD
Department of Pharmacy and Therapeutics, University of Pittsburgh School of Pharmacy, Pittsburgh, Pennsylvania

XIAOCHAO MA, PhD
Department of Pharmaceutical Sciences, University of Pittsburgh School of Pharmacy, Pittsburgh, Pennsylvania

MOHAMMAD KOWSER MIAH, PhD
Department of Pharmaceutical Sciences, University of Pittsburgh School of Pharmacy, Pittsburgh, Pennsylvania

JOSEPH A. ODIN, MD, PhD, FAASLD
Division of Liver Diseases, Icahn School of Medicine at Mount Sinai, New York, New York

K. RAJENDER REDDY, MD
Ruimy Family President's Distinguished Professor of Medicine and Surgery; Director of Hepatology; Director, Liver Transplantation, Viral Hepatitis Center, University of Pennsylvania, Philadelphia, Pennsylvania

HEMAMALA SAITHANYAMURTHI, MD
Department of Medicine, Division of Gastroenterology, Hepatology and Nutrition, University of Pittsburgh Medical Center, University of Pittsburgh School of Medicine, Pittsburgh, Pennsylvania

OBAID S. SHAIKH, MD, FRCP
Section of Gastroenterology, Department of Medicine, Veterans Affairs Pittsburgh Healthcare System; Division of Gastroenterology, Hepatology, and Nutrition, University of Pittsburgh School of Medicine, Pittsburgh, Pennsylvania

AMINA IBRAHIM SHEHU, BS
Department of Pharmaceutical Sciences, University of Pittsburgh School of Pharmacy, Pittsburgh, Pennsylvania

AVERELL H. SHERKER, MD, FRCPC, FAASLD
Liver Diseases Research Branch, Division of Digestive Diseases and Nutrition, National Institute of Diabetes and Digestive and Kidney Diseases, National Institutes of Health, Bethesda, Maryland

JONATHAN G. STINE, MD, MSc, FACP
Division of Gastroenterology and Hepatology, Department of Medicine, University of Virginia, Charlottesville, Virginia

D. LANSING TAYLOR, PhD
Professor, Department of Computational and Systems Biology, University of Pittsburgh Drug Discovery Institute, University of Pittsburgh Cancer Institute, Pittsburgh, Pennsylvania

AMIT TEVAR, MD
Thomas Starzl Transplantation Institute, University of Pittsburgh, Pittsburgh, Pennsylvania

RAMAN VENKATARAMANAN, PhD
Department of Pharmaceutical Sciences, School of Pharmacy; Department of Pathology, University of Pittsburgh Medical Center, Thomas Starzl Transplantation Institute, University of Pittsburgh, Pittsburgh, Pennsylvania

LAWRENCE A. VERNETTI, PhD
Research Associate Professor, Department of Computational and Systems Biology, University of Pittsburgh Drug Discovery Institute, Pittsburgh, Pennsylvania

ANDREAS VOGT, PhD
Associate Professor, Department of Computational and Systems Biology, University of Pittsburgh Drug Discovery Institute, Pittsburgh, Pennsylvania

Contents

Omar Abdulhameed Almazroo, Mohammad Kowser Miah, and
Raman Venkataramanan

Metabolism is a biotransformation process, where endogenous and exogenous compounds are converted to more polar products to facilitate their elimination from the body. The process of metabolism is divided into 3 phases. Phase I metabolism involves functionalization reactions. Phase II drug metabolism is a conjugation reaction. Phase III refers to transporter-mediated elimination of drug and/or metabolites from body normally via liver, gut, kidney, or lung. This review presents basic information on drug-metabolizing enzymes and potential factors that might affect the metabolic capacities of the enzyme or alter drug response or drug-mediated toxicities.

Hemamala Saithanyamurthi and Alison Jazwinski Faust

Drug-induced liver injury (DILI) is a term used to describe a spectrum of clinical presentations and severity that ranges from mild elevation of liver enzymes on routine blood work to acute liver failure and death. Approximately 10% of all patients with DILI develop acute liver failure resulting in death or liver transplantation. DILI may be prolonged with persistence of elevated liver enzymes for longer than 6 months in approximately 5% to 20% of cases. Cirrhosis and long-term liver-related morbidity and mortality have also been described but are rare, occurring in 1% to 3% of cases.

Amina Ibrahim Shehu, Xiaochao Ma, and Raman Venkataramanan

Drug-induced hepatotoxicity (DIH) is a significant cause of acute liver failure and liver transplantation. Diagnosis is challenging due to the idiosyncratic nature, its presentation in the form of other liver disease, and the lack of a definite diagnostic criteria. Generation of reactive metabolites, oxidative stress, and mitochondrial dysfunction are common mechanisms involved in DIH. Certain risk factors associated with a drug and within an individual further predispose patients to DIH.

Jawad Ahmad and Joseph A. Odin

Idiosyncratic drug-induced liver injury (DILI) from prescription medications and herbal and dietary supplements has an annual incidence rate of approximately 20 cases per 100,000 per year. However, the risk of DILI varies greatly according to the drug. In the United States and Europe, antimicrobials are the commonest implicated agents, with amoxicillin/clavulanate the most common, whereas in Asian countries, herbal and dietary supplements predominate. Genetic analysis of DILI is currently limited, but multiple polymorphisms of human leukocyte antigen genes and genes involved in drug metabolism and transport have been identified as risk factors for DILI.

Hepatotoxic adverse drug reactions are associated with significant morbidity and mortality and are the leading cause of postmarketing regulatory action in the United States. They are classified as Type A (intrinsic) or Type B (idiosyncratic). Type A are predictable, dose-related toxicities, often identified in preclinical or clinical trials, and usually occur in overdose settings or with pre-existing hepatic impairment. Type B are not clearly related to increasing dose and are associated with drug-specific and patient-specific characteristics and environmental risks. Rare Type B reactions are often identified postmarketing. Identification and management, including electronic resources, has evolved.

Drug hepatotoxicity can simulate nearly any clinical syndrome or pathologic lesion that may occur in the liver, so clinical and histopathologic diagnosis of drug-induced liver injury may be difficult. Nevertheless, most drugs that are known to idiosyncratic liver injury tend to cause patterns of injury that produce characteristic phenotypes. Recognition of these patterns or phenotypes in liver biopsy material is helpful in evaluation of clinical cases of suspected drug-induced liver injury.

Drug-induced liver injury presents as various forms of acute and chronic liver disease. There is wide geographic variation in the most commonly implicated agents. Smoking can induce cytochrome P450 enzymes but this does not necessarily translate into clinically relevant drug-induced liver injury. Excessive alcohol consumption is a clear risk factor for intrinsic hepatotoxicity from acetaminophen and may predispose to injury from antituberculosis medications. Understanding of the role of infection, proinflammatory states, disorders of coagulation, and the hepatic clock in predisposing patients to drug-induced liver injury is evolving. More study focusing specifically on environmental risk factors predisposing patients to drug-induced liver injury is needed.

Idiosyncratic hepatotoxicity is one of the most common reasons for an approved drug being restricted. This article focuses on hepatotoxicity of selected and recently introduced agents, such as, tyrosine kinase inhibitors, monoclonal antibodies, novel oral anticoagulants, newer antiplatelets, anti-biotics, anti-diabetics, anti-epileptics, anti-depressants, anti-psychotics and anti-retrovirals. Overall, the incidence of clinically relevant hepatotoxic-ity from newer agents seems to be lower than that of the older agents. Nevertheless, cases of severe hepatotoxicity have been reported due to some of these newer agents, including, trastuzumab, ipilimumab, infliximab, imatinib, bosutinib, dasatinib, gefitinib, erlotinib, sunitinib, ponatinib, lapati-nib, vemurafenib, dabigatran, rivaroxaban, felbamate, lamotrigine, levetira-cetam, venlafaxine, duloxetine, darunavir, and maraviroc.

Herbal and Dietary Supplement–Induced Liver Injury

Ynto S. de Boer and Averell H. Sherker

The increase in the use of herbal and dietary supplements (HDSs) over the last decades has been accompanied by an increase in the reports of HDS-associated hepatotoxicity. The spectrum of HDS-induced liver injury is diverse and the outcome may vary from transient liver test increases to fulminant hepatic failure resulting in death or requiring liver transplant. There are no validated standardized tools to establish the diagnosis, but some HDS products have a typical clinical signature that may help to iden-tify HDS-induced liver injury.

Drug-Induced Acute Liver Failure

Shahid Habib and Obaid S. Shaikh

Drug-induced acute liver failure (ALF) disproportionately affects women and nonwhites. It is most frequently caused by antimicrobials and to a lesser extent by complementary and alternative medications, antiepilep-tics, antimetabolites, nonsteroidals, and statins. Most drug-induced liver injury ALF patients have hepatocellular injury pattern. Cerebral edema and intracranial hypertension are the most serious complications of ALF. Other complications include coagulopathy, sepsis, metabolic derange-ments, and renal, circulatory, and respiratory dysfunction. Although ad-vances in intensive care have improved outcome, ALF has significant mortality without liver transplantation. Liver-assist devices may provide a bridge to transplant or to spontaneous recovery.

Management of Acute Hepatotoxicity Including Medical Agents and Liver Support Systems

Humberto C. Gonzalez, Syed-Mohammed Jafri, and Stuart C. Gordon

Drug-induced liver injury (DILI) can be predictable or idiosyncratic and has an estimated incidence of approximately 20 cases per 100,000 persons per year. DILI is a common cause of acute liver failure in the United States. No accurate tests for diagnosing DILI exist, and its diagnosis is based on exclusion of other conditions. Managing DILI includes discontinuing the suspected causative agent and in selected cases administering an anti-dote. Liver support systems are used for long-term support or as a bridge to transplantation and are effective for improving encephalopathy, hyper-bilirubinemia, and other liver-related conditions, but whether they improve survival remains uncertain.

> Living donor liver transplant (LDLT) fills a critically needed gap in the number of livers available for transplant. However, little is known about the functional recovery of the liver in the donor and in the recipient after surgery. Given that both donor and recipients are treated with several drugs, it is important to characterize the time course of recovery of hepatic synthetic, metabolic, and excretory function in these patients. In the absence of data from LDLT, information on the effect of liver disease on the pharmacokinetics of medications can be used as guidance for drug dosing in LDLT patients.

> In this article, we review the past applications of in vitro models in identifying human hepatotoxins and then focus on the use of multiscale experimental models in drug development, including the use of zebrafish and human cell-based, 3-dimensional, microfluidic systems of liver functions as key components in applying Quantitative Systems Pharmacology (QSP). We have implemented QSP as a platform to improve the rate of success in the process of drug discovery and development of therapeutics.

CLINICS IN LIVER DISEASE

Preface

Drug-induced Hepatotoxicity...A Topic Where We Don't Know Enough!

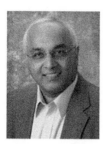

Vinod K. Rustgi, MD, MBA
Editor

Americans filled 4.3 billion prescriptions and spent nearly $374 billion on medicines in 2014. Therefore, it is important that clinicians (and others) have a recognition of drug-induced hepatotoxicity. The LiverTox database maintained by the National Institute of Diabetes and Digestive and Kidney Diseases is an important resource in this arena and will become increasingly so. As of the end of 2013, the US Food and Drug Administration (FDA) had approved 1453 drugs, and only a handful had received approval prior to creation of the FDA in 1938. Among that handful were morphine in 1827 and aspirin in 1899.

In this issue, we attempt to cover the state-of-the-art explaining epidemiology, clinical findings, pathology, and mechanisms. There are important articles on management and the specialized situation encountered in living donor liver transplants. The final article introduces clinicians to newer experimental models of hepatotoxicity, including zebrafish and a "human on a chip."

The contributors have done an excellent job, and I hope you enjoy their hard work.

Vinod K. Rustgi, MD, MBA
Robert Wood Johnson School of Medicine
Robert Wood Johnson School of Public Health
New Brunswick, NJ 08901, USA

E-mail address:
vr262@rwjms.rutgers.edu

Clin Liver Dis 21 (2017) xiii
http://dx.doi.org/10.1016/j.cld.2016.10.001
1089-3261/17/© 2016 Published by Elsevier Inc.

Drug Metabolism in the Liver

Omar Abdulhameed Almazroo, MSc, CCTS[a], Mohammad Kowser Miah, PhD[a],
Raman Venkataramanan, PhD[b,c],*

KEYWORDS

- Drug metabolism • Cytochrome P450 • Conjugation • Drug transporters
- Liver metabolism • Phase I, II, and III metabolism enzyme

KEY POINTS

- Drug metabolism typically results in the formation of a more hydrophilic compound that is readily excreted by the liver, kidney, and/or gut.
- Drug metabolism involves chemical biotransformation of drug molecules by enzymes in the body; in addition, drug transporters facilitate movement of drugs and metabolites in and out of cells/organs.
- In rare cases, a metabolite formed from a drug can cause hepatotoxicity.
- Several disease states and altered physiologic conditions can affect the efficiency of the drug metabolic or transport processes.
- Certain pathophysiologic conditions and use of certain concomitant medications can alter the metabolism or transport of drugs and metabolites and result in altered pharmacokinetic and/or pharmacodynamics of certain drugs.

INTRODUCTION

Drugs are typically small molecules that are generally classified as xenobiotics, which are foreign to the human body. Several endogenous molecules, however, such as steroids and hormones, are also used for the treatment of certain disease conditions and are also referred to as drugs. The term, *metabolism*, refers to the process of transformation of chemicals from one chemical moiety to another by an enzyme. The most well-known drug-metabolizing enzymes are cytochrome P450s (CYP450s), which

The authors have nothing to disclose.
[a] Department of Pharmaceutical Sciences, School of Pharmacy, University of Pittsburgh, 731 Salk Hall, 3501 Terrace Street, Pittsburgh, PA 15261, USA; [b] Department of Pharmaceutical Sciences, School of Pharmacy, University of Pittsburgh, 718 Salk Hall, 3501 Terrace Street, Pittsburgh, PA 15261, USA; [c] Department of Pathology, University of Pittsburgh Medical Center, Thomas Starzl Transplantation Institute, University of Pittsburgh, Pittsburgh, PA, USA
* Corresponding author. Department of Pharmaceutical Sciences, School of Pharmacy, University of Pittsburgh, 718 Salk Hall, 3501 Terrace Street, Pittsburgh, PA 15261.
E-mail address: RV@pitt.edu

are mainly oxidases, reductases, and hydrolases. The primary purpose of metabolism is to clear endogenous and/or exogenous molecules from the body. Typically, the process of metabolism converts lipophilic chemicals to hydrophilic products to facilitate elimination.[1,2] In certain instances, however, drug-metabolizing enzymes convert substances into their pharmacologically active form. For example, prodrugs (pharmacologically inactive) are synthesized to overcome absorption/bioavailability issues and they are converted to activate drug after being absorbed into the body. To overcome the low bioavailability of ampicillin, pivampicillin is synthesized as a prodrug, which can be hydrolyzed into ampicillin after being absorbed into the blood stream. Another important example of a prodrug is the use of mycophenolate mofetil to increase the oral bioavailability of mycophenolic acid.[3] Mycophenolic acid is used as immunosuppressant in transplant recipient to prevent acute rejection.[4]

The by-products of metabolism are known as metabolites; they can be either pharmacologically active or inactive.[5] CYP450 enzymes that play a major role in drug elimination are mainly present on the smooth endoplasmic reticulum (ER) and mitochondria of the hepatocytes and small intestinal epithelia and to a lesser extent in the proximal tubules of the kidneys.[6] The contribution and importance of conjugating enzymes and drug transporters are increasingly appreciated.[7] These pathways interplay during the absorption, distribution, metabolism, and excretion of drugs, and any alterations may result in changes in the pharmacokinetics and pharmacodynamics of a drug.

This article discusses the major drug-metabolizing/eliminating pathways: phase I, phase II, and phase III (**Table 1**). Additionally, the contribution of the primary organs (liver, gut, and kidneys) involved in drug metabolism is reviewed. In the last part, major factors that could affect these pathways are summarized.

DRUG METABOLISM PATHWAYS
Phase I Pathway

The most common phase I drug-metabolizing enzymes are represented by CYP450 superfamily. CYP450s are the major group of enzymes that chemically modify drugs

Table 1
Summary of main role of liver, gut, and kidneys in the 3 drug metabolism pathways

	Liver	Gut	Kidneys
Pathway I	Hepatic CYP450s are very important in metabolism of xenobiotics and endogenous molecules.	Enterocytes contain enzymes that can metabolize xenobiotics.	Minimal metabolism activity but important in steroid metabolism
Pathway II	Liver expresses UGTs and other conjugation enzymes; UGTs metabolize approximately 40%–70% of the xenobiotics.	Intestinal enterocytes participate in phase II drug metabolism as well.	Kidney also makes significant contribution in phase II drug metabolism, but GST is the main conjugating enzyme in kidney.
Pathway III	Drug transporters uptake compounds into hepatocytes and efflux into bile.	P-gp is well known to decrease the bioavailability of several drugs because of efflux mechanism into the gut.	They are important to actively efflux drugs into the urine.

into their water-soluble products to facilitate the excretion by kidney and/or liver.[1] In the late 1980s, Nebert developed and reported a nomenclature system for CYP450 enzymes. Human CYP450 genes comprise more than 115 gene and pseudogene members and are among the most extensively annotated mammalian genes, starting from CYP1A1 and currently ending with CYP51P3.[8,9] In humans, CYP450s are distributed throughout various tissues and organs, including peripheral blood cells, platelets, aorta, adrenal glands, adipose tissues, nasal tissue, vaginal tissues, seminal vesicles, brain, lung, kidneys, gut, and liver. Of all the various tissues, liver and small intestine contribute to the maximum extent to the overall metabolism and elimination of drugs. Among all the CYP450 enzymes in human liver, CYP3A4 is the most abundant, followed by CYP2E1 and CYP2C9, representing approximately 22.1%, 15.3%, and 14.6% of the total CYP450s (based on protein content), respectively (**Fig. 1**).[10] CYP450 enzymes also may be classified based on their major substrates, such as sterols, xenobiotics, fatty acids, eicosanoids, vitamins, and unknown substrates.[8]

CYP450 enzymes catalyze several reactions, including oxidation, sulphoxidation, aromatic hydroxylation, aliphatic hydroxylation, N-dealkylation, O-dealkylation, and deamination. Among all, oxidation is the primary reaction, which leads to addition of 1 or more oxygen atom(s) to the parent drug.[2] The CYP450-mediated oxidation process is chemically represented in the following scheme:

$$NADPH + H^+ + O_2 + RH \xrightarrow{CYP450} NADP^+ + H_2O + ROH \ ,$$

where, *NADPH*, *RH*, and *ROH* are nicotinamide adenine dinucleotide phosphate (a cofactor), any oxidizable substrate, and the oxidized metabolite, respectively.

Reduction of the parent compounds is another pathway of phase I drug metabolism. This type of reaction is coupled with secondary enzymatic system that is known to be either NADH cytochrome-b_5 reductase system or NADPH cytochrome-c reductase. This route is important for metabolizing aromatic nitro, nitroso, azo, and N-oxide compounds. Hydrolysis of the parent compounds is also carried out by certain CYP450s, particularly in case of esters and amides.

CYP450s expression is regulated in different compartments of the cell, nuclei, or cytosol by many factors. Nuclear receptor–mediated regulation of gene expression occurs in the nucleus, which is the most critical regulatory pathway, resulting in

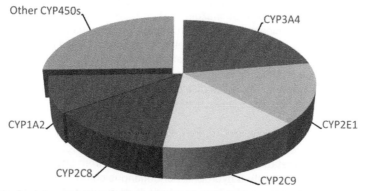

Fig. 1. Pie chart showing the expression of various CYP450 enzymes in the liver in the human. (*Data from* Achour B, Barber J, Rostami-Hodjegan A. Expression of hepatic drug-metabolizing cytochrome p450 enzymes and their intercorrelations: a meta-analysis. Drug Metab Dispos 2014;42(8):1352.)

differential gene transcription. Aryl hydrocarbon receptor is a receptor activated by several endogenous and exogenous ligands, which activates the gene translation and synthesis of various CYP450s.[11] Both pregnane X receptor (PXR) (NR1I2 [nuclear receptor subfamily 1, group I, member 2]) and constitutive androstane receptor (CAR) (NR1I3 [nuclear receptor subfamily 1, group I, member 3]) play similar roles in the regulation of expression of several important CYP450s.[12–16]

In the cytosol, cofactors, such as NADPH-Cytochrome P450 reductase; cytochrome-b_5 reductase; and/or cytochrome-c reductase, are essential to carry out the biotransformation reactions. Iron is important for CYP450s synthesis and is present in the center of the binding site between the enzyme and substrate.[2,17] Thus, the different statuses of all these regulators affect the functional activity of CYP450s, resulting in interindividual and intraindividual variability in the metabolic capacity in a population. Consequently, differences in the pharmacologic responses to the same dose of a drug may result due to differences in metabolism and elimination of drugs.[18]

Apart from CYP450 enzymes, other phase I enzymes can contribute to the clearance of many drugs. Some examples of non-CYP450 enzymes that could metabolize endogenous molecules and xenobiotics include flavin-containing monooxygenases, monoamine oxidases, molybdenum hydroxylases, alcohol dehydrogenases, aldehyde dehydrogenases, aldo-keto reductase, NADPH:quinone reductases, and hydrolytic enzymes.[17]

The expression and activity of CYP450 enzymes can be modulated by several factors. Increased mRNA expression leads to increased protein synthesis and a corresponding increase in the activity of enzymes. Induction of CYP450 enzymes leads to increased clearance of certain drugs, leading to decreased drug exposure and response. On the other hand, CYP450 inducers could decrease the risk of hepatotoxicity of certain drugs. Examples of inducers are rifampin and phenobarbital. Calcineurin inhibitors, such as tacrolimus and cyclosporine, and mammalian target of rapamycin inhibitors, such as sirolimus and everolimus are substrates for CYP3A.[19] Induction of CYP3A by rifampin increases their metabolism and decreases their exposure, requiring an increase in their dose.

Inhibition of CYP450 enzymes by endogenous or exogenous compounds leads to a decreased ability of the enzyme to clear the drug. CYP450 inhibitors can drastically increase the blood levels of various substrates of CYP450 enzymes, leading to toxicity. Inhibitors of CYP450 enzymes include azole antifungals; HIV protease inhibitors, such as ritonavir; and certain hepatitis C virus (HCV) drugs.[19,20] Coadministration of azole antifungals, such as ketoconazole, and protease inhibitors, such as ritonavir, lead to decrease in the clearance of certain drugs due to inhibition of CYP enzymes requiring a decrease in drug dosing. A typical dose of tacrolimus in a transplant patient not on ritonavir is 3 mg, twice a day. In patients on lopinavir and ritonavir (Kaletra, North Chicago, IL), it is sufficient to give less than 1 mg once a week to achieve comparable trough blood concentrations of tacrolimus.[21] (More information about substrates, inhibitors, and inducers is discussed later and in **Table 2**).

Phase II Pathways

During phase II drug metabolism, the drugs or metabolites from phase I pathways are enzymatically conjugated with a hydrophilic endogenous compound with the help of transferase enzymes. The most common phase II drug-metabolizing enzymes are UDP-glucuronosyltransferases (UGTs), sulfotransferases (SULTs), *N*-acetyltransferases (NATs), glutathione S-transferases (GSTs), thiopurine S-methyltransferases (TPMTs), and catechol O-methyltransferases (COMTs).

Table 2
List of well-known substrates, inhibitors, and inducers for phase I, II, and III metabolism pathways

Enzymes	Substrates	Inhibitors	Inducers
Phase I			
CYP3A	Midazolam, buspirone, felodipine, lovastatin, eletriptan, sildenafil, simvastatin, triazolam	Ketoconazole, clarithromycin, itraconazole, saquinavir, fluconazole, grapefruit juice, tipranavir/ritonavir	Phenytoin, rifampin, St. John's wort, efavirenz, etravirine, nafcillin, prednisone
1A2	Alosetron, caffeine, duloxetine, melatonin, ramelteon, tacrine, tizanidine	Ciprofloxacin, enoxacin, fluvoxamine, oral contraceptives, phenylpropanolamine,	Montelukast, phenytoin, smoking components of cigarettes
2C8	Repaglinide, paclitaxel	Gemfibrozil, fluvoxamine, ketoconazole, trimethoprim	Rifampin
2C9	Celecoxib, warfarin, phenytoin	Amiodarone, fluconazole, miconazole, oxandrolone, capecitabine, etravirine, fluvastatin, metronidazole, sulfinpyrazone, tigecycline	Carbamazepine, rifampin, aprepitant, bosentan, phenobarbital, St. John's wort
Phase II			
UGTs	Bilirubin, phenols, estradiols, opiates, and carboxylic acids	Paclitaxel, midazolam, cyclosporine A, ketoconazole, phenobarbital, and phenytoin	Bilirubin, phenobarbitone, rifampin
SULTs	Phenols, alcohols, and amines	Flavonoids, mefenamic acids, salicylic acids, clomiphene, and danazol	Retinoic acid, methotrexate
NATs	Para-aminobenzoic acid, para-aminosalicylic acids, para-aminoglutamate, sulfamethazine, isoniazid, hydralazine, and sulfonamides	Caffeic acid, esculetin, qurcetin, genitin, scopoletin and coumarin	Androgens, aminophylline
GSTs	Epoxides, quinone, sulfoxides, esters, and peroxides	Phenols, quinone, vitamin C derivatives, dopamine, and *trans* retinoic acid	Extracts of broccoli, cabbage, Brussels sprouts, and grapefruits
Phase III			
P-gp	Digoxin, loperamide, vinblastine, talinolol	Amlodarone, azithromycin, cyclosporine, diltiazem, dronedarone, erythromycin, itraconazole, ketoconazole, lopinavir/ritonavir, quinidine, verapamil	Avasimibe, carbamazepine, phenytoin, rifampin, St John's wort, tipranavir/ritonavir

Uridine 5′-diphospho-glucuronosyltransferases

Glucuronidation is the major phase II drug metabolism pathway, with approximately 40% to 70% of human endogenous and exogenous compounds conjugated to glucuronidated end products.[22] Conjugated products are more hydrophilic and are readily excreted from body. In the cytoplasm, glucose-1 phosphate reacts with uridine triphosphate to form uridine diphosphate glucuronic acid (UDPGA), a cosubstrate, and this is transferred into the ER by transmembrane proteins. In the ER, UGT attaches UDPGA to the appropriate substrate by nucleophilic attack, forming glucuronidated compounds. UGTs are members of a superfamily of protein, having a molecular weight in the range of 50 kDa to 60 kDa, and structurally they have a catalytic domain and a C-terminal anchoring domain. Until now, 4 families of UGTs in human have been identified: UGT1, UGT2, UGT3, and UGT8. UGT2s have been subdivided into UGT2A and UGT2B.[23]

UGTs metabolize a wide range of compounds and their substrates also overlap with each other. Based on current knowledge, UGT1A1 is the highly expressed phase II enzyme in human, which preferentially metabolizes bilirubin; UGT1A1 also metabolizes certain phenols and estradiols.[24] Whereas UGT2B7 metabolizes opiates,[25] UGT1A3, UGT1A9, and UGT2A1 metabolize carboxylic acids. Various organs express UGTs; however, UGTs are normally highly expressed in the liver and gut (see **Table 1**).

The functional activity of the UGTs is controlled by the amount of enzymes available and the amount of cosubstrate available to conjugate the drug or the metabolite. There are some drugs, such as phenobarbital and rifampin, which are known to increase the expression of UGTs and decreased drug exposure. On the other hand, competition for UGTs may lead to inhibition of metabolism and increased drug exposure.

Sulfotransferases

SULTs are another important superfamily of phase II drug-metabolizing enzymes. Although they are not as highly expressed in the body as UGTs, they are essential for metabolism of several endogenous compounds. They catalyze the reaction between 3′-phosphoadenosine 5′-phosphosulphate (PAPS) and N, O, or S atoms in targeted compounds. A wide range of endogenous compounds (steroids, catecholamine, serotonin, eicosanoids, retinol, and so forth) as well as exogenous compounds are metabolized by SULTs. An endogenous compound like dopamine is almost entirely metabolized by SULTs. Expression of SULTs in human occurs almost in every organ, most commonly found in liver, gut, breast, lung, adrenal glands, kidney, blood cells, brain, and placenta. SULTs have 2 forms; one is metabolically very important and presents in cytosol, the other one is membrane bound and metabolically less important. The function of the membrane-bound isoforms is to synthesize housekeeping substances rather than to metabolize endogenous or exogenous compounds.

Until now, 13 SULTs have been identified in humans and they have been divided into 4 families: SULT1, SULT2, SULT4, and SULT6. There are 9 members in SULT1 family, which could be further subdivided into 4 subfamilies (1A1, 1A2, 1A3, 1A4; 1B1; 1C1 and 1C2; and 1E1). On the other hand, SULT2 family has been divided into 2 subfamilies, SULT2A and SULT2B. Additionally, the SULT4 and SULT6 family contain only 1 member in each group, SULT4A1 and SULT6B1, respectively.

So far, SULT1A1 is the most extensively studied sulfation enzyme, which metabolizes phenols, alcohols, and amines. SULT1A2 and SULT1A3 also metabolize amines; aromatic amines are the primary substrates for both of these isoforms. SULT1B1 is restricted to the metabolism of thyroids hormones and some small phenolic compounds. SULT1C1 metabolizes iodothyronines, and SULT1C2 metabolizes

4-nitrophenols. Furthermore, SULT1E1 has special preference for the metabolism of estrogens, even though it has affinity for other compounds as well. There are various compounds that are reported to be inhibitors of SULTs. Curcumin is a potent inhibitor of SULT1A1. Additionally, SULT1A1 and SULT1A3 can be inhibited by various fruits juices, such as grape, orange, green tea, and black tea. Nonsteroidal anti-inflammatory drugs also have been reported to be inhibitors of SULT1A1 and SULT1E1.[26,27] Mefenamic acid, salicylic acid, clomiphene, and danazol are also potent inhibitors of SULTs.[26] There are several medications that can induce the expression of SULTs in human cells. Retinoic acid induces SULT1A1, SULT2A1, and SULT1E1 in hepatic carcinoma cells as well as in Caco-2 cells.[28] Methotrexate has been shown to have induction capability for various SULTs enzymes in human cells.

N-acetyltransferases
Unlike other enzymes, products of NATs are sometimes more lipophilic instead of being more hydrophilic (metabolites of sulfonamides). In certain situations, the metabolite itself can become more toxic than the parent compound. There are several enzymes that increase the hydrophilicity of the metabolites as well as perform housekeeping activity, such as histone acetyltransferase that regulates the expression of genes in human and other animals. Acetyltransferases in human are classified into 2 subfamilies: NAT1 and NAT2. All NATs are cytosolic enzymes and they use acetyl coenzyme A as a cofactor for metabolic reaction. Until now, 25 members of NAT1 and 27 members of NAT2 alleles have been identified in humans. NAT1 is ubiquitous enzyme, expressed in almost all tissues.

NATs have different substrate specificity and they do not overlap like other metabolizing enzymes. Para-aminobenzoic acid, para-aminosalicylic acid, and para-aminoglutamate are the main substrates for NAT1 in human. On the other hand, sulfamethazine, isoniazid, hydralazine, and sulfonamides are the common substrates for NAT2. Polyphenolic compounds are believed the main inhibitors of NATs. Compounds like caffeic acid, esculetin, qurcetin, and genitin inhibit NAT1, whereas scopoletin and coumarin are the known inhibitors of NAT2.[29] Additionally, major components of garlic, diallyl sulphide and diallyl disulphide, are the common inhibitors for both enzymes.[30]

Glutathione S-transferases
GSTs are ubiquitously present isozymes, found in almost all animal species. GSTs are also important phase II drug-metabolizing enzymes, involved in the metabolism of exogenous and endogenous compounds. Additionally, GSTs are crucial for the detoxification of endogenously produced free radicals, hence protecting the body from oxidative stress. There are 2 superfamilies of GSTs, and members of both the groups have transferases activity. One group is called soluble GSTs; they are found mostly in the cytosol, and recent studies have shown that mitochondria also contains soluble forms of GSTs. The second group of GSTs are called microsomal transferases, also called membrane-associated proteins in eicosanoid and glutathione metabolism (MAPEG).[31] Soluble GSTs are again divided into 8 families based on their degree of sequence identity, designated α, μ, π, σ, θ, ζ, ω, and κ. On the other hand, there are 6 members in the MAPEG family. These enzymes are distributed throughout the human body; the most heavily expressed organs are liver, kidney, brain, heart, lung, and gut.

Almost all types of compounds are substrate for GSTs, which are capable of reacting with the thiol moiety in glutathione; common compounds are epoxides, quinone, sulfoxides, esters, and peroxides. Up-regulation of GSTs in cancer is one of the reasons for therapeutic failure of certain anticancer drugs (melphalan and doxorubicin). Inhibition of GSTs over expression remains one of the treatment strategies in cancer. Until now, however, there has been no report available showing significant improvement in cancer treatment due to inhibition of GST. The most commonly used inhibitors of GST include phenols, quinone, certain vitamin C derivatives, dopamine, and *trans* retinoic acid. Induction of GSTs may also be beneficial in certain situations, which would help remove oxidative molecules that are generated in the body. There are reports suggesting that broccoli, cabbage, and Brussels sprouts induce GSTs.[32] Acetaminophen-induced hepatic toxicities are well known in toxicology. A glutathione precursor (*N*-acetylcysteine) as well as glutathione itself is used as an antidote to protect the liver from acetaminophen-induced hepatic toxicity.[33]

Thiopurine S-methyltransferases

TPMT is an important enzyme, particularly in cancer chemotherapy; this enzyme catalyzes S-methylation of aromatic heterocyclic sulfhydryl compounds, including anticancer and immunosuppressive medications. Thiopurines 6-mercaptopurine, 6-thioguanine, and azathioprine are prodrugs. These drugs have to be metabolically converted to the active form by hypoxanthine phosphoribosyl transferases. The metabolites of hypoxanthine phosphoribosyl transferases are cytotoxic and exert anticancer activity; however, there has to be a delicate balance between cytotoxicity for anticancer action in cancer cells and normal cells. TPMT metabolizes those compounds to the nontoxic forms by methylation. TMPT is a cytosolic enzyme mostly found in the liver, kidney, and lung; additionally, human red blood cells also have a significant level of TMPT expression. Thiopurines are good substrates for the TPMT, which make them important for cancer chemotherapy. Inhibition of TPMT activity may lead to the accumulation of toxic metabolites in the human body, causing other conditions, such as myelosuppression after azathioprine treatment. Naproxen, mefenamic, and tolfenamic acid are known to inhibit TPMT in noncompetitive manner.[34]

Catechol O-methyltransferases

COMTs are the enzymes responsible for the transfer of a methyl group from S-adenosylmethionine to its substrate. This methylation is one of the major pathways for the metabolism of catecholamines and catechol estrogens, including neurotransmitters, such as dopamine, epinephrine, and norepinephrine as well as drugs that have catechol functional groups attached to their structure.[35] COMT is mostly expressed in the postsynaptic neurons in the mammalian cells. There are 2 forms of COMT: the soluble form, called S-COMT, and the membrane-bound form, called MB-COMT. Structurally, both S-COMT and MB-COMT share almost similar sequences, however, their substrate affinity and specificity vary significantly. For example, MB-COMT has approximately 10 times more affinity for dopamine and noradrenaline compared with S-COMT. There are several inhibitors of COMT but the most commonly used are entacapone, tolcapone, and flavonoids (found in green tea). Inhibition of COMT leads to the accumulation of its substrate, which is used as treatment strategies for Parkinson diseases.[36]

Phase III Pathways

Drug transporters are generally transmembrane proteins that facilitate the transport of large and/or ionized molecules in and out of the cells. Phase III pathway is classified into 2 main superfamilies: ATP-binding cassette (ABC) and solute carrier (SLC) transporters. ABC transporters are dependent on the energy (ATP) consumption to actively uptake or efflux the drug from one side of the cell membrane to another, whereas SLCs facilitate the passage of certain solutes (eg, sugars and amino acids) across the membrane and actively transport other solutes against their electrochemical gradients by coupling the process with other solute or ion. They are present in many locations, such as liver, kidney, intestine, and brain. Conceptually, uptake transporters help in transferring the molecules into the cells and efflux transporters pump them outside the cell. In the liver, the main uptake transporters are Na^+-taurocholate cotransporting polypeptide (NTCP) (SLC10A1), organic cation transporter 1 (OCT1) (SLC22A1), organic anion transporter 2 (OAT2) (SLC22A7), and organic anion-transporting polypeptides (OATP1B1, OATP1B3, OATP2B1; SLCO1B1, SLCO1B3, and SLCO2B1, respectively). The hepatic efflux transporters are multidrug resistance protein 1 (MDR1) (also known as P-glycoprotein [P-gp] and ABC subfamily B member 1 [ABCB1]), bile salt export pump (BSEP) (also known as ABC subfamily B member 11 [ABCB11]), and multidrug resistance-associated protein (MRP) 2 (also known as ABC subfamily C member 2 [ABCC2])[37-39] (**Fig. 2**).

SITES OF DRUG METABOLISM
Liver

The liver is the major organ for phase I and phase II drug metabolic processes. Nevertheless, drug transporters also play an important role in facilitating the entry of molecules into the hepatocytes and out into the bile. Large and charged compounds are normally transported by drug transporters. **Fig. 2** demonstrates the interplay between phase I, II, and III pathways in the hepatocyte. Some drugs secreted in the bile are reabsorbed back from the intestine; some metabolites secreted in the bile can be converted back to the drug by β-Glucuronidase in the gut and can be reabsorbed. This phenomenon is known as enterohepatic circulation, a process that prolongs the residence of a drug in the body.

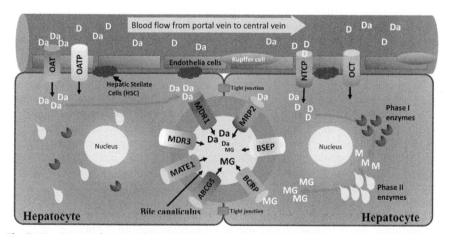

Fig. 2. Hepatocyte showing the main components and transporters. D and Da are 2 different drugs that have different clearance pathways. (1) Drug D is uptaken by transporter then metabolized by phase I pathway to M (main metabolic product) followed by conjugation process by phase II enzymes and finally effluxed into biliary system by transporter. (2) In this scenario, drug Da is transported into the hepatocyte through OAT then pumped out by MDR1 without any chemical modification to the drug molecule. D, drug; Da, drug a; M, metabolite; MG, metabolite glucuronide.

Liver and gut play a dominant role in the first-pass metabolism of orally administered medications.[40] The oral bioavailability of various drugs is increased with liver diseases. In patients with liver cirrhosis there is an increase in the severity of drug-induced liver injury. In HCV patient population, it is advised to closely monitor drug dosing after liver transplantation, especially when HCV therapies are used to prevent any recurrence.[19]

Gut

The primary function of intestinal tract is to serve as an absorptive organ for nutrients, electrolytes, and drug molecules. The gut also has metabolic functions, however, which can have an impact on the systemic bioavailability of certain therapeutic agents. Any medication that is taken orally has to be absorbed from gut lumen into the enterocytes, then move into the portal circulation, then to the liver, and finally into the systemic circulation. The systemic availability (*F*) of a drug is the product of fraction absorbed (*Fab*), fractions escaping gut metabolism (*Fg*), and the fraction escaping hepatic metabolism (*Fh*) before reaching the systemic circulation; this can be expressed as, $F = Fab \times Fg \times Fh$.[41] Human gut expresses most of the phase I and phase II drug-metabolizing enzymes, including CYP450s and UGTs.

Human small intestine expresses appreciable amounts of various CYP450 enzymes, contributing to the oxidation of several xenobiotics. Among all the CYP450s, CYP3A4 is the more prominent CYP450 enzyme, affecting the bioavailability of several therapeutic agents. In addition to CYP3A, the human small intestine also expresses CYP2C9, CYP2C19, CYP1A1, CYP2D6, and CYP2J2. The amount of CYP450 expression in the intestine varies from 20 pmol/g to 210 pmol/g of the tissues, indicating a large interpersonal variability. Additionally, the expression of the enzymes also is not uniform throughout the intestine. The duodenum, jejunum, and ileum are the places where expression is maximum; the expression level goes down further down in the intestine. CYP3A (CYP3A3/CYP3A4, CYP3A5, CYP3A7, and CYP3A43) is the predominant CYP450 family enzymes, which represent almost approximately 70% to 80% of the total CYP450 enzymes expressed in the intestine.[42]

UGTs are one of the major phase II drug-metabolizing enzymes expressed in human intestine in addition to the liver and kidney. Human intestine expresses several UGTs, including UGT1A1, UGT1A6, UGT1A7, UGT1A8, UGT1A9, and UGT1A10. Bioavailability of drugs could be affected by UGTs significantly; raloxifene is an estrogen receptor modulator, used for the treatment of osteoporosis and breast cancer. Unfortunately, oral bioavailability of raloxifene is only approximately 2%, where intestinal UGT1A8 and UGT1A10 play a significant role in lowering the systemic availability of the compound.[43]

In addition to the drug-metabolizing enzymes, the gut expresses a wide range of transporters including both influx and efflux transporters (**Fig. 3**). The intricate interplay between drug-metabolizing enzymes and transporters could significantly alter overall systemic availability of some drugs. Among all the efflux transporters, human gut expresses P-gp (MDR1), MRPs, and BCRP (breast cancer resistance protein), which are known to be responsible for most of the efflux function. Overexpression of the efflux transporters at the luminal site could lead to lower bioavailability of the drug, whereas overexpression at the abluminal site may increase systemic availability.[44,45] Transporters are mainly gate keepers at the gut, preventing toxins or unwanted substances from entering into blood. Most of the influx transporters are expressed at the luminal site, playing an important role in drug uptake. OATP3A1, OATP4A1, OCT1, and OCT2 are expressed at the abluminal site as well.[46,47] P-gp expressed luminally limits the absorption of cyclosporine, and the expression of P-gp is inversely correlated with the

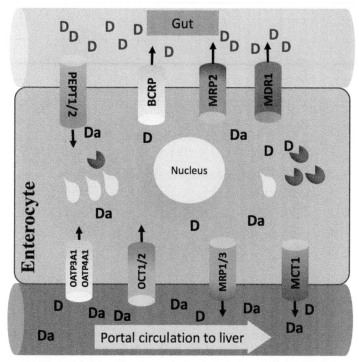

Fig. 3. Drug-metabolizing enzymes and transporters in gut, enterocyte. The drug (D) is transported from gut into enterocyte and then to the circulation. Metabolite (Da) also can be affected by transporters either by efflux or uptake transports.

oral bioavailability of its substrates. Ironically, the efflux transporters may be responsible for the development of drug resistance as well as causing therapeutic failure.

Kidney

Kidneys play an important role in clearing toxins but contribute to a lesser extent in terms of overall drug metabolism. Nephrons are the main functional unit of kidney and drugs are normally filtered excreted based on glomerular filtration, secreted at the proximal tubules, and reabsorbed by the tubules. Phase III transporters play a critical role in actively secreting drug molecules against their electrochemical gradients.[1] Kidneys do contribute to the metabolism of some endogenous compounds and xenobiotics. For example, kidneys activate 25-hydroxyvitamin D to the hormone 1,25-dihydroxyvitamin D_3 by CYP27B1, then deactivate it by CYP24A1.[48] Cyclosporine is converted to its metabolites in the kidney by CYP3A enzymes in the kidney and this may contribute to cyclosporine mediated nephrotoxicity.[49,50]

FACTORS AFFECTING THE METABOLISM OF DRUGS

Metabolism of drugs in human is not constant or immune to various internal and external factors. Metabolism could be affected by age, gender, pregnancy, different disease states, solid organ transplantation, medications, and genetic polymorphism **(Fig. 4)**.

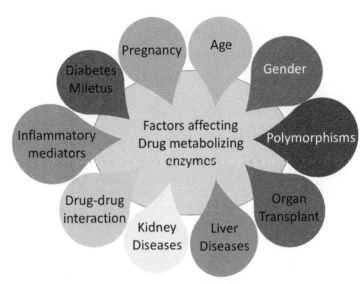

Fig. 4. Factors affecting the drug-metabolizing enzymes expression and functions.

Age

Age is known to have an impact on hepatic drug metabolism. In infants, lower expression of the enzyme may lead to decreased drug metabolism. The fetal liver expresses CYP3A7, which metabolizes endogenous compounds and some exogenous substrates of CYP3A4. Typically, the neonatal expression of CYP2C, CYP2E1, and CYP1A2 are approximately 10 times lower than adults. The activity of CYP450 enzymes in neonates is less than half that in adult human, which results in the inability of neonates to clear most of the medication at earlier life. The clearance of caffeine is approximately 6 times lower in newborn compared with adults. As neonates mature, the drug metabolic capacity increases. Young children tend to have higher clearance of certain drugs compared with young adults. Conjugation reactions can also be affected by age. In neonates, the clearance of bilirubin is low because UGTs are not well expressed at that age and in some cases can lead to neonatal jaundice. Overall, the maturation of the conjugative enzymes is slower than other biotransformation pathways. The expression and function of the enzymes are not significantly affected in elderly subjects compared with adults. The function of most CYP450 enzymes does not decline with advanced age, except CYP2D6 and CYP1A2. In the elderly, however, a combination of disruptive hepatic blood flow and use of multiple drugs (polypharmacy) may modify drug metabolism. With age, the liver volume decreases at a rate of 0.5% to 1% per year. Additionally, decrease in hepatic blood flow and oxygenation and increase in the fat deposition could lead to reduced overall metabolism of drug in elderly.[51–53]

Gender

Adverse drug reaction is 1.5 to 2 times more common in women compared with men.[54] This difference in side effects of drugs may be due to impact of sex hormones, body weight, body fat composition, and volume of distribution. It has been reported that while the activity of certain enzymes is higher in men than women, other enzymatic pathways are increased in women. The activities of CYP2D6 and CYP1A2 have been reported to be higher in men than women. CYP3A4 activity has been reported to be higher in women than in men.[55]

Pregnancy

Pregnancy is associated with several physiologic changes. These changes in body water, fat content, and hormones can potentially alter absorption, distribution, metabolism, and elimination of drugs.[56,57] In the United States, more than 60% pregnant women take at least 1 medication and many of these are metabolized.[58] The activities of CYP2D6, CYP3A4, CYP2B6, and CYP2C9 increase during pregnancy. As a result, the half-life of drugs those are substrate for these enzymes are shorter compared with nonpregnant women (phenytoin, midazolam, and metoprolol). On the other hand, the activity of CYP1A2 and CYP2C19 decreases during pregnancy, which leads to decrease in the clearance of drugs, which are substrates for the enzymes (caffeine-CYP1A2). Additionally, the activity of conjugating enzyme is altered during pregnancy. There are reports suggest that the activity of UGT1A4 is significantly increased during pregnancy, whereas the activity of UGT2B7 remains unaffected, and NATs are reduced.

Liver Diseases

Various liver diseases are known to affect the metabolism of drugs as well as endogenous compounds. There are several reasons for the observed changes in drug metabolism in patients with liver disease. Altered hepatic blood flow, altered expression of drug-metabolizing enzymes, altered availability of cosubstrates, and altered binding of drugs to plasma proteins can account for the observed changes in drug metabolism in patients with liver disease.

Plasma concentrations of midazolam are more than 2-fold higher in patients with nonalcoholic steatohepatitis (NASH) compared with normal health subjects. The observed increase in plasma concentration of midazolam is due to NASH-mediated decrease in hepatic drug metabolism. Additionally, more than 50% reduction in the plasma concentration of 4β-hydroxycholesterol, which is used as an endogenous biomarker for CYP3A4 activity, was reported in patients with simple steatosis.[59] The clearance of several drugs that are metabolized in the liver is decreased in cirrhosis. Liver cirrhosis decreases the clearance of voriconazole, a drug that is completely metabolized in the liver. Patients with hepatic insufficiency must be closely monitored when dosed with voriconazole to prevent any drug-associated toxicities[60,61] **(Table 3)** includes a list of hepatic diseases and their effect on drug-metabolizing enzymes.[62–66]

Table 3
List of hepatic diseases and their common effect on drug-metabolizing enzymes and drugs

Liver Diseases	Affected Enzymes	Selected Drugs Affected
Cirrhosis	CYP2E1, CYP2C9, CYP3A, CYP1A2, and UGTs	Isavuconazole, tacrolimus, sirolimus cyclosporine, chlorzoxazone, midazolam, dacarbazine, enflurane, diazepam
Hepatitis	CYP2E1, CYP3A, and CYP2C19	Isavuconazole, sirolimus, tacrolimus, cyclosporine, chlorzoxazone, midazolam, dacarbazine, omeprazole, phenytoin, lansoprazole
NASH	CYP2E1, CYP3A, UGTs, and SULTs	Isavuconazole, sirolimus, cyclosporine, tacrolimus, chlorzoxazone, midazolam, dacarbazine, midazolam
Cholestasis	CYP1A2, CYP2E1, CYP3A4, and UGTs	Acetaminophen, caffeine, verapamil, sirolimus, Cyclosporine, tacrolimus, midazolam, isavuconazole

Data from Refs.[62–66]

Kidney Diseases

Multiple molecular mediators and mechanisms can cause a reduction in the functionality of the nonrenal excretion pathways, mainly hepatic metabolism in patients with kidney diseases. As an example, the systemic exposure of intravenously given midazolam, a CYP3A4 probe, in chronic kidney disease before hemodialysis had increased 6-fold in comparison to healthy subjects.[67,68] There is a direct association between accumulation of circulating uremic toxins and reduction in the levels of mRNA, protein, and activity of some CYP450s. Two months after successful kidney transplant or directly after hemodialysis, however, the enzymatic activity appears to be restored. Most of the effect seems correlated with the accumulation of parathyroid hormone and proinflammatory cytokines (eg, interleukin [IL]-6, tumor necrosis factor [TNF], and IL-1β). The mechanism is believed to be reduced binding of the nuclear receptor PXR complex to CYP450 promoter region and, indirectly, by activation of the nuclear factor κB that depresses CYP450 transcription.[68] Furthermore, alteration of drug transporters activity as measured half-life of fexofenadine (3 times longer), which is a nonspecific transporter probe, has been documented in patients with glomerulonephritis compared with control subjects.[69]

Diabetes Mellitus

Diabetes mellitus has been an increasingly recognized problem worldwide and affects several systems in the body, such as the cardiovascular and nervous systems. Drug metabolism plays a major role in the regulation of glucose, lipoproteins, and lipid metabolism. Drug-metabolizing enzymes have been reported to be altered in diabetes. Dostalek and colleagues[70] investigated the effect of diabetes on the expression and activity of CYP3A4 and CYP2E1. They have shown that the protein levels and mRNA expressions in liver tissue were significantly decreased in diabetic patient compared with healthy individuals. In addition, CYP3A4 activity was tested using midazolam and testosterone as probes in human liver microsomes. It was concluded that diabetes significantly decreased CYP3A4 activity, resulting in lower metabolite(s) production (1'-hydroxymidazolam, 4-hydroxymidazolam, and 6β-hydroxytestosterone).[70] Patients with diabetes have a greater risk of having side effects and toxicities due to decreased metabolism. Therefore, modification of the dose of hepatically metabolized medications with narrow therapeutic index should be considered in diabetic population.

Solid Organ Transplantation

Liver transplantation is the only cure for patients with end-stage liver disease. Many factors that are inherent after liver transplantation can affect all 3 pathways. In cases of living donor liver transplantation, the size of transplanted graft is much smaller than normal livers and livers in deceased donor liver transplantation. Consequently, the intrinsic metabolic capacity is significantly reduced. The hepatic blood flow is higher per unit weight of liver in the liver donor and transplant recipient.[71]

In the deceased donor liver transplantation population, liver grafts are more susceptible to ischemia/reperfusion injury because of the longer duration of cold preservation and lack of oxygen and nutrients. Additionally, this injury is worsened when the hepatic blood flow is re-established. Ischemia/reperfusion injury is also associated with higher proinflammatory cytokines that lead to lower activity of drug-metabolizing enzymes. Metabolizing enzymes and transporters can be altered when graft rejection occurs, either acutely or chronically. It is documented that the expression of P-gp (MDR1) transporter and CYP3A4 in the intestine is decreased when there is chronic rejection of the liver graft with an increase in proinflammatory cytokines (cyclooxygenase-2, IL-2, IL-6, IL-8, IL-10, and TNF-α).[72]

Commonly used immunosuppressants in solid organ transplantation are cyclosporine, tacrolimus, and mycophenolic acids.[73] Cyclosporine A is a well-known inhibitor of P-gp and can potentially alter the bioavailability of drugs that are P-gp substrate.[74]

Medication (Drug-Drug Interactions)

Concomitant administration of medications can affect metabolism of each other. The Food and Drug Administration requires all drugs under development to be tested for any possible interaction as substrate, inhibitors, and/or inducers.[75] Inhibitors mainly work on the enzyme levels where they block or compete at the site of metabolism. Types of inhibitors are competitive (binds to the active site of free enzyme), uncompetitive (binds to the drug-enzyme complex to inhibit), noncompetitive (binds to different site other than site of the metabolism), and mixed. Inducers act by increasing the gene transcription that result in higher enzyme content. Some drugs can increase and stabilize the enzyme to be more active. Both of these processes increase the overall metabolic rate. **Table 2** lists different inhibitors and inducers that are clinically relevant. Usually in the presence of inhibitors drug exposure increases and that requires a decrease in the dose, dosing interval, or both and vice versa for the inducers.[76–78]

Polymorphism

Polymorphism in drug-metabolizing enzymes and transporters is known to influence the kinetics of several drugs. For example, CYP3A has several polymorphisms, including CYP3A4*1G, CYP3A5 6986A > G, and CYP3A5*1. Also, MDR1 (P-gp) has been identified as having several polymorphisms that affect the clearance of many drugs.[71] Warfarin is an oral anticoagulant used to treat thrombotic disorders. The effective dose of warfarin varies from 0.5 mg to 60 mg daily; this wide range is mainly because of interindividual variability in metabolism of warfarin. Warfarin is primarily metabolized by CYP2C9, and genetic polymorphism in this enzyme leads to variation in the metabolism of the drug.[79] Patients who carry various alleles of CYP2C9, such as CYP2C9*2 and CYP2C9*3, tend to have lower metabolism of warfarin leading to higher plasma concentrations.[80,81] Both of these alleles have impaired hydroxylation activity of S-warfarin when tested in vitro. Voriconazole metabolism is mainly affected by CYP2C19 polymorphisms. Patients can be either homozygous poor metabolizer, heterozygous extensive metabolizer, or homozygous extensive metabolizer; voriconazole levels can be 4 to 5 times higher in poor metabolizers in comparison to extensive metabolizers. Poor phenotype varies based on ethnicity from less than 7% to 20%.[61]

SUMMARY

Drug metabolism is an important process for the removal of unwanted substances from the body. Abnormal drug metabolism profile could lead to life-threatening complications. Both phase I (mainly CYP450s) and phase II (mainly UGTs) enzymes play a significant role in drug metabolism. Although metabolites in general are expected to be not active and not toxic, certain metabolites can cause hepatotoxicity. Various diseases may potentially change the metabolic profile of a drug by altering the expression and function of key enzymes. Additionally, coadministration of multiple drugs may also lead to drug-drug interaction and adverse reaction due to competitive binding to the same metabolizing enzyme. Care must be exercised while prescribing multiple medications to patients with certain diseases, which can alter drug pharmacokinetics/pharmacodynamics profiles.

REFERENCES

1. Benedetti MS, Whomsley R, Poggesi I, et al. Drug metabolism and pharmacokinetics. Drug Metab Rev 2009;41(3):344–90.
2. Ionescu C, Caira MR. Drug metabolism: current concepts. Dordrecht (Netherlands): Springer; 2005.
3. Lee WA, Gu L, Miksztal AR, et al. Bioavailability improvement of mycophenolic acid through amino ester derivatization. Pharm Res 1990,7(2).101–0.
4. Bullingham RE, Nicholls AJ, Kamm BR. Clinical pharmacokinetics of mycophenolate mofetil. Clin Pharmacokinet 1998;34(6):429–55.
5. Olsen L, Oostenbrink C, Jorgensen FS. Prediction of cytochrome P450 mediated metabolism. Adv Drug Deliv Rev 2015;86:61–71.
6. Mittal B, Tulsyan S, Kumar S, et al. Cytochrome P450 in cancer susceptibility and treatment. Adv Clin Chem 2015;71:77–139.
7. Terada T, Hira D. Intestinal and hepatic drug transporters: pharmacokinetic, pathophysiological, and pharmacogenetic roles. J Gastroenterol 2015;50(5):508–19.
8. Ortiz de Montellano PR. Cytochrome P450: structure, mechanism, and biochemistry. 3rd edition. New York: Kluwer Academic/Plenum Publishers; 2005.
9. Nelson DR. The cytochrome p450 homepage. Hum Genomics 2009;4(1):59–65.
10. Achour B, Barber J, Rostami-Hodjegan A. Expression of hepatic drug-metabolizing cytochrome p450 enzymes and their intercorrelations: a meta-analysis. Drug Metab Dispos 2014;42(8):1349–56.
11. Guenthner TM, Nebert DW. Cytosolic receptor for aryl hydrocarbon hydroxylase induction by polycyclic aromatic compounds. Evidence for structural and regulatory variants among established cell cultured lines. J Biol Chem 1977;252(24):8981–9.
12. Kliewer SA, Moore JT, Wade L, et al. An orphan nuclear receptor activated by pregnanes defines a novel steroid signaling pathway. Cell 1998;92(1):73–82.
13. Bertilsson G, Heidrich J, Svensson K, et al. Identification of a human nuclear receptor defines a new signaling pathway for CYP3A induction. Proc Natl Acad Sci U S A 1998;95(21):12208–13.
14. Forman BM, Tzameli I, Choi HS, et al. Androstane metabolites bind to and deactivate the nuclear receptor CAR-beta. Nature 1998;395(6702):612–5.
15. Honkakoski P, Zelko I, Sueyoshi T, et al. The nuclear orphan receptor CAR-retinoid X receptor heterodimer activates the phenobarbital-responsive enhancer module of the CYP2B gene. Mol Cell Biol 1998;18(10):5652–8.
16. Kohle C, Bock KW. Coordinate regulation of human drug-metabolizing enzymes, and conjugate transporters by the Ah receptor, pregnane X receptor and constitutive androstane receptor. Biochem Pharmacol 2009;77(4):689–99.
17. Khojasteh SC, Wong H, Hop CECA, et al. Drug metabolism and pharmacokinetics quick guide. New York: Springer Science+Business Media, LLC; 2011. Available at: http://dx.doi.org/10.1007/978-1-4419-5629-3.
18. Dvorak Z, Pavek P. Regulation of drug-metabolizing cytochrome P450 enzymes by glucocorticoids. Drug Metab Rev 2010;42(4):621–35.
19. Parikh ND, Levitsky J. Hepatotoxicity and drug interactions in liver transplant candidates and recipients. Clin Liver Dis 2013;17(4):737–47, x–xi.
20. Tischer S, Fontana RJ. Drug-drug interactions with oral anti-HCV agents and idiosyncratic hepatotoxicity in the liver transplant setting. J Hepatol 2014;60(4):872–84.

21. Jain AB, Venkataramanan R, Eghtesad B, et al. Effect of coadministered lopinavir and ritonavir (Kaletra) on tacrolimus blood concentration in liver transplantation patients. Liver Transpl 2003;9(9):954–60.
22. Wang Q, Jia R, Ye C, et al. Glucuronidation and sulfation of 7-hydroxycoumarin in liver matrices from human, dog, monkey, rat, and mouse. In Vitro Cell Dev Biol Anim 2005;41(3–4):97–103.
23. Iyer KR, Sinz MW. Characterization of Phase I and Phase II hepatic drug metabolism activities in a panel of human liver preparations. Chem Biol Interact 1999;118(2):151–69.
24. Iyer L, King CD, Whitington PF, et al. Genetic predisposition to the metabolism of irinotecan (CPT-11). Role of uridine diphosphate glucuronosyltransferase isoform 1A1 in the glucuronidation of its active metabolite (SN-38) in human liver microsomes. J Clin Invest 1998;101(4):847–54.
25. Coffman BL, King CD, Rios GR, et al. The glucuronidation of opioids, other xenobiotics, and androgens by human UGT2B7Y(268) and UGT2B7H(268). Drug Metab Dispos 1998;26(1):73–7.
26. Wang LQ, James MO. Inhibition of sulfotransferases by xenobiotics. Curr Drug Metab 2006;7(1):83–104.
27. Harris RM, Waring RH. Sulfotransferase inhibition: potential impact of diet and environmental chemicals on steroid metabolism and drug detoxification. Curr Drug Metab 2008;9(4):269–75.
28. Maiti S, Chen X, Chen G. All-trans retinoic acid induction of sulfotransferases. Basic Clin Pharmacol Toxicol 2005;96(1):44–53.
29. Kukongviriyapan V, Phromsopha N, Tassaneeyakul W, et al. Inhibitory effects of polyphenolic compounds on human arylamine N-acetyltransferase 1 and 2. Xenobiotica 2006;36(1):15–28.
30. Lin JG, Chen GW, Su CC, et al. Effects of garlic components diallyl sulfide and diallyl disulfide on arylamine N-acetyltransferase activity and 2-aminofluorene-DNA adducts in human promyelocytic leukemia cells. Am J Chin Med 2002; 30(2–3):315–25.
31. Jakobsson PJ, Morgenstern R, Mancini J, et al. Common structural features of MAPEG – a widespread superfamily of membrane associated proteins with highly divergent functions in eicosanoid and glutathione metabolism. Protein Sci 1999; 8(3):689–92.
32. Perez JL, Jayaprakasha GK, Valdivia V, et al. Limonin methoxylation influences the induction of glutathione S-transferase and quinone reductase. J Agric Food Chem 2009;57(12):5279–86.
33. Saito C, Zwingmann C, Jaeschke H. Novel mechanisms of protection against acetaminophen hepatotoxicity in mice by glutathione and N-acetylcysteine. Hepatology 2010;51(1):246–54.
34. Oselin K, Anier K. Inhibition of human thiopurine S-methyltransferase by various nonsteroidal anti-inflammatory drugs in vitro: a mechanism for possible drug interactions. Drug Metab Dispos 2007;35(9):1452–4.
35. Zhang J, Kulik HJ, Martinez TJ, et al. Mediation of donor-acceptor distance in an enzymatic methyl transfer reaction. Proc Natl Acad Sci U S A 2015;112(26): 7954–9.
36. Antonini A, Abbruzzese G, Barone P, et al. COMT inhibition with tolcapone in the treatment algorithm of patients with Parkinson's disease (PD): relevance for motor and non-motor features. Neuropsychiatr Dis Treat 2008;4(1):1–9.
37. International Transporter Consortium, Giacomini KM, Huang SM, et al. Membrane transporters in drug development. Nat Rev Drug Discov 2010;9(3):215–36.

38. Hediger MA, Romero MF, Peng JB, et al. The ABCs of solute carriers: physiological, pathological and therapeutic implications of human membrane transport proteinsIntroduction. Pflugers Arch 2004;447(5):465–8.

39. Morrissey KM, Wen CC, Johns SJ, et al. The UCSF-FDA TransPortal: a public drug transporter database. Clin Pharmacol Ther 2012;92(5):545–6.

40. Ding X, Kaminsky LS. Human extrahepatic cytochromes P450: function in xenobiotic metabolism and tissue-selective chemical toxicity in the respiratory and gastrointestinal tracts. Annu Rev Pharmacol Toxicol 2003;43:149–73.

41. Peters SA, Jones CR, Ungell AL, et al. Predicting drug extraction in the human gut wall: assessing contributions from drug metabolizing enzymes and transporter proteins using preclinical models. Clin Pharmacokinet 2016;55(6):673–96.

42. Pavek P, Dvorak Z. Xenobiotic-induced transcriptional regulation of xenobiotic metabolizing enzymes of the cytochrome P450 superfamily in human extrahepatic tissues. Curr Drug Metab 2008;9(2):129–43.

43. Mizuma T. Intestinal glucuronidation metabolism may have a greater impact on oral bioavailability than hepatic glucuronidation metabolism in humans: a study with raloxifene, substrate for UGT1A1, 1A8, 1A9, and 1A10. Int J Pharm 2009; 378(1–2):140–1.

44. Lown KS, Mayo RR, Leichtman AB, et al. Role of intestinal P-glycoprotein (mdr1) in interpatient variation in the oral bioavailability of cyclosporine. Clin Pharmacol Ther 1997;62(3):248–60.

45. Fricker G, Drewe J, Huwyler J, et al. Relevance of p-glycoprotein for the enteral absorption of cyclosporin A: in vitro-in vivo correlation. Br J Pharmacol 1996; 118(7):1841–7.

46. Shugarts S, Benet LZ. The role of transporters in the pharmacokinetics of orally administered drugs. Pharm Res 2009;26(9):2039–54.

47. Chan LM, Lowes S, Hirst BH. The ABCs of drug transport in intestine and liver: efflux proteins limiting drug absorption and bioavailability. Eur J Pharm Sci 2004;21(1):25–51.

48. Jovicic S, Ignjatovic S, Majkic-Singh N. Biochemistry and metabolism of vitamin D. J Med Biochem 2012;31(4):309–15.

49. Dai Y, Iwanaga K, Lin YS, et al. In vitro metabolism of cyclosporine A by human kidney CYP3A5. Biochem Pharmacol 2004;68(9):1889–902.

50. Zheng S, Tasnif Y, Hebert MF, et al. CYP3A5 gene variation influences cyclosporine A metabolite formation and renal cyclosporine disposition. Transplantation 2013;95(6):821–7.

51. Wynne HA, Cope LH, Mutch E, et al. The effect of age upon liver volume and apparent liver blood flow in healthy man. Hepatology 1989;9(2):297–301.

52. Woodhouse KW, Wynne HA. Age-related changes in liver size and hepatic blood flow. The influence on drug metabolism in the elderly. Clin Pharmacokinet 1988; 15(5):287–94.

53. Wynne H. Drug metabolism and ageing. J Br Menopause Soc 2005;11(2):51–6.

54. Kando JC, Yonkers KA, Cole JO. Gender as a risk factor for adverse events to medications. Drugs 1995;50(1):1–6.

55. Zhou S, Yung Chan S, Cher Goh B, et al. Mechanism-based inhibition of cytochrome P450 3A4 by therapeutic drugs. Clin Pharmacokinet 2005;44(3):279–304.

56. Zhao Y, Hebert MF, Venkataramanan R. Basic obstetric pharmacology. Semin Perinatol 2014;38(8):475–86.

57. Feghali M, Venkataramanan R, Caritis S. Pharmacokinetics of drugs in pregnancy. Semin Perinatol 2015;39(7):512–9.

58. Isoherranen N, Thummel KE. Drug metabolism and transport during pregnancy: how does drug disposition change during pregnancy and what are the mechanisms that cause such changes? Drug Metab Dispos 2013;41(2):256–62.

59. Woolsey SJ, Mansell SE, Kim RB, et al. CYP3A Activity and expression in nonalcoholic fatty liver disease. Drug Metab Dispos 2015;43(10):1484–90.

60. Weiler S, Zoller H, Graziadei I, et al. Altered pharmacokinetics of voriconazole in a patient with liver cirrhosis. Antimicrob Agents Chemother 2007;51(9):3459–60.

61. Pasqualotto AC, Xavier MO, Andreolla HF, et al. Voriconazole therapeutic drug monitoring: focus on safety. Expert Opin Drug Saf 2010;9(1):125–37.

62. Weltman MD, Farrell GC, Hall P, et al. Hepatic cytochrome P450 2E1 is increased in patients with nonalcoholic steatohepatitis. Hepatology 1998;27(1):128–33.

63. Schuck RN, Zha W, Edin ML, et al. The cytochrome P450 epoxygenase pathway regulates the hepatic inflammatory response in fatty liver disease. PLoS One 2014;9(10):e110162.

64. Tsunedomi R, Iizuka N, Hamamoto Y, et al. Patterns of expression of cytochrome P450 genes in progression of hepatitis C virus-associated hepatocellular carcinoma. Int J Oncol 2005;27(3):661–7.

65. Hardwick RN, Ferreira DW, More VR, et al. Altered UDP-glucuronosyltransferase and sulfotransferase expression and function during progressive stages of human nonalcoholic fatty liver disease. Drug Metab Dispos 2013;41(3):554–61.

66. Chen J, Zhao KN, Chen C. The role of CYP3A4 in the biotransformation of bile acids and therapeutic implication for cholestasis. Ann Transl Med 2014;2(1):7.

67. Thomson BK, Nolin TD, Velenosi TJ, et al. Effect of CKD and dialysis modality on exposure to drugs cleared by nonrenal mechanisms. Am J Kidney Dis 2015;65(4):574–82.

68. Ladda MA, Goralski KB. The effects of CKD on cytochrome P450-mediated drug metabolism. Adv Chronic Kidney Dis 2016;23(2):67–75.

69. Joy MS, Frye RF, Nolin TD, et al. In vivo alterations in drug metabolism and transport pathways in patients with chronic kidney diseases. Pharmacotherapy 2014;34(2):114–22.

70. Dostalek M, Court MH, Yan B, et al. Significantly reduced cytochrome P450 3A4 expression and activity in liver from humans with diabetes mellitus. Br J Pharmacol 2011;163(5):937–47.

71. Li M, Zhao Y, Humar A, et al. Pharmacokinetics of drugs in adult living donor liver transplant patients: regulatory factors and observations based on studies in animals and humans. Expert Opin Drug Metab Toxicol 2016;12(3):231–43.

72. Masuda S, Goto M, Kiuchi T, et al. Enhanced expression of enterocyte P-glycoprotein depresses cyclosporine bioavailability in a recipient of living donor liver transplantation. Liver Transpl 2003;9(10):1108–13.

73. Liu Z, Chen Y, Tao R, et al. Tacrolimus-based versus cyclosporine-based immunosuppression in hepatitis C virus-infected patients after liver transplantation: a meta-analysis and systematic review. PLoS One 2014;9(9):e107057.

74. Liow JS, Lu S, McCarron JA, et al. Effect of a P-glycoprotein inhibitor, Cyclosporin A, on the disposition in rodent brain and blood of the 5-HT1A receptor radioligand, [11C](R)-(-)-RWAY. Synapse 2007;61(2):96–105.

75. Food and Drug Administration-Center for Drug Evaluation and Research. Guidance for industry: drug interaction studies — study design, data analysis, implications for dosing, and labeling recommendations. Rockville, MD: Food and Drug Administration; 2012. p. 79.

76. Gubbins PO, Amsden JR. Drug-drug interactions of antifungal agents and implications for patient care. Expert Opin Pharmacother 2005;6(13):2231–43.

77. Bruggemann RJ, Alffenaar JW, Blijlevens NM, et al. Clinical relevance of the pharmacokinetic interactions of azole antifungal drugs with other coadministered agents. Clin Infect Dis 2009;48(10):1441–58.

78. Lin JH, Lu AY. Inhibition and induction of cytochrome P450 and the clinical implications. Clin Pharmacokinet 1998;35(5):361–90.

79. Daly AK, Day CP, Aithal GP. CYP2C9 polymorphism and warfarin dose requirements. Br J Clin Pharmacol 2002;53(4):408–9.

80. Goldstein JA. Clinical relevance of genetic polymorphisms in the human CYP2C subfamily. Br J Clin Pharmacol 2001;52(4):349–55.

81. Furuya H, Fernandez-Salguero P, Gregory W, et al. Genetic polymorphism of CYP2C9 and its effect on warfarin maintenance dose requirement in patients undergoing anticoagulation therapy. Pharmacogenetics 1995;5(6):389–92.

Drug-Induced Liver Disease

Clinical Course

Hemamala Saithanyamurthi, MD, Alison Jazwinski Faust, MD, MHS*

KEYWORDS

- Drug-induced liver injury • Acute liver failure • Chronic drug-induced liver injury

KEY POINTS

- Most patients with suspected drug-induced liver injury (DILI) have uneventful recovery after the withdrawal of implicated agent.
- Approximately 10% of patients with DILI progress to acute liver failure leading to death or liver transplantation.
- 5% to 20% of patients with DILI will have persistent abnormalities at 6 months.
- Cirrhosis as a result of DILI is rare but described and can be associated with decompensated disease and liver-related death months to years after DILI is recognized.

INTRODUCTION

Despite the crucial role of the liver in the metabolism of many medications, drug-induced liver injury (DILI) is a relatively infrequent event. DILI accounts for less than 1% of patients hospitalized for jaundice.[1] However, DILI is a leading cause of medications not making it to the market during the investigational stage. Population-based studies from France and Iceland have estimated an incidence rate of 13.9 and 19 per 100,000 persons.[2,3]

DILI can range from mild elevation of transaminases detected on routine blood work to acute liver failure (ALF) requiring liver transplantation or death. Many drugs can cause mild elevation of liver enzymes that resolve with continued exposure by a process of adaptation. Idiosyncratic DILI is a result of complex interaction between a drug or metabolites and host immune response. Defective adaptation potentially related to T-cell response can lead to severe liver injury.[4] Idiosyncratic DILI differs from intrinsic DILI, which occurs in a predictable fashion from known hepatotoxins, such as acetaminophen. Chronic liver enzyme elevation may result from DILI, and in rare cases, cirrhosis and its complications can develop with resultant liver-related morbidity and mortality.[5–7]

The authors have nothing to disclose.
Department of Medicine, Division of Gastroenterology, Hepatology and Nutrition, University of Pittsburgh Medical Center, University of Pittsburgh School of Medicine, 200 Lothrop Street, Pittsburgh, PA 15213, USA
* Corresponding author. 3471 Fifth Avenue, Kaufman Building Suite 916, Pittsburgh, PA 15213.
E-mail address: jazwinskiab@upmc.edu

Most information on the clinical course of DILI has come from the Drug-Induced Liver Injury Network in the United States (DILIN) and the Spanish Group for the Study of Drug-Induced Liver Injury in Europe. Each of these networks has prospectively collected data on the natural history of DILI. In addition, there is a large cohort of patients that were reported to the Swedish Adverse Drug Reactions Committee that has provided insight into the natural history of DILI through retrospective review. Data from these networks are reviewed in this article, with a focus on the clinical course of idiosyncratic DILI. **Table 1** describes the outcomes from each of the 3 large DILI cohorts.

DISCUSSION
Diagnosis

The diagnosis of DILI can be quite difficult to make, although it only requires evidence that liver injury resulted from a drug or herbal supplement. Several challenges to making the diagnosis are described in later discussion. **Fig. 1** outlines the steps to make the diagnosis of DILI, including a reasonable diagnostic workup to rule out alternative causes of liver injury.

DILI may be found incidentally on routine blood work; however, patients that develop severe DILI generally present with symptoms such as jaundice, pruritus, abdominal pain, nausea/vomiting, and malaise. Fever, rash, and eosinophilia may be seen in cases of hypersensitivity reactions.

An accurate diagnosis of DILI depends on an accurate list of all prescription medications (PMs), over-the-counter medications, and herbal/dietary supplements that the patient is taking. The diagnosis of DILI can be limited by patient history and may require corroboration from family members or a phone call to the patient's pharmacy to obtain accurate records. A good understanding of the most common offending agents, latency periods, and pattern of injury can help determine which drug caused the episode. However, many drugs and herbal/dietary supplements can cause DILI, so it may be necessary for the clinician to examine the literature for cases of DILI for each medication that a patient is taking. The National Institutes of Health has developed a

Table 1
Results of drug-induced liver injury registries

Study	Total Number of Cases[a]	Pattern of Injury (%)			ALF (%)		Chronic DILI (%)[b]
		Hepatocellular	Mixed	Cholestatic	Death	LT	
US DILI Network	899	53	22	23	6	4	18.9
Spanish DILI Registry	805	61	16	20	2.5	1.5	5.7
Swedish Adverse Drug Reactions Committee	784	52	22	26	7.5	1.7	3.4

Numbers were taken from the most recent publication as of May 2016 for each group.
Abbreviation: LT, liver transplantation.
[a] Only cases determined to be possible, probable, or highly probable were included in the study analyses.
[b] The definition of Chronic DILI varied by study. In the US DILIN, chronic DILI was defined as elevation of ALT, AST, ALP, or bilirubin, histologic or radiologic findings that persisted for more than 6 months from the original DILI episode. The Spanish DILI registry defined chronic hepatocellular injury as elevated enzymes 3 months after the original DILI episode and chronic cholestatic injury as elevated enzymes 6 months after the original DILI episode. The Swedish Registry did not use a predefined definition of DILI; this number reflects the number of patients hospitalized with a diagnosis of liver disease after the original episode of DILI.

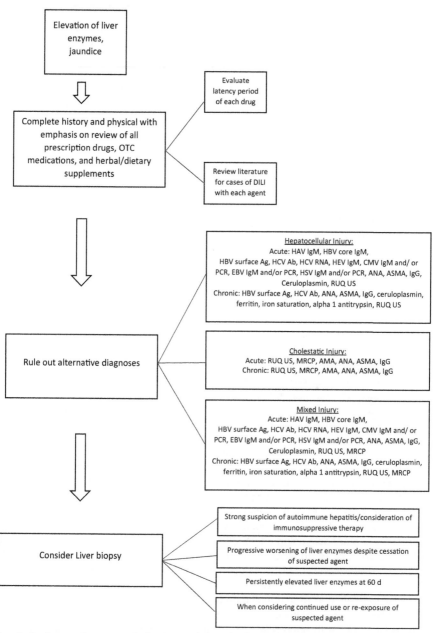

Fig. 1. A diagnostic approach for DILI. Ab, antibody; ANA, antinuclear antibody; ASMA, anti-smooth muscle antibody; CMV, cytomegalovirus; EBV, Epstein-Barr virus; HAV, hepatitis A virus; HBV, hepatitis B virus; HCV, hepatitis C virus; HEV, hepatitis E virus; HSV, herpes simplex virus; IgG, Immunoglobulin G; MRCP, magnetic resonance cholangiopancreatography; PCR, polymerase chain reaction; RUQ US, right upper quadrant ultrasound.

Web site, http://www.livertox.nih.gov/, to index all case reports of DILI for a large number of drugs and which is a good resource for this purpose.[8] The most common drugs associated with DILI are antimicrobials, followed by herbal/dietary supplements, cardiovascular drugs, and central nervous system agents.[9–11]

It can be difficult to make the association between liver injury and a specific agent in the case of polypharmacy, which is frequently encountered. Complicating matters further, in 10% to 20% of cases, more than one drug is suspected to be responsible for DILI.[9,12] In the US DILIN, most of the patients had DILI as a result of a single PM (73%), although DILI in some patients was attributed to use of herbal supplements (9%) or multiple PMs and herbal supplements (18%).[13]

The time from exposure to the suspected agent to the development of elevated liver enzymes or clinical symptoms (latency period) varies substantially. In the US DILIN, the median duration between the first exposure to the implicated agent and DILI was 42 days, with a range of 20 to 117 days.[10] Some agents have been described to have a very short latency period (<7 days). In the US DILIN, these agents included moxifloxacin, azithromycin, and ciprofloxacin. Other drugs, such as nitrofurantoin, minocycline, statins, and amiodarone, have the potential for a long latency period of 1 to 3 years.[13] In the US DILI cohort, no differences were seen in clinical presentation between those drugs with short or long latency periods, but there was a trend toward slower resolution and higher likelihood of chronic DILI in cases of DILI from drugs with a long latency.[13]

DILI may occur more frequently in the elderly, women, obese individuals, and those with human immunodeficiency virus, diabetes, or chronic liver disease. However, the data are mixed and confounded by other factors, such as multiple medical comorbidities. In addition, some risk factors may be drug specific.[14] In the clinical practice of Hepatology, it is common to see other prescribers avoid specific medications because of perceived risk of hepatotoxicity. Dr Hyman Zimmerman,[15] the father of modern-day drug hepatotoxicity, has said that most drugs can be safely used in patients with underlying chronic liver disease. However, if a patient with underlying chronic liver disease develops hepatotoxicity, they may tolerate it less well than a patient without underlying liver disease. Therefore, it is reasonable to avoid drugs with a significant potential for hepatotoxicity in patients with chronic liver disease. In the DILI network, about 10% of patients had preexisting CLD, which were mainly hepatitis C virus (HCV) and nonalcoholic fatty liver disease. More severe liver injury and higher mortality (16% vs 5.2%) were seen compared with those without preexisting liver disease.[13]

To make the diagnosis of DILI, alternative causes of acute or chronic liver injury must be ruled out (see **Fig. 1**), including viral hepatitis, autoimmune hepatitis, biliary obstruction/primary sclerosing cholangitis, metabolic/genetic diseases, vascular abnormalities such as Budd Chiari or portal vein thrombosis, primary biliary cirrhosis, and alcoholic and nonalcoholic steatohepatitis. The pattern of liver enzyme elevation will help to direct the appropriate testing. In prospective studies of DILI, a substantial number of patients that were not ultimately diagnosed with DILI had acute hepatitis C (1.3%) or hepatitis E (3%) infection; thus, in the right clinical setting, these conditions must be ruled out with appropriate serologic tests (HCV RNA and hepatitis E virus [HEV] immunoglobulin M [IgM], respectively).[10,16]

A liver biopsy is not required to make the diagnosis of DILI; however, it can be helpful in certain circumstances, which are detailed in **Fig. 1**. Although there is not a single classic histologic pattern of injury seen on biopsy that confirms DILI, there are several well-described patterns of injury that in the right clinical setting provide more evidence for the presence of DILI. Furthermore, a biopsy can be helpful in determining the severity of the liver injury and can determine whether chronic changes such as significant fibrosis are present.

Several classification systems have been developed to aid in making the diagnosis of DILI. The Roussel Uclaf Causality Assessment Method (RUCAM) score is the most frequently cited. The diagnostic elements included in the RUCAM score are detailed in **Table 2** with point values assigned to each. The RUCAM score ranges from −9 to +10; higher scores indicate higher likelihood of DILI. Scores are often grouped

Table 2
Roussel Uclaf Causality Assessment Method score for diagnosis of drug-induced liver injury

Criteria	Hepatocellular Injury	Points	Cholestatic Injury	Points
Time from drug start	5–90 d <5, >90 d	+2 +1	5–90 d <5, >90 d	+2 +1
Time from drug stop	≤15 d	+1	≤30 d	+1
Course	ALT decrease ≥50% in 8 d	+3	ALP/bili decrease ≥50% in 180 d	+2
	ALT decrease ≥50% in 30 d ALT decrease ≥50% in >30 d ALT decrease <50% in 30 d	+2 0 −2	Decrease <50% in 180 d Persistence or increase or no info	+1 0
Risk factor: Alcohol	Yes No	+1 0	Yes or pregnancy No	+1 0
Age ≥50	Yes No	+1 0	Yes No	+1 0
Other drugs	None or no info Drug with suggestive timing Known hepatotoxin with suggestive timing Drug with other evidence for a role	0 −1 −2 −3	None or no info Drug with suggestive timing Known hepatotoxin with suggestive timing Drug with other evidence for a role	0 −1 −2 −3
Competing causes	Rule out HAV, HBV, HCV, biliary obstruction, alcoholism, recent hypotension, CMV, EBV, HSV	+2	Rule out HAV, HBV, HCV, biliary obstruction, alcoholism, recent hypotension, CMV, EBV, HSV	+2
	Rule out HAV, HBV, HCV, biliary obstruction, alcoholism, recent hypotension	+1	Rule out HAV, HBV, HCV, biliary obstruction, alcoholism, recent hypotension	+1
	Rule out 4 or 5: HAV, HBV, HCV, biliary obstruction, alcoholism, recent hypotension	0	Rule out 4 or 5: HAV, HBV, HCV, biliary obstruction, alcoholism, recent hypotension	0
	Rule out <4: HAV, HBV, HCV, biliary obstruction, alcoholism, recent hypotension	−2	Rule out <4: HAV, HBV, HCV, biliary obstruction, alcoholism, recent hypotension	−2
	Nondrug cause highly probable	−3	Nondrug cause highly probable	−3
Previous information	Reaction in product label Reaction published, no product label Reaction unknown	+2 +1 0	Reaction in product label Reaction published, no product label Reaction unknown	+2 +1 0
Rechallenge	Positive Compatible Negative Not done	+3 +1 −2 0	Positive Compatible Negative Not done	+3 +1 −2 0

into likelihood levels of the following: excluded (score ≤0), unlikely (1–2), possible (3–5), probable (6–8), and highly probable (>8).

Although the RUCAM assessment was intended for use in clinic or at the bedside, it can be cumbersome. Hyman Zimmerman advised maintaining some flexibility in the assessment. Elements of the RUCAM assessment that have been criticized include the following: (1) The risk factors cited have not been well defined. For example, many cases of DILI occur in patients that are under the age of 55. Additionally, alcohol and pregnancy have not been reliably determined to increase the risk of DILI. (2) There is a narrow latency period and the score does not account for delayed responses occurring greater than 15 days after stopping the drug. (3) The RUCAM assessment requires response to a "rechallenge", which most practitioners would be hesitant to try for concern of a more severe reaction. (4) Histology is not accounted for. (5) The nondrug exclusions are not complete.[17]

The US DILIN used a structured expert opinion process that incorporated elements from RUCAM. Three reviewers independently assess the cases, and discussions among the reviewers occur in the case of discrepancies. A percentage probability score is used to define cases as definite (>95%, beyond any reasonable doubt), highly likely (75%–95%, clear and convincing data, but not definite), probable (50%–74%, most data support causal relationship), possible (25%–49%, most data suggest no causal relationship but possibility remains), unlikely (<25%, causal relationship very unlikely).[10]

Pattern of Injury

Once a diagnosis of DILI is made, the episode should be classified into one of following patterns of injury: hepatocellular, cholestatic, or mixed. The classification is made by determining R, which is calculated as serum alanine aminotransferase (ALT)/upper limit of normal (ULN) for ALT divided by serum alkaline phosphatase (ALP)/ULN for ALP. If the R is >5, the DILI is classified as hepatocellular injury. If the R is <2, the DILI is classified as cholestatic injury, and if the R is between 2 and 5, the DILI is classified as mixed injury.

This classification system helps to determine the risk of developing ALF or chronic liver disease and can help guide the diagnostic workup (see **Fig. 1**). Studies have indicated that patients with hepatocellular pattern of injury and jaundice are more likely to have severe and fatal disease and those with cholestatic pattern may be more likely to have persistent laboratory abnormalities.[5,7,9,11] The mixed pattern of injury appears to have the most favorable outcomes, having roughly half the incidence of death and liver transplantation compared with those having hepatocellular or cholestatic pattern. Preexisting liver disease is less common in those with mixed pattern for some unknown reasons, but it may explain the better outcomes.[10,13] As seen in **Table 1**, hepatocellular pattern of injury was the most common pattern observed in the major DILI studies.

Clinical Course

Table 3 describes the clinical course of the first 300 patients enrolled in the US DILIN. Patients that had severe or fatal/transplant courses were compared with patients with mild to moderate courses to assess for any factors that may predispose to more severe disease. On univariate analyses, significant associations were seen for use of alcohol (32% vs 57%, $P = .001$), days between exposure and DILI recognition (65.5 days vs 35.5 days, $P = .006$), presentation serum ALT, bilirubin, and international normalized ratio (INR), and peak serum ALT, bilirubin, and INR. However, on multivariable modeling, the only independent associations with severe or fatal/transplant were presence of diabetes (odds ratio [OR] 2.69, 95% confidence interval [CI] 1.14–6.45)

Table 3
Clinical course in first 300 patients enrolled in US drug-induced liver injury

Clinical Course	Definition	Cases (%)
Mild	Serum enzyme elevations but bilirubin <2.5 mg/dL	27
Moderate	Bilirubin >2.5 or INR >1.5 without the need for hospitalization	19
Moderate—hospitalized	Bilirubin >2.5 or INR >1.5 with the need for hospitalization	33
Severe	Bilirubin >2.5 and signs of hepatic or other organ failure	15
Fatal/transplant	Death from liver disease or the need for liver transplantation	6

and alcohol use in the preceding 12 months, which was a negative predictor (OR 0.33, 95% CI 0.15–0.76).[10]

In this cohort of patients, the peak mean serum chemistries were ALT 985 ± 1168 U/L, ALP 390 ± 382 U/L, total bilirubin 11.4 ± 10.2 mg/dL, and INR 1.6 ± 1.4. The median duration between DILI recognition and peak value for ALT was 1 (0–7) days, ALP 4 (0–16) days, and total bilirubin 7 (0–17) days. The median time from DILI recognition to peak bilirubin level was 7 days; from peak bilirubin level to 50% reduction was 13 days, and from peak bilirubin level to bilirubin less than 2.5 mg/dL was 26.5 days. No differences were seen by patient age, pattern of injury, or whether the injury was from PMs or dietary supplements. Therefore, it is important to note when counseling patients that time to jaundice resolution is on average about 1 month. Although not statistically significant, the interval to resolution was longer in patients that were elderly, had cholestatic forms of DILI, and had DILI from dietary supplements.[10]

Acute Liver Failure, Death, Liver Transplantation

Idiosyncratic DILI is a self-limiting disease in most patients. However, idiosyncratic DILI was the suspected cause in 13% to 15% of cases of ALF in reports from the United States and Sweden.[18,19]

The Acute Liver Failure Study Group published prospective data on 133 cases of ALF from DILI. All of the patients had coagulopathy (INR >1.5) with encephalopathy that developed within 26 weeks as well as no evidence of underlying chronic liver disease. The reported outcomes at 21 days were transplant-free survival, liver transplantation, or death. The majority (70.6%) of the patients were women, and the average age was 43.8 years. Ethnic minorities were overrepresented in this cohort, because 57.1% of the patients were white, 15.8% African American, 15.0% Hispanic, and 12% other. The patients were generally overweight with median body mass index (BMI) of 28.7. The mean bilirubin level was 20.8 mg/dL, median aspartate aminotransferase (AST) 551 IU/L, median ALT 574, median INR 2.6, and mean Model for End-Stage Liver Disease (MELD) score 33. Hepatocellular injury was the most common presenting pattern of injury (77.8%), followed by cholestatic injury (12.6%) and mixed injury (9.5%). In this cohort, 27.1% of subjects spontaneously recovered, 42.1% underwent liver transplantation, and 23.3% died while awaiting liver transplantation. Baseline factors associated with a good outcome included lower coma grade, bilirubin, INR, creatinine, and MELD scores but not age, gender, BMI, blood pressure, drug class, type of DILI reaction, or liver enzyme elevation. In comparison with those that underwent liver transplantation or died, transplant-free survivors had lower bilirubin (20.5 mg/dL, 23.3 mg/dL, and

12.6 mg/dL, respectively). Subjects that did not undergo transplantation but died had worse renal compromise than survivors that did not undergo transplantation and subjects undergoing transplantation (creatinine 2.1 mg/dL, 1.1 mg/dL, and 1.0 mg/dL, respectively). In this cohort, outcome was not different if the subjects discontinued the agent before or after symptoms/jaundice.[20]

Hillman and colleagues[21] subsequently published an analysis from the Acute Liver Failure Study comparing ALF from complementary/alternative medicine (CAM) with ALF from PM. The study size had increased to a total of 253 cases of DILI. Of these cases, 210 (83.7%) were due to PMs and 41 (16.3%) were due to CAM, of which more than half (n = 26) were herbal supplements. Between 1998 and July 7, 2007, there were 154 cases of DILI, 17 of which were due to CAM (12.4%). From July 8, 2007 to 2015, there were 138 cases of DILI, 24 of which were attributed to CAM (21.1%), which was a statistically significant increase in the percent of DILI cases due to CAM (P = .047). No differences existed between the CAM and PM groups with respect to age, sex, BMI, or race. Both groups were predominantly men, Caucasian, and overweight. Overall, there were less medical comorbidities in the patients in the CAM group. There was no difference in presenting symptoms between the groups. Jaundice was the most common presenting symptom for both groups and occurred in greater than 90% of patients. Malaise and nausea/vomiting were the next most frequent presenting complaints. There was no difference in the type of liver injury (hepatocellular, mixed, cholestatic) between groups. Hepatocellular injury was the most common pattern of injury in both groups (80% in CAM group and 73% in PM group). The only laboratory value that was statistically different between the 2 groups at presentation was ALP, which was higher in PM-induced DILI than CAM-induced DILI (mean 215.1 IU/L vs 156.2 IU/L, P = .005). There were no differences between the groups in median ALT/AST, INR, platelets, bilirubin, MELD score, or coma grade. A higher percentage of patients with CAM-induced DILI were listed for liver transplantation compared with those with PM-induced DILI (65.9% vs 47.1% P = .28) but this was not statistically significant. However, at 21 days, more CAM patients than PM patients did undergo liver transplantation (56.1 vs 31.9%, P<.005). Mortality was not statistically different between the groups (22% in CAM and 32.9% in PM). The increase in transplants for patients with CAM-induced liver injury could be related to less frequent comorbidities in this group; however, CAM-induced liver failure had a lower 21-day transplant-free survival than those with PM-induced ALF (17.4% vs 34.4%, P = .044). Therefore, these data suggest that CAM-induced liver injury can be as severe as or more severe than DILI from PMs.

Other studies have also shown that survival of patients with ALF secondary to DILI is poor without liver transplantation with mortality in the range of 60% to 80%.[22,23] Given the high mortality with ALF and significant consequences of death or liver transplantation, a major clinical dilemma is to identify those patients at highest risk for this outcome.

Hyman Zimmerman made the observation that elevation of transaminases in combination with jaundice suggests serious liver injury with fatalities (10%–50% mortality). Zimmerman's observation is recognized as Hy's Law for monitoring DILI and states that elevation of liver enzymes, AST, or ALT more than 3× ULN or ALP more than 1.5× ULN in combination with elevated bilirubin >3× ULN at any time after starting a new drug may imply serious liver injury, and the suspected drug should be stopped.[15] More recently, Hy's Law cases have been defined as DILI resulting an ALT value >3× ULN and total bilirubin levels >2× ULN after excluding other potential causes. This definition has been used by US Food and Drug Administration to identify potential hepatotoxic drugs during clinical drug development.[24]

In large cohort studies of DILI, ALF leading to death or liver transplantation occurs in about 10% of patients (**Table 1**). In the Swedish study, a total of 72 (9.2%) patients died of liver failure or underwent liver transplantation. Patients with hepatocellular injury had the highest mortality (12.7%) compared with 7.8% of the patients with cholestatic injury and 2.4% of those with mixed injury. A total of 13 patients, all of which presented with hepatocellular injury, underwent liver transplantation. The patients that died or underwent liver transplantation were older than those who recovered (65 years vs 58 years, $P = .04$). There was a similar proportion of women and men, and no difference in the duration of treatment was seen. Serum bilirubin was higher in those patients who died or underwent transplantation (18.7 vs 5.5, $P<.0001$), as were serum AST, ALT, and AST/ALT ratio. Serum ALP levels were not significantly different. In multivariable analysis, AST and bilirubin were found to independently predict death or transplantation in the study population with an OR of 1.013 for each increase × ULN of AST and an OR of 1.092 for each increase × ULN of bilirubin.[11]

Fontana and colleagues[7] studied a group of 660 patients with DILI from 2004 to 2011 in the US DILI network. Of those patients, 30 patients (4.5%) underwent liver transplantation and 32 (5%) died. Of the patients that died, 53% of the deaths were deemed to be liver related. More patients with early death or liver transplantation had acute hepatocellular injury compared with mixed or cholestatic injury (13% vs 6%). Several demographic and clinical variables were evaluated to determine factors associated with an early severe outcome. The variables that were significant included Asian race, underlying diabetes, lung disease, kidney disease, and malignancy. More patients in the early death or transplant group had preexisting liver disease (24.2% vs 10.7%, $P<.01$). In addition, those patients had higher white blood cell counts at presentation (7.9 vs 6.3, $P<.01$), but lower mean eosinophil counts (65 vs 147, $P<.01$). Serum ALT (1051 U/L vs 466 U/L $P<.01$), total bilirubin (9.5 mg/dL vs 4.9 mg/dL, $P<.01$), INR (1.8 vs 1.1, $P<.01$), and MELD scores (24 vs 16, $P<.01$) were higher at presentation. More patients that had early death or transplant met Hy's law criteria compared with survivors (45.8% vs 26.2%, $P<.01$). Patients that died or were transplanted were also more likely to have received corticosteroids than those that survived (82% vs 36.6%, $P<.01$). A significantly longer duration of medication use was seen in the early death/transplant group compared with survivors (67 vs 31 days, $P = .02$). On multivariate modeling, predictors of both time to death/transplantation and time to liver-related death/transplantation included Asian race, lower serum albumin and platelet counts at presentation, higher serum ALT and bilirubin levels at presentation, underlying pulmonary disease, and lack of itching.

Robles-Diaz and colleagues[24] evaluated cases of ALF from the Spanish DILI network between April 1994 and August 2012. A total of 805 DILI episodes were analyzed, and 32 episodes (4%) led to ALF and/or liver transplantation. Of the patients with ALF, 38% underwent liver transplantation, 59% died, and 3% recovered. Ten additional patients died within 6 months of the DILI episode from non-liver-related causes. The mean time between recognition of DILI by abnormal laboratory tests and death/liver transplantation in the ALF group was 26.6 days. There was a preponderance of women in the ALF group (64%), and more patients in the non-ALF group had dyslipidemia (14% vs 0%, $P = .027$). More patients with hepatocellular injury developed ALF than cholestatic injury (5.3% vs 1.4%). Three time points were analyzed and included DILI recognition, ALT peak, and bilirubin peak. Significant factors on multivariable regression included total bilirubin and AST/ALT ratio at the 3 time points, hepatocellular injury at DILI recognition and bilirubin peak, female sex at DILI recognition, and ALT peak.

The Spanish group aimed to develop a new prognostic algorithm to identify patients at highest risk for ALF at presentation. Most cases that meet the Hy's Law criteria do not go on to develop ALF; thus, it has poor specificity. They found that AST levels greater than 17.3 × ULN and bilirubin levels greater than 6.6 × ULN have a higher risk of ALF/OLT (orthotopic liver transplantation) progression than those without these 2 parameters. Having an AST/ALT ratio of greater than 1.5 further increased the risk of ALF/OLT. Using this algorithm, they identified 20% of cases as having a higher risk of ALF and 15% of those cases developed ALF resulting in 82% specificity and 80% specificity (AUROC [area under the receiver operating curve] 0.8). The prognostic algorithm was then tested on a group of DILI cases from Latin America and showed similar sensitivity (80%) and specificity (82%), although the number of cases of ALF was very small (5 of 97 cases), precluding true validation.[24]

Although serum ALT is a component of Hy's Law, several studies have shown that AST may have more prognostic importance. In the Swedish study, where stepwise logistic regression was performed to identify risk factors for death/transplantation, AST but not ALT was significant.[11] Other studies have also shown that AST levels were higher in those that progressed to fulminant hepatic failure compared with those that did not.[25]

In summary, DILI comprises a significant portion of cases of ALF and has high mortality without liver transplantation. Approximately 10% of patients with DILI will have ALF and die or require liver transplantation. Women may be more predisposed to ALF from DILI, but the data are mixed. Hepatocellular pattern of injury more commonly leads to ALF than cholestatic or mixed injury, and AST or AST/ALT ratio may be a better prognostic marker than ALT. However, there are no well-validated predictive scores to determine which patients will progress to ALF at the present time.

Persistent Liver Abnormalities/Chronic Drug-Induced Liver Injury

Although previously thought to be an "all or none" phenomenon, with patients either progressing to death or liver transplantation or completely recovering, several studies have described the development of chronic liver disease that is thought to be a result of DILI.

The Spanish DILI registry defined chronic DILI as persistent liver enzyme abnormalities 3 months after stopping the offending drug. If the injury was cholestatic/mixed, the abnormality needed to be persistent for more than 6 months following drug withdrawal. This study found that 28 patients of 493 (5.7%) met criteria for chronic DILI. They found that cholestatic/mixed type of damage was more prone to chronic outcome than hepatocellular injury (9% vs 4%, P<.031). Ten patients had chronic hepatocellular-type injury, 8 of which underwent a liver biopsy. Of these patients, 3 had cirrhosis and 2 had chronic hepatitis. Only 1 of these patients had complete normalization of liver tests after 26 months of follow-up. Eighteen patients with cholestatic injury had chronic enzyme elevations, and 7 were biopsied but only 1 had cirrhosis. Per the authors, an appropriate workup was performed and none of the patient with chronic hepatitis or cirrhosis had an alternative cause for chronic liver disease. In 6 of 10 patients with chronic hepatocellular damage, continued exposure to the offending drug was documented despite the development of symptoms of DILI over a median period of 23.5 days. Similarly, 10 of the 18 patients with chronic cholestatic damage continued the drug after symptoms had appeared (median 36 days). Nine patients exhibited chronic changes with a mixed pattern of injury. The patients with chronic DILI were compared between hepatocellular, cholestatic, and mixed groups. The patients with cholestatic injury were older (64 years vs 54 years for hepatocellular and 48 years for mixed). **Table 4** lists the drug classes that were associated with chronic injury and those associated with self-limited injury. There was a different

Table 4
Drug classes associated with chronic and self-limited drug-induced liver injury in Spanish registry

Chronic DILI	Cases (%)	Self-Limited DILI	Cases (%)
Cardiovascular	28.5	Anti-infectious	33
Central nervous system	25	Musculoskeletal	14
Anti-infectious	21	Central nervous system	13
Musculoskeletal	14	Cardiovascular	10
Gastrointestinal	11		

Cardiovascular drugs included angiotensin-converting enzyme inhibitors, angiotensin II antagonists, statins, fibrates.
    Central nervous system drugs included antidepressants, antiepileptics, anxiolytics.
    Anti-infectious agents included β-lactamase inhibitor penicillins, broad spectrum penicillins, macrolides.
    Musculoskeletal agents included nonsteroidal anti-inflammatory drugs.
    Gastrointestinal agents included histamine 2 inhibitors.

distribution, with cardiovascular drugs being the most common class in the group that developed chronic DILI and antimicrobials the most common class in those that had self-limited DILI. The authors also describe 2 cases of cirrhosis and portal hypertension that developed after the liver tests had nearly normalized and suggested that the true incidence of chronic liver injury could be underestimated if liver enzyme elevation is the only criteria used as a marker of chronic disease. Of the 3 patients that developed cirrhosis in the hepatocellular group, 2 were related to ebrotidine, a histamine 2 receptor antagonist that is no longer in use. The third case of cirrhosis in the hepatocellular group was attributed to unintentional re-exposure to amoxicillin-clavulanate. The case of cirrhosis in the cholestatic group was attributed to tamoxifen-induced hepatotoxicity with voluntary positive rechallenge.[5]

A study performed retrospectively using the Swedish registry evaluated a total of 784 patients that presented with acute idiosyncratic DILI. The cohort of patients with DILI was reported to the Swedish Adverse Drug Reactions Committee between the years of 1970 and 2004. Follow-up in the original study was only a few months, although in most cases patients were followed to the resolution of liver enzymes. This study used the National Cause of Death Register and Swedish Hospital Discharge Register to identify patients that were hospitalized after the DILI episode. They evaluated whether the subjects were hospitalized for liver disease and/or died of liver disease since the original study. Of the 784 patients that were in the cohort, 72 patients died of the DILI and 27 reports could not be retrieved. Thus, 685 patients could be included for analysis. Of these patients, 23 (3%) were diagnosed with a liver disorder during follow-up of a median of 11 years (range 3–23 years). Seven patients were admitted for a protracted DILI course with liver injury that required additional investigation with liver biopsy and/or endoscopic retrograde cholangiopancreatography. The patients with protracted liver injury were predominantly those with cholestatic reactions at the original DILI event (6 of 7 cases, 86%). Of those patients, only 1 patient still had abnormal liver tests at the last follow-up. Five patients were diagnosed with autoimmune hepatitis during follow-up. Six patients were hospitalized because they experienced another episode of DILI: 2 patients with the same offending drug and 4 patients with other drugs. Two patients developed serious liver disease during follow-up and were hospitalized for complications of cirrhosis. One of the patients had features of the metabolic syndrome, and thus fatty liver may have played a role. In total, 5 cases of "cryptogenic cirrhosis" were diagnosed in the total study cohort

(0.73%). Five patients died of liver disease according to the death certificate, and an additional 2 patients with liver disorder died of non-liver-related causes. The only factor that was associated with liver-related morbidity and mortality after DILI was longer duration of treatment with the offending medication (mean 135 days vs 53 days, P<.0001). There was no association of gender, age, type of liver injury, or degree of liver enzyme elevation. The major limitation of this study is that it is retrospective and relies on diagnosis codes from hospital registries. However, the authors report that 98% of the original cohort had a subsequent admission during their follow-up period; thus, any clinically significant liver disease should have been identified.[6]

In the US DILI network, chronic DILI was defined as having a persistently elevated serum AST, ALT, ALP, or total bilirubin level, histologic evidence of ongoing liver injury, or radiologic evidence of persistent liver injury (ie, ascites on imaging) at 6 months or more after the initial DILI onset date. When the US DILIN published their results, a total of 598 patients had data available for review at 6 months after their presentation with DILI. Of those patients, 113 (18.9%) met at least one of the protocol defined criteria for chronic DILI. The only demographic factor that was associated with the development of chronic DILI was African American race (18.6% vs 8.7%, P<.01). Chronic DILI patients were more likely to have a malignancy requiring treatment, and the median duration of medication use was longer in those that developed chronic DILI compared with those that did not (51 days vs 30 days, P<.01). Chronic DILI patients were more likely to have cholestatic liver injury at presentation compared with patients that did not develop chronic DILI (42.5% vs 21.9% P<.01). Peak bilirubin (13.7 mg/dL vs 7.9 mg/dL, P<.01) and INR (1.2 vs 1.1, P <.01) levels were higher in patients that developed chronic DILI compared with those that did not. Corticosteroids were more commonly used in patients that developed chronic DILI compared with those that did not (45.5% vs 34.4%, P<.01). On multivariable modeling, independent predictors of chronic DILI included presenting serum ALP, African American race, active malignancy and heart disease.[7]

In summary, liver enzyme elevations can persist for months to years after the episode of DILI in a significant portion of patients. Risk factors for chronic DILI appear to be cholestatic pattern of injury and longer duration of exposure to the offending agent. Age and African American race may also predispose to chronic DILI. The development of cirrhosis and liver-related morbidity and longer-term mortality has also been described but is rare.

SUMMARY

DILI is an important cause of abnormal liver tests in the population. The diagnosis requires a complete history and physical examination and exclusion of other causes of liver disease. The most common offending agents are antimicrobials and herbal/dietary supplements. Withdrawal of the offending agents leads to resolution of injury in most patients, although some patients will progress to ALF or develop chronic liver injury. Patients that present with hepatocellular injury with markedly elevated AST levels and jaundice are at the highest risk for developing ALF. Patients that present with cholestatic injury may develop a protracted course and are more likely to develop chronic DILI. Continued research to identify predictors of outcomes is necessary to help clinicians determine prognosis in patients that present with DILI.

REFERENCES

1. Meier Y, Cavallaro M, Roos M, et al. Incidence of drug-induced liver injury in medical inpatients. Eur J Clin Pharmacol 2005;61(2):135–43.

2. Bjornsson ES, Bergmann OM, Bjornsson HK, et al. Incidence, presentation, and outcomes in patients with drug-induced liver injury in the general population of Iceland. Gastroenterology 2013;144(7):1419–25.

3. Sgro C, Clinard F, Ouazir K, et al. Incidence of drug-induced hepatic injuries: a French population-based study. Hepatology 2002;36(2):451–5.

4. Dara L, Liu ZX, Kaplowitz N. Mechanisms of adaptation and progression in idiosyncratic drug induced liver injury, clinical implications. Liver Int 2016;36(2): 158–65.

5. Andrade RJ, Lucena MI, Kaplowitz N, et al. Outcome of acute idiosyncratic drug-induced liver injury: long-term follow-up in a hepatotoxicity registry. Hepatology 2006;44(6):1581–8.

6. Bjornsson E, Davidsdottir L. The long-term follow-up after idiosyncratic drug-induced liver injury with jaundice. J Hepatol 2009;50(3):511–7.

7. Fontana RJ, Hayashi PH, Gu J, et al. Idiosyncratic drug-induced liver injury is associated with substantial morbidity and mortality within 6 months from onset. Gastroenterology 2014;147(1):96–108.e104.

8. Available at: http://www.livertox.nih.gov/. Accessed May 1, 2016.

9. Andrade RJ, Lucena MI, Fernandez MC, et al. Drug-induced liver injury: an analysis of 461 incidences submitted to the Spanish registry over a 10-year period. Gastroenterology 2005;129(2):512–21.

10. Chalasani N, Fontana RJ, Bonkovsky HL, et al. Causes, clinical features, and outcomes from a prospective study of drug-induced liver injury in the United States. Gastroenterology 2008;135(6):1924–34.

11. Bjornsson E, Olsson R. Outcome and prognostic markers in severe drug-induced liver disease. Hepatology 2005;42(2):481–9.

12. Jinjuvadia K, Kwan W, Fontana RJ. Searching for a needle in a haystack: use of ICD-9-CM codes in drug-induced liver injury. Am J Gastroenterol 2007;102(11): 2437–43.

13. Chalasani N, Bonkovsky HL, Fontana R, et al. Features and outcomes of 899 patients with drug-induced liver injury: the DILIN prospective study. Gastroenterology 2015;148(7):1340–52.e1347.

14. Chalasani NP, Hayashi PH, Bonkovsky HL, et al. ACG Clinical Guideline: the diagnosis and management of idiosyncratic drug-induced liver injury. Am J Gastroenterol 2014;109(7):950–66 [quiz: 967].

15. Zimmerman HJ. Hepatotoxicity: the adverse effects of drugs and other chemicals on the liver. 2nd edition. Philadelphia: Lippincott Williams & Wilkins; 1999.

16. Davern TJ, Chalasani N, Fontana RJ, et al. Acute hepatitis E infection accounts for some cases of suspected drug-induced liver injury. Gastroenterology 2011; 141(5):1665–72.e1661–1669.

17. Lewis JH. Causality assessment: which is best—expert opinion or RUCAM? Clin Liver Dis 2014;4(1):4–8.

18. Ostapowicz G, Fontana RJ, Schiodt FV, et al. Results of a prospective study of acute liver failure at 17 tertiary care centers in the United States. Ann Intern Med 2002;137(12):947–54.

19. Wei G, Bergquist A, Broome U, et al. Acute liver failure in Sweden: etiology and outcome. J Intern Med 2007;262(3):393–401.

20. Reuben A, Koch DG, Lee WM, Acute Liver Failure Study Group. Drug-induced acute liver failure: results of a U.S. multicenter, prospective study. Hepatology 2010;52(6):2065–76.

21. Hillman L, Gottfried M, Whitsett M, et al. Clinical features and outcomes of complementary and alternative medicine induced acute liver failure and injury. Am J Gastroenterol 2016;111(7):958–65.

22. O'Grady JG, Alexander GJ, Hayllar KM, et al. Early indicators of prognosis in fulminant hepatic failure. Gastroenterology 1989;97(2):439–45.

23. Hoofnagle JH, Carithers RL Jr, Shapiro C, et al. Fulminant hepatic failure: summary of a workshop. Hepatology 1995;21(1):240–52.

24. Robles-Diaz M, Lucena MI, Kaplowitz N, et al. Use of Hy's law and a new composite algorithm to predict acute liver failure in patients with drug-induced liver injury. Gastroenterology 2014;147(1):109–18.e105.

25. Ohmori S, Shiraki K, Inoue H, et al. Clinical characteristics and prognostic indicators of drug-induced fulminant hepatic failure. Hepatogastroenterology 2003; 50(53):1531–4.

Mechanisms of Drug-Induced Hepatotoxicity

Amina Ibrahim Shehu, BSᵃ, Xiaochao Ma, PhDᵃ, Raman Venkataramanan, PhDᵇ,*

KEYWORDS

- Hepatotoxicity • Reactive metabolites • Mitochondria • Hepatocellular • Cholestasis

KEY POINTS

- Drug-induced hepatotoxicity (DIH) is an important clinical problem and a leading cause of liver failure in adults.
- Multiple mechanisms and factors contribute to the etiology and pathology of DIH.
- Generation of reactive metabolites, oxidative stress, and mitochondrial dysfunction are common mechanisms of DIH.

Drug-induced hepatotoxicity (DIH) is an important clinical problem in the United States and around the world. It is one of the primary reasons for failure of drug candidates during preclinical drug development, early-phase clinical trials, and Food and Drug Administration drug withdrawal from the market after drug approval (examples in **Tables 1** and **2**).[1] Previous reports have shown that drug-mediated hepatotoxicity is responsible for more than 50% of reported cases of acute liver failure in the United States.[2] Although acetaminophen (APAP) accounts for a majority of cases of DIH, other drugs also account for acute liver failure more frequently than viral hepatitis and other causes.[2] In a population-based study in Iceland, the incidence of DIH was reported to be as high as 19 cases per 100,000 people.[3] DIH can present as acute liver failure or chronic liver failure, which makes it difficult to distinguish DIH from other liver diseases.

DIH usually appears as elevations of serum liver enzymes with or without an increase in bilirubin. DIH is defined as an increase in alanine aminotransferase (ALT) 5 times above the upper limit of normal or baseline value; alkaline phosphatase (ALP) 2 times above the upper limit of normal; or a combination of ALT 3 times above the upper limit of normal and bilirubin 2 times above the upper limit of normal.[4] The pattern of liver enzyme increase is further classified into 3 subtypes based on the R value, which is defined as the ratio of ALT to ALP expressed in multiples of the

The authors have nothing to disclose.
ᵃ Department of Pharmaceutical Sciences, School of Pharmacy, University of Pittsburgh, 3rd Floor Salk Pavillion, Pittsburgh, PA 15261, USA; ᵇ Department of Pharmaceutical Sciences, School of Pharmacy, University of Pittsburgh, 718 Salk Hall, 3501 Terrace Street, Pittsburgh, PA 15261, USA
* Corresponding author.
E-mail address: RV@pitt.edu

Clin Liver Dis 21 (2017) 35–54
http://dx.doi.org/10.1016/j.cld.2016.08.002
1089-3261/17/

Table 1
Drugs withdrawn from the market due to hepatotoxicity (United States, European Union, United Kingdom, and France)

Drug	Class	Mechanism of Toxicity
Troglitazone	Antidiabetic/anti-inflammatory	Reactive metabolites
Benoxaprofen	NSAID	Reactive metabolites
Bromfenac	NSAID	Reactive metabolites
Ibufenac	NSAID	Reactive metabolites
Temafloxacin	Fluoroquinoline antibiotic	Not clear
Alatrofloxacin	Fluoroquinoline antibiotic	Not clear
Trovafloxacin	Fluoroquinoline antibiotic	Mitochondrial dysfunction, inflammatory stress
Benzarone	Thrombolytic	Reactive metabolites
Ximelagatran	Anticoagulant	Immune mediated
Clomacron	Psychotropic drug	Not clear
Nafazodone	Antidepressant	Reactive metabolites
Cyclofenil	Antiestrogen	Not clear
Dilevalol	Antihypertensive	Immune mediated
Sitaxentan	Antihypertensive	Mitochondrial dysfunction Covalent binding to liver proteins
Tienilic acid	Antihypertensive	Reactive metabolites Immune response
Pemoline	CNS stimulant	Partly immune mediated Not completely clear

Abbreviations: CNS, central nervous system; NSAID, nonsteroidal anti-inflammatory drug.
   Data from Refs.[115–119]

upper limit of normal. An R value greater than 5 denotes hepatocellular injury; R value of 2 to 5 is mixed; and R value less than 2 is cholestatic type of injury. Hepatocellular pattern of liver injury is characterized by cellular necrosis and inflammation with little or no elevation of bilirubin. ALT and aspartate aminotransferase (AST) levels are usually high whereas ALP levels are mildly increased. Patients usually present with malaise and exhaustion. The cholestatic pattern of injury is typified by accumulation of bile in the hepatocytes due an insult to the bile ducts, increased levels of bilirubin and ALP, and jaundice with itching on the skin. The mixed pattern of injury is often encountered in DIH and combines the features of hepatocellular and cholestatic pattern of liver injury. Patients may present with both exhaustion and itching, elevated levels of ALT and ALP, and bile accumulation. DIH can also appear in the form of other liver diseases, like acute or cholestatic hepatitis, steatosis, acute necrosis, chronic hepatitis, and nonalcoholic fatty liver disease (http://livertox.nih.gov/Phenotypes_enzy.html).

DIH can be dose dependent and predictable or it can be idiosyncratic, which occurs only in specific individuals and is not strictly drug dose dependent. Many efforts have been made in understanding the mechanisms that drive DIH. General mechanisms involved in DIH include cell death, metabolism-mediated reactive metabolite formation, immune-mediated reaction, and mitochondrial dysfunction. Multiple mechanisms together seem to contribute to clinically observed DIH (**Fig. 1**).

Table 2
Examples of drugs currently used in the clinic that can cause hepatotoxicity

Drug/Class	Pattern of Injury	Mechanism of Toxicity
Amoxicillin-clavulanate (antibiotic)	Cholestasis, mixed, or hepatocellular	Immunoallergic
INH (antibiotic)	Hepatocellular	Reactive metabolites immunoallergic
KTE (antifungal)	Hepatocellular, cholestatic	Reactive metabolites?
Ibuprofen (analgesic)	Mixed or cholestatic	Immunoallergic
Nitrofurantoin (antibiotic)	Hepatocellular	Reactive metabolites, autoimmune mediated
[a]Propylthiouracil (antithyroid)	Hepatocelluar, cholestatic, or mixed	Immunoallergic
Carbamazepine (anti-epileptic)	Cholestatic, mixed, or hepatocellular	Reactive metabolites, immunoallergic
[a]Valproate (antiepileptic)	Mixed or hepatocellular	Mitochondrial dysfunction
Asparaginase (anticancer)	Cholestatic	Mitochondrial dysfunction
Azathioprine (immunosuppressant)	Cholestatic, mixed	Reactive metabolites, immunoallergic
Infliximab	Hepatocellular, cholestatic	Autoimmune mediated
Diclofenac	Hepatocellular	Immunoallergic
Flutamide	Hepatocellular	Reactive metabolites?

[a] Drugs show a high incidence of hepatotoxicity in the pediatric population.
Data from Refs.[3,38,95], and http://livertox.nlm.nih.gov/index.html.

CELL DEATH (APOPTOSIS AND NECROSIS)

The hallmark of DIH is death of hepatocytes or sometimes cholangiocytes and endothelial cells. Different modes of cell death are encountered with different drugs. The 2 most common forms of cell death in DIH are apoptosis and necrosis. Apoptosis, also known as programmed cell death, is an ATP-dependent process characterized by shrinking of the cell, condensation of chromatin, and extensive distortion of the extracellular membrane blebbing but without the release of cellular contents to the extracellular medium.[5] Surrounding phagocytes immediately clear the dying cells. In this mode of cell death, inflammation is limited because cellular contents are not released into the surrounding cells.[5] The proteolytic enzymes caspases are responsible for the controlled degradation of cells during apoptosis. Apoptosis can occur through intrinsic or extrinsic pathways. The intrinsic pathway is activated by intracellular stimuli, such as toxins, radiation, or depletion of growth factors in the cell. This results in the activation of proapoptotic mitochondrial proteins, like Bax, Bid, and Bim, that guide the opening of the outer mitochondrial membrane and the release of cytochrome c, endoribonuclease G, and other mitochondrial proteins. The release of cytochrome c leads to the activation of initiator caspase 9 and eventually caspase 3 that executes apoptosis.[5] On the other hand, the extrinsic pathway of apoptosis is induced by ligand binding to death receptors of the tumor necrosis factor (TNF)-α family present on the transmembrane surface of a cell. Some examples of death receptors and their ligands that transmit lethal stimuli to intracellular signaling pathways include fatty acid synthase receptor and ligand and the TNF receptor 1 and TNF-α. Activation of death receptors leads to the subsequent activation of caspase 8 and the

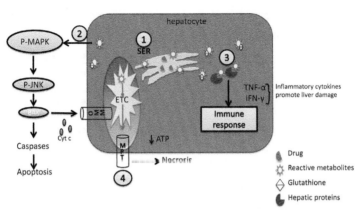

Fig. 1. General mechanisms of DIH death. (1) Drug is metabolized in the ER by P450s or other enzymes to reactive metabolites. (2) RM can lead to the activation of stress signaling pathways like the JNK pathway to induce apoptosis through the recruitment of Bax to the OMM. Insertion of Bax to the OMM leads to the permeability of the OMM and the release of mitochondrial proteins like Cyt c. Cyt c release can lead to the activation of caspases and the induction of apoptosis. (3) RMs is usually detoxified by antioxidants like glutathione. Depletion of glutathione, however, can allow RM to covalently bind to hepatic proteins. This can lead to an immune response through the activation of cytotoxic T cells. (4) Generation of ROS in the mitochondria can also lead to the inhibition of ECT chain and opening of MPT pore. This can lead to the collapse of mitochondrial respiration, inhibition of ATP synthesis and cell death via necrosis. Cyt c, cytochrome c; ETC, electron transport chain; MPT, mitochondria permeability transition; OMM, outer mitochondrial membrane; RM, reactive metabolite.

executioner caspase 3, which leads to cell death.[5] Diclofenac is a drug that induces apoptosis in hepatocytes.[6]

Necrotic cell death, on the other hand, involves swelling of the endoplasmic reticulum (ER) and mitochondria, complete dissolution of the nuclear fragment, and rupture of the cell membrane to release cellular contents.[7] Unlike apoptosis, necrosis is usually accompanied by inflammation due to the recruitment of chemotactic signals resulting from the release of cellular contents to the neighboring cells.[5] Also, there is loss of mitochondrial membrane potential due ion gradient collapse and ATP depletion.[8] Necrosis used to be considered an unregulated process until recent years, when studies have shown its regulation by activation of receptor-interacting protein kinases 1 and 3 and involves the mitochondria.[9] APAP is a classic example of a drug that induces necrosis in hepatocytes.

REACTIVE METABOLITE FORMATION (BIOACTIVATION)

The metabolism of drugs normally involves the breakdown of lipophilic compounds to more water-soluble substances that can be readily excreted out of the body. Drug biotransformation, however, can sometimes lead to the formation of reactive chemical metabolites that can bind to nucleic acids, cellular proteins, and lipids, thus leading to DNA damage, loss of protein function, and lipid peroxidation.[10] Reactive metabolite generation can also activate the adaptive immune response and induce stress in the ER and mitochondria, which all together contribute to liver damage.[11] The formation of reactive metabolites as a mechanism for hepatotoxicity is reported for drugs like APAP, halothane, and tienilic acid.

DRUG TRANSPORTER–MEDIATED DRUG-INDUCED HEPATOTOXICITY

Hepatic drug transporters are involved in the uptake and efflux of endogenous compounds and certain drugs into and out of hepatocytes, respectively. Altered expression (genetic polymorphism) or inhibition of these transporters can predispose patients to DIH.[12] Polymorphism in the uptake transporter, organic anionic transporting polypeptide (OATP1B1), predisposes patients to rifampin-mediated liver injury.[13] Also, polymorphism in the canalicular transporter multidrug resistance-associated protein (MRP) 2 is associated with elevated levels of bilirubin and jaundice.[14] Certain drugs, like cyclosporine, estradiol, and bosentan, can alter the activity of the biliary transporter bile salt excretory pump (BSEP) and lead to cholestatic or mixed type of liver injury.[14] Transporters, like MRP2 and MRP3, are involved in secretion of drugs and metabolites into bile. Altered expression of these transporters have been reported in patients with drug-induced liver injury.[15]

IMMUNE-MEDIATED RESPONSE

Injury to hepatocytes can trigger the release of chemicals that can activate cells of the innate immune system that are resident in the liver. The Kupffer cells, natural killer cells, and natural killer T cells exist in large numbers in the liver to protect it from harm by viral or bacterial toxins and xenobiotics. Activation of these cells, however, promotes DIH through the recruitment of proinflammatory cytokines, such as TNF-α, interferon (IFN)-γ, and interleukin (IL)-Iβ, that potentiate the inflammatory response resulting in further tissue damage.[11] Genome-wide association studies have shown a connection between various HLA haplotypes and DIH. For example, abacavir is generally well tolerated, but hypersentivity reactions take place in 5% to 8% of patients due to the activation of HLA-B*5701.[16,17] DIH associated with the adaptive immune response presents with allergic reaction–related symptoms, like skin rash, fever, eosinophilia, and detection of antibodies directed against modified or native hepatic proteins indicative of an immune-mediated response. In addition, rechallenge with the drug causes toxicity. Examples of drugs that show such reactions are halothane and phenytoin.[18]

MITOCHONDRIAL DYSFUNCTION

The mitochondria are the powerhouse of the cell where energy is produced for normal cellular function. Many drugs used clinically target this organelle to cause toxicity by interfering with different functions of the mitochondria, such as fatty acid β-oxidation, mitochondrial permeability transition pore formation (MPTP), oxidative phosphorylation, and mitochondrial DNA replication. The MPTP is a protein pore that is located in the inner membrane of the mitochondria. MPTP pore induction increases mitochondrial permeability to molecules greater than 1.5 kDa, which in turn allows the inflow of water and ions like calcium into mitochondria and the escape of protons. As a result, mitochondria can undergo swelling and rupture of the outer mitochondrial membrane.[19] This leads to disruption of the electrochemical gradient, loss of membrane potential, generation of reactive oxygen species (ROS), and ATP depletion due to collapse of the electron transport chain.[20] IFN-α and nucleoside analog drugs can affect the replication of mitochondrial DNA,[21] and ibuprofen can inhibit fatty acid β oxidation.[22] Mitochondrial toxicity can lead to cell death via necrosis (due to ATP depletion) and apoptosis (through the release of mitochondrial proteins like cytochrome c).[23] Mitochondrial dysfunction leads to the activation of other stress pathways that are discussed in the following section.

ACTIVATION OF STRESS SIGNALING PATHWAYS

The c-jun N-terminal kinase (JNK) serves diverse functions in hepatocytes, including cell death, regeneration, and differentiation.[24] JNK is activated by a wide variety of stress signals, like ROS, drugs, radiation, cytokines, and pathogens. JNK is regulated upstream by 2 successive mitogen-activated protein kinases (MAPKs). The MAP kinase kinase kinases (MAP3Ks [eg, ASK1 and MLK]) activates MAP kinase kinases (MAP2Ks [eg, MKK4 and MKK7]), which then activate JNK (MAPK) at the threonine tyrosine residue.[25] Once JNK is activated, it induces its protein substrates downstream to execute its functions. JNK activates mitochondrial proteins, like antiapoptotic Bcl2 and Bcl-XL; proapoptotic Bad, Bim, and Bid; and other nonmitochondrial proteins, like Bax, c-jun, p53, and c-Myc.[24]

TNF-α is one of the common cytokines induced during hepatocyte injury that serves as a stimulus for JNK activation. Sustained JNK activation and its interaction with diverse signaling pathways have been implicated in the pathology of many liver diseases, including but not limited to ischemia and reperfusion liver injury, nonalcoholic liver disease, hepatocellular carcinoma, APAP-induced hepatotoxicity, and liver fibrosis.[24] TNF-related apoptosis–inducing ligand potentiates Fas-induced hepatocyte apoptosis through JNK activation that to leads to the phosphorylation of Bim and subsequent mitochondrial dysfunction.[26]

ER stress is another stress pathway that can lead to the induction of JNK to mediate cell death via apoptosis.[24] The ER is the organelle where the cytochrome P450 (CYP450) metabolizing enzymes are located. The ER is also responsible for proper protein folding, secretion, and transportation to other target organs.[27] Hepatocytes are rich in ER. Misfolding or accumulation of proteins in the ER due to stress signals, like ROS, drugs, calcium depletion, and toxins, can trigger the unfolded protein response (UPR) to help restore proper ER function. Three signal transducers that are located on the ER membrane control the UPR. This includes inositol-requiring protein 1 (IRE1), protein kinase RNA-like ER kinase, and activating transcription factor ATF-6.[27] They act by inhibiting global protein synthesis, induction of chaperones, and degradation pathways to increase protein folding and clearing of accumulated proteins. The IRE1 pathway can activate JNK through its interaction with TRAF-2 to induce apoptosis when the UPR is not able to restore normal ER homeostasis.[27]

FACTORS THAT CONTRIBUTE TO DRUG-INDUCED LIVER INJURY
Age

Age has an important effect on DIH (**Fig. 2**). People greater than 40 years are normally more susceptible to liver injury due to altered drug disposition, excretion, and the intake of multiple drugs at the same time. On the contrary, children are at more risk of DIH with drugs like valproate and aspirin. Also, 1 study conducted using cases of DIH in a Spanish registry reported that older patients experienced more cholestatic type of liver injury compared with a younger population who experienced hepatocellular type of injury.[28]

Gender

Gender might influence differences in susceptibility to DIH in men and women. Women are more susceptible to autoimmune-mediated DIH and to liver injury caused by drugs like isoniazid (INH), halothane, and erythromycin.[29] Women with DIH were also reported to have a worse outcome that results in fulminant liver injury and transplantation.[28] Men are more susceptible to liver injury caused by azathioprine and amoxicillin-clavunate.[28,30,31]

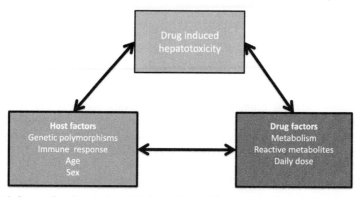

Fig. 2. Risk factors for developing DIH. Most DIH is idiosyncratic; thus, the genetic make-up of individuals as well as their health condition and the interplay of other factors increase the susceptibility to a drugs toxic effect.

Genetic Factors

Genetic factors, such as mutations in CYP450 or phase II enzyme genes, mitochondrial DNA, and antioxidant genes, are believed to contribute significantly to DIH, especially idiosyncratic drug reactions. For example, mutations in CYP2E1 (CYP2E1 c1/c1) and *N*-acetyltransferase (NAT [NAT *5, *6, *7]) both enzymes associated with isoniazid (INH) metabolism, increase susceptibility to INH hepatotoxicity. In patients with NAT slow acetylator phenotype, the conversion of INH to acetyl-INH and acetyl hydrazine to diacetyl hydrazine, that is required for normal breakdown of INH to non-toxic metabolites, is decreased. This results in formation of toxic by-products that are believed to mediate INH hepatotoxicity.[32] Polymorphisms associated with detoxification and antioxidant enzymes like glutathione S transferase (GST), and mitochondrial superoxide dismutase are reported to be associated with increased risk of DIH. Genetic variation in the expression of the bile salt export pump (BSEP) transporter has been associated with increased susceptibility to cholestatic DIH caused by drugs like troglitazone.[33] In addition to genes regulating drug metabolism and transport, genes regulating human leukocyte antigens, cytokines, and oxidative stress may also impact DIH.

Immune Response

Immune response in individuals is a major determinant of idiosyncratic DIH. The presence of preexisting inflammatory response, polymorphisms in cytokine-encoding genes, and HLA class II antigens contributes to how the body responds to drugs and the occurrence of immune-mediated DIH. For example, genetic variants of the anti-inflammatory cytokine IL-10 were found more in individuals who had diclofenac-induced hepatotoxicity compared with those who were on diclofenac but did not develop DIH or their healthy controls.[34] Also, a genome-wide association study showed that flucloxacillin DIH was associated with the HLA-B*5701 genotype.[35] Reactive metabolites covalently bind to hepatic proteins and may serve as antigens that falsely trigger an immune response and that leads to the formation of antibodies against the modified or native proteins and the induction of cytotoxic response to clear antigens.[34] This may contribute to the pathogenesis of DIH although a direct causal relationship has not been established.

Daily Dose of Drug and Metabolism

In 2 studies conducted using data on oral prescription drugs most commonly prescribed in the United States, drugs administered at a dose of greater than 50 mg a day and are extensively metabolized by the liver are more likely to cause DIH compared to those administered at lower doses or less hepatic metabolism.[36,37]

Other factors, such as preexisting diseases, like viral hepatitis and diabetes, increase the risk of DIH. The consumption of alcohol and concomitant use of other hepatotoxic drugs is also associated with increased susceptibility to DIH. Furthermore, the duration of exposure to the drug may determine the severity of hepatotoxicity.[38] A combination of these factors predisposes individuals to DIH (see **Fig. 2**). In the following section, DIH associated with selected drugs is discussed in detail.

Acetaminophen

APAP-induced hepatotoxicity is one of the most well studied DIHs and provides a model for studying and understanding DIH. APAP accounts for greater than 50% of acute liver failure in the United States.[2,39] APAP is an example of a drug that induces predictable hepatotoxicity because it is dose dependent and clinical symptoms are well characterized. The maximum daily dose of APAP is less than 4 g. Doses greater than 4 g daily increase the risk of APAP-induced hepatotoxicity. In some cases, however, doses less than 4 g have also been reported to cause toxicity.

Mechanism

Reactive metabolites APAP is primarily metabolized by glucuronidation and sulfation. It is also metabolized by CYP2E1 and to a lesser extent by CYP1A2, and CYP3A4.[40,41] At normal doses, APAP is metabolized to the reactive metabolite N-acetyl-p-benzoquinone amine (NAPQI) that is efficiently detoxified through conjugation with glutathione.[42,43] At toxic doses, increased amounts of NAPQI are produced that lead to the depletion of reduced glutathione by 80% to 90%. An insufficient level of reduced glutathione needed for detoxification of NAPQI causes covalent binding of the reactive metabolite to cellular proteins, DNA, and leads to increased levels of ROS.[44]

Covalent binding was shown in an elegant study in mice using radiolabeled APAP. Mice dosed with 300 mg/kg to 750 mg/kg of APAP showed a dose-dependent increase in covalent binding of APAP metabolite to mouse liver protein in the microsome and cytoplasm. Furthermore, covalent binding correlated with the severity of hepatic necrosis.[44] Activation of the nuclear receptor pregnane X receptor (PXR) that regulates the induction of CYP3A4, one of the enzymes that contributes to APAP metabolism, has also been reported to increase APAP toxicity in a humanized PXR and CYP3A4 mouse model.[45] Mitchell and colleagues[43] also reported that administration of cysteine in mice receiving toxic doses of APAP reduced toxicity and covalent binding of toxic metabolite to mouse liver proteins. This study formed the basis for use of N-acetylcysteine (NAC) as antidote in APAP-induced hepatotoxicity.[46,47] The activation of liver X receptor (LXR) has also been proposed as a potential target for ameliorating APAP-induced hepatotoxicity because transgenic mice with LXR activation were resistant to APAP toxicity compared with transgenic mice with LXR deficiency.[48]

Oxidative stress Covalent binding of NAPQI to proteins, especially mitochondrial proteins, has been recognized as an important source of oxidative stress in APAP-induced hepatotoxicity.[49] Glutathione disulfide, which is the oxidized form of glutathione and a marker for increased formation of hydrogen peroxide, was increased greater than 20% in the mitochondria of mice treated with toxic doses of APAP compared with their controls.[49] Another study in mice also showed similar elevations of glutathione disulfide and the formation of peroxynitrite, a by-product of superoxide and nitric oxide reaction, evidenced by an increased staining for nitro tyrosine in centrilobular hepatocytes.[50,51] Furthermore, cells stained for APAP-protein adduct also contained nitrated proteins and correlated with necrosis.[51] These studies support the hypothesis that there is an increased generation of superoxide and peroxynitrite in the mitochondria, which causes glutathione and ATP depletion in APAP toxicity.[49,50] These effects can be reversed by administration of NAC and glutathione.[52]

Mitochondrial injury Mitochondrial dysfunction plays an important role in APAP toxicity. Livers from mice treated with toxic doses of APAP showed altered mitochondrial morphology and decreased mitochondrial respiration.[53,54] High doses of APAP cause mitochondrial dysfunction through the induction of the MPTP, which leads to the depolarization and permeability of inner mitochondria membrane, ATP depletion, and swelling of the mitochondria due accumulation of calcium.[55,56] Oxidative stress and peroxynitrite formation occur downstream of the mitochondrial permeability transition, which together mediate APAP-induced hepatic necrosis.[57] In a study of human subjects with APAP-induced hepatotoxicity, biomarkers for mitochondrial dysfunction-glutamate dehydrogenase and mitochondrial DNA and fragments of nuclear DNA were elevated in the plasma of these patients compared with their healthy controls and controls that ingested APAP but showed no signs of liver injury.[58] This study further confirmed the importance of mitochondrial injury in APAP-induced hepatotoxicity in both humans and mice.

Activation of signaling kinase-c-jun N-terminal kinase activation Sustained JNK activation is observed in APAP-induced hepatotoxicity both in vitro and in vivo in mice. JNK activation mediates APAP toxicity through the recruitment of Bax and Sab to the mitochondrial outer membrane and the potentiation of oxidative stress and peroxynitrite formation in the mitochondria. Treatment with JNK inhibitor or knockout of JNK in mice abrogated APAP toxicity.[59–61]

Isoniazid

INH remains one of the first-line drugs used in the treatment of tuberculosis since its introduction into the clinic.[62,63] It is used in combination with other antituberculosis drugs or alone for the treatment of active or latent tuberculosis disease, respectively.[64] INH was reported to cause hepatitis in a small number of patients shortly after its use in the clinic and thus acquired black box warning for DIH in 1967.[64] Elevation of ALT above 5 times the upper limit of normal is seen in approximately 3% to 5% of patients, whereas severe hepatotoxicity occurs in less than 1% of patients (http://livertox.nlm.nih.gov/Isoniazid.htm). A pattern of INH-induced hepatotoxicity seen in patients is hepatocellular injury with inflammation and mutilobular necrosis, in some patients.[65] Mechanisms of INH-induced hepatotoxicity are still poorly understood due to the lack of correlation of phenotype seen in human to phenotype seen in animal models.[64] Significant efforts have been made, however, to understand the mechanisms involved. Mechanisms proposed for INH-induced liver injury include the following.

Metabolism and reactive metabolites
INH is metabolized by NAT and acyl amidase to acetyl-INH and acetylhydrazine, respectively. The oxidation of acetylhydrazine to toxic metabolites that can covalently bind to liver proteins is believed to be a key player in INH-induced hepatotoxicity.[66]

Hydrazine has been reported to cause ATP depletion both in vivo and in vitro in rats, mega mitochondria in rats, glutathione depletion, inhibition of catalase activity, and lactate dehydrogenase.[67–69] Other proposed mechanisms for INH toxicity are the bioactivation of INH itself to form metabolites that can directly react with lysine groups in liver proteins[70] and auto-oxidation of INH, independent of metabolism, to form free radicals that form adducts with human serum albumin in vitro; similar adducts were found in patients in INH therapy.[30] Recently, the activation of the nuclear receptor PXR was shown to modulate INH combined with rifampicin-induced hepatotoxicity through the disturbance of the heme biosynthesis pathway and the induction of protoporphyrin IX (a hepatotoxin) accumulation in the liver.[71]

Immune-mediated mechanisms

Clinical studies have highlighted the role of the immune system in INH-induced hepatotoxicity, although most patients who develop hepatotoxicity on INH do not present with symptoms, like fever, rash, and reoccurrence, on rechallenge with the drug (indicative of an allergic reaction). Early work on developing a clinical test that could be used to identify patients with a higher risk of developing INH hepatotoxicity showed that patients who tested positive for lymphocyte transformation test had an increased risk compared with patients who tested negative, suggesting the role of T cells in mediating INH-induced hepatotoxicity.[72] In a recent study of patients who developed liver injury on INH therapy, antibodies against INH and CYP2E1, CYP3A4, and CYP2C9 were detected in the sera of these patients compared with a control group of patients on INH therapy but with mild liver injury.[73] Another study in patients on INH for treatment of latent tuberculosis who developed mild increase in ALT levels reported an increase in T helper 17 cells and T cells that produce IL-10. T helper 17 cells secrete IL-17 that is proinflammatory and has been associated autoimmune diseases as well as liver injury whereas IL-10 is an anti-inflammatory cytokine. The conclusion from this study was that the increased production of IL-10 in these patients was a protective mechanism to prevent the development of more severe hepatotoxicity.[74] These findings support the hypothesis that those patients on INH with mild elevations of ALT that does not progress to fatal hepatotoxicity develop an immune tolerance to protect them. In a small percentage of patients where immune tolerance fails, severe hepatotoxicity ensues.

Risk factors associated with isoniazid -induced hepatotoxicity

Many host factors are considered important in INH-induced hepatotoxicity. Increasing age, alcohol consumption, malnutrition, female gender, and pregnancy are associated with an increased risk of INH-induced liver toxicity.[75–77] Patients with an NAT slow acetylator phenotype have increased blood levels of acetylhydrazine and INH, which increase their exposure and risk of developing liver injury. Genetic variations in other enzymes, like CYP2E1, GST M1, and manganese superoxide dismutase, that contribute less to INH metabolism may also increase risk.[78,79]

Nevirapine

Nevirapine (NVP) is a non-nucleoside reverse transcriptase inhibitor used in combination with other drugs for the treatment of HIV disease. NVP is associated with serious hypersensitivity skin reactions and hepatotoxicity, which occurs either alone or concomitantly. Reports about incidence of hepatotoxicity with NVP treatment range from 1% to 6% and in severe cases can lead to death.[80] Toxicity usually ensues within 5 weeks of starting NVP therapy and is usually preceded by elevations of amino transaminase liver enzymes.[80] The lack of animal models that mimic clinical features of

NVP-induced hepatotoxicity has made understanding the mechanism difficult. The 2 major mechanisms proposed, however, are metabolic activation to reactive metabolites and immune-mediated reactions.

Reactive metabolites in nevirapine hepatotoxicity

NVP is metabolized mainly by CYP3A4 and CYP2B6 to its hydroxyl metabolites that undergo glucuronidation. A study on NVP using anti-NVP antiserum has shown the ability of NVP to covalently bind to hepatic proteins through one of its toxic metabolites, quinone methide, in rats, mice, and humans. Covalent binding in mice and rats in vivo, however, did not correlate with induction of liver injury.[81] In addition, another study in human liver microsomes showed that the quinone methide, an intermediate generated by NVP metabolism, could react with the sulfhydryl group in glutathione to form glutathione conjugates.[82] This supports the hypothesis that NVP undergoes bioactivation to form reactive metabolites that may initiate NVP hepatotoxicity. Increased levels of NVP and its metabolites with continuous dosing have been proposed as a risk factor for NVP hepatotoxicity. A clinical study in patients, however, could not find any correlation between plasma levels of NVP and its metabolites to hepatotoxicity.[83] Furthermore, a gender-dependent metabolism of NVP has been reported in a clinical study where women were found to have increased proportion NVP metabolites 3–hydroxy-NVP and 12–hydroxy-NVP compared men. The investigators concluded the difference in metabolism might be responsible for sex dimorphism in NVP hepatotoxicity, with women showing greater risk.[84]

Immune-mediated reactions

NVP use is limited by a hypersentivity reaction that presents itself within the first few weeks of starting therapy. Rash and hepatotoxicity occurs in approximately 6% of patients who start NVP-based therapy.[85] NVP-induced hypersensitivity reaction is thought to be immune mediated because of the delayed onset of the reaction, remediation on discontinuation of the drug, and reoccurrence on rechallenge. A higher rate of NVP-induced hepatotoxicity is reported in treatment-naïve or treatment-experienced patients with higher CD4 cell counts starting NVP-based antiretroviral therapy or HIV-negative patients taking NVP for postexposure prophylaxis.[86] Furthermore, various genetic variants of the HLA class I and II are reportedly associated with NVP-induced hepatitis among different populations.[87]

Azoles—ketoconazole

The incidence of acute liver injury with ketoconazole (KET) ranges from 0.1% to 1%.[88] In 2013, the Food and Drug Administration issued a black box warning of hepatotoxicity associated with the use of KET.[89] Hepatotoxicity is not associated with clinically used dose and is usually mild and reversible on discontinuation of the drug. Few cases of fatal injury have been reported.[90] Pattern of injury is mostly hepatocellular. Exact mechanism of hepatotoxicity is not known; however, in vitro studies in animals suggest involvement of reactive metabolite(s). Studies in rat postnatal hepatocytes showed that KET was cytotoxic in a dose and time-dependent manner.[91] Furthermore, KET is metabolized by flavin monooxygenases and other enzymes to N-deacetyl- KET, which is more toxic than the parent drug and can undergo further metabolism to generate reactive aldehyde that can induce toxicity.[92] In vivo studies in rats also showed that KET can lead to the depletion of glutathione and covalently bind to hepatic proteins in microsomes.[93] In another study in rabbits, elevation of serum transaminases correlated to the area under the curve of KET not the dose or maximum concentration of the drug.[94] This suggests that the concentration as well as the duration of exposure to KET may be key factors in toxicity. Overall, there are few clinical data in humans that highlight the mechanism of KET toxicity; nonetheless, studies in animals suggest KET and N-deacetyl-KET to be the hepatotoxicants.

Amoxicillin-Clavulanic Acid

Amoxicillin-clavulanic acid (ACA) is the leading cause of DIH resulting from prescription medications, as published by different prospective studies from the United States, Spain, and Iceland.[3,38,95] The incidence of ACA-induced hepatotoxicity is estimated to be approximately 1 in 2500 prescriptions (http://livertox.nih.gov/AmoxicillinClavulanate. htm).

The mechanism of hepatotoxicity is believed to be immunoallergic due to the presence of rash and eosinophilia observed in some patients.[31] Hepatotoxicity is causally linked to clavulanic acid and not amoxicillin.[96] In a prospective study using data from a Spanish registry on ACA-induced hepatotoxicity, hepatocellular injury was common with younger age whereas older age and longer duration predisposed more to cholestatic/mixed type of injury. ACA-induced hepatotoxicity is predominant in men compared with women and is associated with the HLA class II variant DRB1*1501 and its extended haplotype.[31,97,98] Sometimes toxicity is delayed up to 24 weeks after discontinuation of treatment, which makes it difficult to diagnose ACA as the offending agent (http://livertox.nih.gov/AmoxicillinClavulanate.htm).

Ursodeoxycholic acid, a hydrophilic bile acid with antioxidant properties used for the treatment of primary biliary cirrhosis, was reported to protect against ACA-induced hepatotoxicity in rats and relieved ACA-induced cholestasis in human patients.[99,100]

Troglitazone

TGZ is a thiazolidinedione antidiabetic drug that was withdrawn from the market because of its hepatotoxic effect. The hepatotoxicity was hepatocellular or mixed (hepatocellular + cholestasis) type of injury. Injury was manifest with elevation of serum aminotransferase levels more than 10 times the upper limit of normal, which was observed a few months after starting therapy with TGZ in a small number of patients.[101] There was no rash, fever, or eosinophilia associated with toxicity, which ruled out the possibility of an immune-mediated reaction to the drug. TGZ-induced hepatotoxicity was reported to progress long term in some patients even after discontinuation of the drug.[102]

Studies in vitro using animal or human hepatocytes suggest the formation of reactive metabolites, mitochondrial dysfunction, and inhibition of the BSEP to be the key mechanisms involved in TGZ-induced hepatotoxicity. The role of reactive metabolites and covalent binding to hepatic proteins in TGZ toxicity remains controversial, because there is no direct evidence linking the formation of metabolites and hepatotoxicity.[103] On the contrary, both in vivo and in vitro studies in mice, rats, and human hepatocytes have shown that TGZ itself is cytotoxic to cells and can cause mitochondrial swelling and calcium accumulation as well as opening of MPTP.[103–106] Mitochondrial dysfunction has also been confirmed in clinical reports from human patients who had TGZ therapy.[102] Furthermore, studies have shown that TGZ is an inhibitor of BSEP; this results in the accumulation of toxic bile salt that is lethal to hepatocytes, leading to cholestasis. This may explain why some patients with TGZ-induced hepatotoxicity present with a mixed (hepatocellular + cholestatic) type of injury.[107]

Herbal Medicines and Dietary Supplements

Herbs and dietary supplements are consumed as over-the-counter medications all over the world. In the United States, reports show that up to 50% of the older adult population use one form of herbal drug or dietary supplements.[108] Although some of these products may be associated with some benefits, several of them are also associated with DIH. Recent reports from the US Drug-Induced Liver Injury Network (DILIN), using data from 839 patients enrolled into their registry between 2004 and 2013, revealed that herbs and supplements accounted for 15.5% of DIH and showed a trend toward an increase in the incidence of DIHs compared with normal medications.[109] Furthermore, it was reported that non–body-building herbals and supplements caused a higher percentage (65%) of hepatotoxicity, with unfavorable outcomes of death and liver transplantation compared with body-building herbs and supplements (35%).[109] Hepatotoxicity due to body-building supplements was associated with cholestasis and more common in younger men. On the contrary, non–body-building supplements caused DIH more in middle-aged women and hepatocellular type of injury.[109] The diagnosis of hepatotoxicity in patients on herbs and supplements is complex because clinicians are usually not aware that patients are on such medications, and supplements usually contain a combination of active ingredients, which make it difficult to discern the actual hepatotoxicant. Other examples of prominent herbals and supplements that are reported to cause DIH include green tea; garcinia cambogia, a weight loss supplement; vitamin A; and linoleic acid.[110]

ROUSSEL UCLAF CAUSALITY ASSESSMENT METHOD

Roussel Uclaf Causality Assessment Method (RUCAM) is a diagnostic scoring assessment tool founded by experts in DIH more than 20 years ago for establishing a causal link between a medication and DIH. The RUCAM classifies the possibility of DIH into 4 categories based on the final number obtained from scoring all criteria. These include definite or highly probable, greater than 8; probable, 6 to 8; possible, 3 to 5; unlikely, 1 to 2, and excluded, less than or equal to 1.[111] RUCAM takes into account information in 7 categories: type of injury (hepatocellular, cholestatic or mixed), duration in days (period of drug use, onset of event, and time to withdrawal of drug and event), risk factors like age, alcohol use, and pregnancy (for cholestatic liver injury), concomitant use of other drugs, previous information on a drug's hepatotoxicity potential, differential diagnosis from other liver diseases, and response on re-exposure.[111]

RUCAM provides a framework of important criteria that physicians can use to narrow down identification of DIH and remains the most widely used tool for diagnosis of DIH by experts in the field.[112] Its use has been limited by a lack of coherence among raters; vague definitions of risk factors like age and alcohol; exclusion of other important risk factors like genetic polymorphisms; a list of other etiologies of liver disease that is not exhaustive but does account for delayed DIH reactions; unclear definition of response to reexposure to a drug; liver biopsy not listed as a criteria for diagnosis; not accommodating for identification of adaptive response with continued use of a drug; and a narrow definition of duration of drug use and discontinuation.[111,113] Based on limitations of RUCAM, it is clear that diagnosis of DIH remains a challenge in clinical practice. In a publication, authors proposed a revised form of the original RUCAM that can be used to better diagnose DIH with decreased user variability and a clearer definition of key components in RUCAM. The DILIN also proposed the use of more definite instructions, a reliable central reference for reports of previous DIH events, and an exclusive list of competing causes of DIH to improve the reliability of RUCAM.[114]

More importantly, there is a need to develop a better tool as well as a computerized algorithm to reduce subjectivity in diagnosing DIH.[114] Other scales used for specific diagnosis of DIH include the Maria and Victorino scale and Digestive Disease Week–Japan scale.

SUMMARY

DIH is an important and complex clinical problem for which more research is needed. Prospective and population-based studies from the DILIN, Spanish DILI Registry, and the Swedish Adverse Drug Reactions Advisory Committee have provided insights into the incidence, severity, risk factors, and commonly used drugs and herbs that cause DIH. The lack of appropriate animal models for idiosyncratic drug reactions and more definitive diagnostic and prognostic markers, however, still limits understanding of the mechanisms that propel DIH.

REFERENCES

1. Lee WM. Drug-induced hepatotoxicity. N Engl J Med 2003;349(5):474–85.
2. Ostapowicz G, Fontana RJ, Schiødt FV, et al. Results of a prospective study of acute liver failure at 17 tertiary care centers in the United States. Ann Intern Med 2002;137(12):947–54.
3. Björnsson ES, Bergmann OM, Björnsson HK, et al. Incidence, presentation, and outcomes in patients with drug-induced liver injury in the general population of Iceland. Gastroenterology 2013;144(7):1419–25, 1425.e1-3.
4. Aithal G, Watkins P, Andrade R, et al. Case definition and phenotype standardization in drug-induced liver injury. Clin Pharmacol Ther 2011;89(6):806–15.
5. Elmore S. Apoptosis: a review of programmed cell death. Toxicol Pathol 2007; 35(4):495–516.
6. Gómez-Lechón MJ, Ponsoda X, O'Connor E, et al. Diclofenac induces apoptosis in hepatocytes by alteration of mitochondrial function and generation of ROS. Biochem Pharmacol 2003;66(11):2155–67.
7. Yuan L, Kaplowitz N. Mechanisms of drug-induced liver injury. Clin Liver Dis 2013;17(4):507–18.
8. Eguchi Y, Shimizu S, Tsujimoto Y. Intracellular ATP levels determine cell death fate by apoptosis or necrosis. Cancer Res 1997;57(10):1835–40.
9. Vandenabeele P, Declercq W, Van Herreweghe F, et al. The role of the kinases RIP1 and RIP3 in TNF-induced necrosis. Sci Signal 2010;3(115):re4.
10. Park B, Laverty H, Srivastava A, et al. Drug bioactivation and protein adduct formation in the pathogenesis of drug-induced toxicity. Chem Biol Interact 2011; 192(1):30–6.
11. Holt MP, Ju C. Mechanisms of drug-induced liver injury. AAPS J 2006;8(1): E48–54.
12. Corsini A, Bortolini M. Drug-induced liver injury: the role of drug metabolism and transport. J Clin Pharmacol 2013;53(5):463–74.
13. Li LM, Chen L, Deng GH, et al. SLCO1B1* 15 haplotype is associated with rifampin-induced liver injury. Mol Med Rep 2012;6(1):75–82.
14. Dawson S, Stahl S, Paul N, et al. In vitro inhibition of the bile salt export pump correlates with risk of cholestatic drug-induced liver injury in humans. Drug Metab Dispos 2012;40(1):130–8.
15. Zollner G, Thueringer A, Lackner C, et al. Alterations of canalicular ATP-binding cassette transporter expression in drug-induced liver injury. Digestion 2014; 90(2):81–8.

16. Chessman D, Kostenko L, Lethborg T, et al. Human leukocyte antigen class I-restricted activation of CD8+ T cells provides the immunogenetic basis of a systemic drug hypersensitivity. Immunity 2008;28(6):822–32.

17. Mallal S, Nolan D, Witt C, et al. Association between presence of HLA-B* 5701, HLA-DR7, and HLA-DQ3 and hypersensitivity to HIV-1 reverse-transcriptase inhibitor abacavir. Lancet 2002;359(9308):727–32.

18. Zimmerman HJ. Drug-induced liver disease. Clin Liver Dis 2000;4(1):73–96.

19. Lemasters JJ, Nieminen AL, Qian T, et al. The mitochondrial permeability transition in cell death: a common mechanism in necrosis, apoptosis and autophagy. Biochim Biophys Acta 1998;1366(1):177–96.

20. Lemasters JJ. V. Necrapoptosis and the mitochondrial permeability transition: shared pathways to necrosis and apoptosis. Am J Physiol 1999;276(1):G1–6.

21. Hargreaves IP, Al Shahrani M, Wainwright L, et al. Drug-induced mitochondrial toxicity. Drug Saf 2016;39(7):661–74.

22. Jaeschke H, Gores GJ, Cederbaum AI, et al. Mechanisms of hepatotoxicity. Toxicol Sci 2002;65(2):166–76.

23. Wang C, Youle RJ. The role of mitochondria in apoptosis*. Annu Rev Genet 2009;43:95–118.

24. Seki E, Brenner DA, Karin M. A liver full of JNK: signaling in regulation of cell function and disease pathogenesis, and clinical approaches. Gastroenterology 2012;143(2):307–20.

25. Davis RJ. Signal transduction by the JNK group of MAP kinases. Cell 2000; 103(2):239–52.

26. Corazza N, Jakob S, Schaer C, et al. TRAIL receptor–mediated JNK activation and Bim phosphorylation critically regulate Fas-mediated liver damage and lethality. J Clin Invest 2006;116(9):2493–9.

27. Ron D, Walter P. Signal integration in the endoplasmic reticulum unfolded protein response. Nat Rev Mol Cell Biol 2007;8(7):519–29.

28. Lucena MI, Andrade RJ, Kaplowitz N, et al. Phenotypic characterization of idiosyncratic drug-induced liver injury: the influence of age and sex. Hepatology 2009;49(6):2001–9.

29. Chalasani N, Björnsson E. Risk factors for idiosyncratic drug-induced liver injury. Gastroenterology 2010;138(7):2246–59.

30. Meng X, Maggs JL, Usui T, et al. Auto-oxidation of isoniazid leads to isonicotinic-lysine adducts on human serum albumin. Chem Res Toxicol 2014;28(1):51–8.

31. Larrey D, Vial T, Micaleff A, et al. Hepatitis associated with amoxycillin-clavulanic acid combination report of 15 cases. Gut 1992;33(3):368–71.

32. Huang YS, Chern HD, Su WJ, et al. Cytochrome P450 2E1 genotype and the susceptibility to antituberculosis drug-induced hepatitis. Hepatology 2003; 37(4):924–30.

33. Russmann S, Kullak-Ublick GA, Grattagliano I. Current concepts of mechanisms in drug-induced hepatotoxicity. Curr Med Chem 2009;16(23):3041–53.

34. Andrade RJ, Robles M, Ulzurrun E, et al. Drug-induced liver injury: insights from genetic studies. Pharmacogenomics 2009;10(9):1467–87.

35. Daly AK, Donaldson PT, Bhatnagar P, et al. HLA-B* 5701 genotype is a major determinant of drug-induced liver injury due to flucloxacillin. Nat Genet 2009; 41(7):816–9.

36. Lammert C, Bjornsson E, Niklasson A, et al. Oral medications with significant hepatic metabolism at higher risk for hepatic adverse events. Hepatology 2010;51(2):615–20.

37. Lammert C, Einarsson S, Saha C, et al. Relationship between daily dose of oral medications and idiosyncratic drug-induced liver injury: search for signals. Hepatology 2008;47(6):2003–9.

38. Chalasani N, Fontana RJ, Bonkovsky HL, et al. Causes, clinical features, and outcomes from a prospective study of drug-induced liver injury in the United States. Gastroenterology 2008;135(6):1924–34, 1934.e1-4.

39. Russo MW, Galanko JA, Shrestha R, et al. Liver transplantation for acute liver failure from drug induced liver injury in the United States. Liver Transpl 2004; 10(8):1018–23.

40. Manyike PT, Kharasch ED, Kalhorn TF, et al. Contribution of CYP2E1 and CYP3A to acetaminophen reactive metabolite formation. Clin Pharmacol Ther 2000; 67(3):275–82.

41. Raucy JL, Lasker JM, Lieber CS, et al. Acetaminophen activation by human liver cytochromes P450IIE1 and P450IA2. Arch Biochem Biophys 1989;271(1): 270–83.

42. Jollow DJ, Thorgeirsson S-S, Potter WZ, et al. Acetaminophen-induced hepatic necrosis. VI. Metabolic disposition of toxic and nontoxic doses of acetaminophen. Pharmacology 1973;12(4–5):251–71.

43. Mitchell J, Jollow D, Potter W, et al. Acetaminophen-induced hepatic necrosis. IV. Protective role of glutathione. J Pharmacol Exp Ther 1973;187(1):211–7.

44. Jollow D, Mitchell J, Potter W, et al. Acetaminophen-induced hepatic necrosis. II. Role of covalent binding in vivo. J Pharmacol Exp Ther 1973;187(1):195–202.

45. Cheng J, Ma X, Krausz KW, et al. Rifampicin-activated human pregnane X receptor and CYP3A4 induction enhance acetaminophen-induced toxicity. Drug Metab Dispos 2009;37(8):1611–21.

46. Peterson RG, Rumack BH. Treating acute acetaminophen poisoning with acetylcysteine. JAMA 1977;237(22):2406–7.

47. Piperno E, Berssenbruegge D. Reversal of experimental paracetamol toxicosis with N-acetylcysteine. Lancet 1976;308(7988):738–9.

48. Saini SP, Zhang B, Niu Y, et al. Activation of liver X receptor increases acetaminophen clearance and prevents its toxicity in mice. Hepatology 2011;54(6): 2208–17.

49. Jaeschke H. Glutathione disulfide formation and oxidant stress during acetaminophen-induced hepatotoxicity in mice in vivo: the protective effect of allopurinol. J Pharmacol Exp Ther 1990;255(3):935–41.

50. Knight TR, Kurtz A, Bajt ML, et al. Vascular and hepatocellular peroxynitrite formation during acetaminophen toxicity: role of mitochondrial oxidant stress. Toxicol Sci 2001;62(2):212–20.

51. Hinson JA, Pike SL, Pumford NR, et al. Nitrotyrosine-protein adducts in hepatic centrilobular areas following toxic doses of acetaminophen in mice. Chem Res Toxicol 1998;11(6):604–7.

52. Saito C, Zwingmann C, Jaeschke H. Novel mechanisms of protection against acetaminophen hepatotoxicity in mice by glutathione and N-acetylcysteine. Hepatology 2010;51(1):246–54.

53. Placke ME, Ginsberg GL, Wyand DS, et al. Ultrastructural changes during acute acetaminophen-induced hepatotoxicity in the mouse: a time and dose study. Toxicol Pathol 1987;15(4):431–8.

54. Meyers LL, Beierschmitt WP, Khairallah EA, et al. Acetaminophen-induced inhibition of hepatic mitochondrial respiration in mice. Toxicol Appl Pharmacol 1988; 93(3):378–87.

55. Kon K, Kim JS, Jaeschke H, et al. Mitochondrial permeability transition in acetaminophen-induced necrosis and apoptosis of cultured mouse hepatocytes. Hepatology 2004;40(5):1170–9.
56. Masubuchi Y, Suda C, Horie T. Involvement of mitochondrial permeability transition in acetaminophen-induced liver injury in mice. J Hepatol 2005;42(1): 110–6.
57. Ramachandran A, Lebofsky M, Baines CP, et al. Cyclophilin D deficiency protects against acetaminophen-induced oxidant stress and liver injury. Free Radic Res 2011;45(2):156–64.
58. McGill MR, Sharpe MR, Williams CD, et al. The mechanism underlying acetaminophen-induced hepatotoxicity in humans and mice involves mitochondrial damage and nuclear DNA fragmentation. J Clin Invest 2012;122(4): 1574–83.
59. Gunawan BK, Liu ZX, Han D, et al. c-Jun N-terminal kinase plays a major role in murine acetaminophen hepatotoxicity. Gastroenterology 2006;131(1):165–78.
60. Saito C, Lemasters JJ, Jaeschke H. c-Jun N-terminal kinase modulates oxidant stress and peroxynitrite formation independent of inducible nitric oxide synthase in acetaminophen hepatotoxicity. Toxicol Appl Pharmacol 2010;246(1):8–17.
61. Win S, Than TA, Han D, et al. c-Jun N-terminal kinase (JNK)-dependent acute liver injury from acetaminophen or tumor necrosis factor (TNF) requires mitochondrial Sab protein expression in mice. J Biol Chem 2011;286(40):35071–8.
62. Randolph H, Joseph S. Toxic hepatitis with jaundice occurring in a patient treated with isoniazid: report of a case in a patient with hereditary hemorrhagic telangiectasia. J Am Med Assoc 1953;152(1):38–40.
63. Gellis SN, Murphy RV. Hepatitis following isoniazid. Dis Chest 1955;28(4):462–4.
64. Boelsterli UA, Lee KK. Mechanisms of isoniazid-induced idiosyncratic liver injury: emerging role of mitochondrial stress. J Gastroenterol Hepatol 2014; 29(4):678–87.
65. Maddrey WC, Boitnott JK. Isoniazid hepatitis. Ann Intern Med 1973;79(1):1–12.
66. Nelson S, Timbrell J, Snodgrass W, et al. Isoniazid and iproniazid: activation of metabolites to toxic intermediates in man and rat. Science 1976;193(4256): 901–3.
67. Preece NE, Ghatineh S, Timbrell JA. Course of ATP depletion in hydrazine hepatotoxicity. Arch Toxicol 1990;64(1):49–53.
68. Wakabayashi T, Teranishi MA, Karbowski M, et al. Functional aspects of megamitochondria isolated from hydrazine-and ethanol-treated rat livers. Pathol Int 2000;50(1):20–33.
69. Hussain SM, Frazier JM. Cellular toxicity of hydrazine in primary rat hepatocytes. Toxicol Sci 2002;69(2):424–32.
70. Metushi IG, Nakagawa T, Uetrecht J. Direct oxidation and covalent binding of isoniazid to rodent liver and human hepatic microsomes: humans are more like mice than rats. Chem Res Toxicol 2012;25(11):2567–76.
71. Li F, Lu J, Cheng J, et al. Human PXR modulates hepatotoxicity associated with rifampicin and isoniazid co-therapy. Nat Med 2013;19(4):418–20.
72. Warrington R, Mcphilips-Feener S, Rutherford W. The predictive value of the lymphocyte transformation test in isoniazid-associated hepatitis. Clin Exp Allergy 1982;12(3):217–22.
73. Metushi IG, Sanders C, Lee WM, et al. Detection of anti-isoniazid and anti–cytochrome P450 antibodies in patients with isoniazid-induced liver failure. Hepatology 2014;59(3):1084–93.

74. Metushi IG, Zhu X, Chen X, et al. Mild isoniazid-induced liver injury in humans is associated with an increase in Th17 cells and T cells producing IL-10. Chem Res Toxicol 2014;27(4):683–9.

75. Nolan CM, Goldberg SV, Buskin SE. Hepatotoxicity associated with isoniazid preventive therapy: a 7-year survey from a public health tuberculosis clinic. JAMA 1999;281(11):1014–8.

76. Franks AL, Binkin NJ, Snider DE Jr, et al. Isoniazid hepatitis among pregnant and postpartum Hispanic patients. Public Health Rep 1989;104(2):151.

77. Saukkonen JJ, Cohn DL, Jasmer RM, et al. An official ATS statement: hepatotoxicity of antituberculosis therapy. Am J Respir Crit Care Med 2006;174(8):935–52.

78. Huang YS. Recent progress in genetic variation and risk of antituberculosis drug-induced liver injury. J Chin Med Assoc 2014;77(4):169–73.

79. Singla N, Gupta D, Birbian N, et al. Association of NAT2, GST and CYP2E1 polymorphisms and anti-tuberculosis drug-induced hepatotoxicity. Tuberculosis 2014;94(3):293–8.

80. Pollard RB, Robinson P, Dransfield K. Safety profile of nevirapine, a nonnucleoside reverse transcriptase inhibitor for the treatment of human immunodeficiency virus infection. Clin Ther 1998;20(6):1071–92.

81. Sharma AM, Li Y, Novalen M, et al. Bioactivation of nevirapine to a reactive quinone methide: implications for liver injury. Chem Res Toxicol 2012;25(8): 1708–19.

82. Wen B, Chen Y, Fitch WL. Metabolic activation of nevirapine in human liver microsomes: dehydrogenation and inactivation of cytochrome P450 3A4. Drug Metab Dispos 2009;37(7):1557–62.

83. Hall DB, MacGregor TR. Case-control exploration of relationships between early rash or liver toxicity and plasma concentrations of nevirapine and primary metabolites. HIV Clin Trials 2007;8(6):391–9.

84. Marinho AT, Rodrigues PM, Caixas U, et al. Differences in nevirapine biotransformation as a factor for its sex-dependent dimorphic profile of adverse drug reactions. J Antimicrob Chemother 2014;69(2):476–82.

85. Wit FW, Kesselring AM, Gras L, et al. Discontinuation of nevirapine because of hypersensitivity reactions in patients with prior treatment experience, compared with treatment-naive patients: the ATHENA cohort study. Clin Infect Dis 2008; 46(6):933–40.

86. Patel SM, Johnson S, Belknap SM, et al. Serious adverse cutaneous and hepatic toxicities associated with nevirapine use by non–HIV-infected individuals. J Acquir Immune Defic Syndr 2004;35(2):120–5.

87. Castro EMC, Carr DF, Jorgensen AL, et al. HLA-allelotype associations with nevirapine-induced hypersensitivity reactions and hepatotoxicity: a systematic review of the literature and meta-analysis. Pharmacogenet Genomics 2015; 25(4):186–98.

88. Tyle JH. Ketoconazole. Mechanism of action, spectrum of activity, pharmacokinetics, drug interactions, adverse reactions and therapeutic use. Pharmacotherapy 1984;4(6):343–73.

89. Greenblatt HK, Greenblatt DJ. Liver injury associated with ketoconazole: review of the published evidence. J Clin Pharmacol 2014;54(12):1321–9.

90. Lake-Bakaar G, Scheuer P, Sherlock S. Hepatic reactions associated with ketoconazole in the United Kingdom. Br Med J (Clin Res Ed) 1987;294(6569): 419–22.

91. Rodriguez RJ, Acosta D. Comparison of ketoconazole-and fluconazole-induced hepatotoxicity in a primary culture system of rat hepatocytes. Toxicology 1995; 96(2):83–92.
92. Rodriguez RJ, Acosta D. N-deacetyl ketoconazole-induced hepatotoxicity in a primary culture system of rat hepatocytes. Toxicology 1997;117(2):123–31.
93. Rodriguez R, Buckholz C. Hepatotoxicity of ketoconazole in Sprague-Dawley rats: glutathione depletion, flavin-containing monooxygenases-mediated bioactivation and hepatic covalent binding. Xenobiotica 2003;33(4):429–41.
94. Ma YM, Ma ZQ, Gui CQ, et al. Hepatotoxicity and toxicokinetics of ketoconazole in rabbits. Acta Pharmacol Sin 2003;24(8):778–82.
95. Andrade RJ, Lucena MI, Fernández MC, et al. Drug-induced liver injury: an analysis of 461 incidences submitted to the Spanish registry over a 10-year period. Gastroenterology 2005;129(2):512–21.
96. Salvo F, Polimeni G, Moretti U, et al. Adverse drug reactions related to amoxicillin alone and in association with clavulanic acid: data from spontaneous reporting in Italy. J Antimicrob Chemother 2007;60(1):121–6.
97. Lucena MI, Andrade RJ, Fernández MC, et al. Determinants of the clinical expression of amoxicillin-clavulanate hepatotoxicity: a prospective series from Spain. Hepatology 2006;44(4):850–6.
98. O'Donohue J, Oien K, Donaldson P, et al. Co-amoxiclav jaundice: clinical and histological features and HLA class II association. Gut 2000;47(5):717–20.
99. El-Sherbiny GA, Taye A, Abdel-Raheem IT. Role of ursodeoxycholic acid in prevention of hepatotoxicity caused by amoxicillin-clavulanic acid in rats. Ann Hepatol 2009;8(2):134–40.
100. Katsinelos P, Vasiliadis T, Xiarchos P, et al. Ursodeoxycholic acid (UDCA) for the treatment of amoxycillin-clavulanate potassium (Augmentin (R))-induced intrahepatic cholestasis: report of two cases. Eur J Gastroenterol Hepatol 2000; 12(3):365.
101. Watkins PB, Whitcomb RW. Hepatic dysfunction associated with troglitazone. N Engl J Med 1998;338(13):916–7.
102. Julie N, Julie I, Kende A, et al. Mitochondrial dysfunction and delayed hepatotoxicity: another lesson from troglitazone. Diabetologia 2008;51(11):2108–16.
103. Masubuchi Y. Metabolic and non-metabolic factors determining troglitazone hepatotoxicity: a review. Drug Metab Pharmacokinet 2006;21(5):347–56.
104. Masubuchi Y, Kano S, Horie T. Mitochondrial permeability transition as a potential determinant of hepatotoxicity of antidiabetic thiazolidinediones. Toxicology 2006;222(3):233–9.
105. Okuda T, Norioka M, Shitara Y, et al. Multiple mechanisms underlying troglitazone-induced mitochondrial permeability transition. Toxicol Appl Pharmacol 2010;248(3):242–8.
106. Kostrubsky VE, Sinclair JF, Ramachandran V, et al. The role of conjugation in hepatotoxicity of troglitazone in human and porcine hepatocyte cultures. Drug Metab Dispos 2000;28(10):1192–7.
107. Pauli-Magnus C, Meier PJ, Stieger B. Genetic determinants of drug induced cholestasis and intrahepatic cholestasis of pregnancy. Semin Liver Dis 2010; 30(2):147–59.
108. Bailey RL, Gahche JJ, Lentino CV, et al. Dietary supplement use in the United States, 2003–2006. J Nutr 2011;141(2):261–6.
109. Navarro VJ, Barnhart H, Bonkovsky HL, et al. Liver injury from herbals and dietary supplements in the US drug-induced liver injury network. Hepatology 2014; 60(4):1399–408.

110. García-Cortés M, Robles-Díaz M, Ortega-Alonso A, et al. Hepatotoxicity by dietary supplements: a tabular listing and clinical characteristics. Int J Mol Sci 2016;17(4):537.
111. García-Cortés M, Stephens C, Lucena MI, et al. Causality assessment methods in drug induced liver injury: strengths and weaknesses. J Hepatol 2011;55(3): 683–91.
112. Danan G, Teschke R. RUCAM in drug and herb induced liver injury: the update. Int J Mol Sci 2015;17(1):14.
113. Lewis JH. Causality assessment: which is best—expert opinion or RUCAM? Clin Liver Dis 2014;4(1):4–8.
114. Rochon J, Protiva P, Seeff LB, et al. Reliability of the Roussel Uclaf causality assessment method for assessing causality in drug-induced liver injury. Hepatology 2008;48(4):1175–83.
115. Fung M, Thornton A, Mybeck K, et al. Evaluation of the characteristics of safety withdrawal of prescription drugs from worldwide pharmaceutical markets-1960 to 1999*. Drug Inf J 2001;35(1):293–317.
116. Qureshi ZP, Seoane-Vazquez E, Rodriguez-Monguio R, et al. Market withdrawal of new molecular entities approved in the United States from 1980 to 2009. Pharmacoepidemiol Drug Saf 2011;20(7):772–7.
117. McNaughton R, Huet G, Shakir S. An investigation into drug products withdrawn from the EU market between 2002 and 2011 for safety reasons and the evidence used to support the decision-making. BMJ Open 2014;4(1):e004221.
118. Guengerich FP, MacDonald JS. Applying mechanisms of chemical toxicity to predict drug safety. Chem Res Toxicol 2007;20(3):344–69.
119. Kenna JG, Stahl SH, Eakins JA, et al. Multiple compound-related adverse properties contribute to liver injury caused by endothelin receptor antagonists. J Pharmacol Exp Ther 2015;352(2):281–90.

Epidemiology and Genetic Risk Factors of Drug Hepatotoxicity

Jawad Ahmad, MD, FRCP*, Joseph A. Odin, MD, PhD

KEYWORDS

- Drug-induced liver injury (DILI) • Epidemiology • Genetics

KEY POINTS

- Idiosyncratic drug-induced liver injury (DILI) is an uncommon event.
- Antimicrobials are the commonest class of drugs associated with DILI.
- Herbal and dietary supplements are increasingly recognized as causes of DILI, particularly in Asian countries.
- Several epidemiologic factors influence the risk, severity, and outcome of DILI.
- Genetic analysis of DILI is currently limited, but multiple polymorphisms of HLA genes and genes involved in drug metabolism and transport have been identified as risk factors for DILI.

INTRODUCTION

Drug-induced liver injury (DILI) is the leading reason drugs are withdrawn from the marketplace in the United States.[1] An accurate assessment of the frequency of DILI is difficult because it mainly relies on voluntary case reports to national registries without an appreciation of the population at risk, leading to underreporting. In addition, the vast majority of DILI cases are idiosyncratic, and the presentation, pattern of injury, latency, and severity differ widely between drugs and sometimes even with the same drug. Despite these limitations, the last 2 decades have seen several advances in the understanding of the epidemiology and genetic risk factors associated with DILI, which are discussed in this article.

EPIDEMIOLOGY
Incidence

Several large studies have tried to determine the incidence of DILI but encountered several methodological issues, leading to a wide range of figures. In addition, the

The authors have nothing to disclose.
Division of Liver Diseases, Icahn School of Medicine at Mount Sinai, 1 Gustave L. Levy Place, Box 1104, New York, NY 10029, USA
* Corresponding author.
E-mail address: jawad.ahmad@mountsinai.org

data are limited to only a handful of countries (**Fig. 1**). **Table 1** lists some of these studies based on their country or region.

Perhaps the most accurate study to date was performed in Iceland using outpatient and inpatient prescription databases, allowing an estimate of the population at risk.[2]

- The crude annual incidence rate of DILI was 19.1 cases per 100,000 patients per year, but there was a very wide range depending on the implicated drug, with
  ○ 43 per 100,000 for amoxicillin-clavulanate
  ○ 11 per 100,000 for diclofenac
  ○ 752 per 100,000 for azathioprine
  ○ 675 per 100,000 for infliximab

An earlier French population-based study suggested a crude annual incidence rate of 13.9 per 100,000 per year and was some 16-fold higher than would be expected by spontaneous reporting to local authorities.[3] A recent study from Korea found a crude rate of 12 per 100,000 per year but only looked at patients that were hospitalized, meaning the true incidence of DILI should be higher.[4]

The higher incidence rate of DILI when assessed prospectively is illustrated by examining retrospective studies. Using general practice databases in the United Kingdom and Spain, the crude incidence rate ranged from 1.35 to 3 cases per 100,000 per year,[5,6] which in part could be explained by only identifying DILI if the patient was hospitalized or referred to a specialist. Similar figures were noted in a hepatology outpatient setting in Sweden of 2.3 per 100,000 per year.[7]

A crucial point to note in these studies is how DILI was diagnosed and which laboratory criteria were used to establish a diagnosis. Typically, an elevation in transaminase level (alanine aminotransferase [ALT] or aspartate aminotransferase), alkaline phosphatase, or bilirubin is required with some multiple of the upper limit of normal for these tests. However, this is not uniform between studies. Attributing causality

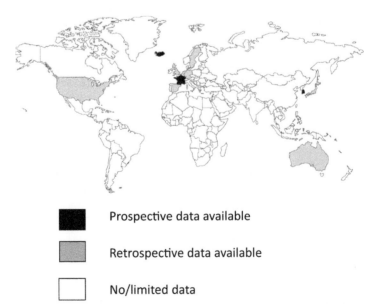

☐ Prospective data available

☐ Retrospective data available

☐ No/limited data

Fig. 1. World map illustrating countries with DILI incidence data. Most of the world lacks any reliable data on DILI incidence.

Table 1
National studies of drug-induced liver injury incidence

Country	Iceland	France	Korea	United Kingdom	Spain	Sweden
Years of study	2010–2011	1997–2000	2005–2007	1994–1999	2004–2009	1995–2005
Study type	Prospective	Prospective	Prospective	Retrospective	Retrospective	Retrospective
Number of DILI cases	96	34	371	128	57	77
Crude DILI incidence rate/ 100,000 per year	19.1	13.9	12	2.4	3.01	2.3

The incidence of DILI varies from 2 to 19 cases per 100,000 per year but appears to be an underestimate in retrospective studies.

to the implicated drug is also heterogeneous, relying on the exclusion of other causes such as viral hepatitis and autoimmune disease, a temporal relationship to the drug, and occasionally using consensus criteria or validated scoring systems, such as the Roussel Uclaf Causality Assessment Method.

DILI registries exist in several countries and have the advantage of collecting very detailed data on each DILI case with a formal causality adjudication process, but they are limited by the lack of information on the number of patients exposed to each agent. Nevertheless, these registries provide information on the types of drugs that cause DILI, the pattern of injury, and the risk of mortality and morbidity. **Table 2** details some of these registries and gives some comparison of the types of drugs involved in each country.

In the United States, the National Institutes of Health has funded the DILI Network (DILIN) since 2004, which is a consortium of several academic centers that collect data on patients with DILI in a prospective and a retrospective study. This group recently published their findings on almost 900 patients that were prospectively enrolled.[8] Antimicrobials accounted for 45% of all the cases, and a further 16% were due to herbal and dietary supplements (HDS). The nature of these registries

Table 2
Drug-induced liver injury registries across the world

Country	United States	Spain	Korea
Years of study	2004–2013	1994–2004	2005–2007
Study type	Prospective	Prospective	Prospective
Number of DILI cases	899	461	371
Antimicrobials (% of total)	45.3%	32%	—
HDS (% of total)	16.1%	—	73%

There are few large prospective DILI registries, but there is a striking difference comparing the United States and Spain with Korea in terms of the implicated drugs with almost all the cases in the latter related to HDS, while prescription antimicrobials are common in the former.

with a bias toward hospitalized patients is reflected in that 10% of patients died or underwent liver transplant and 17% developed chronic DILI. Similar findings were noted in the Spanish DILI Registry with a death or transplant rate of 11.7% in jaundiced patients and 32% of all cases related to the use of anti-infectious drugs.[9] The contrast with Asian studies is marked when considering the type of agents that cause DILI. In a prospective Korean cohort of 371 DILI patients, more than 70% were thought to be related to HDS.[4] In Japan, an analysis of 1676 DILI cases demonstrated that 10% were related to dietary supplements and 7.1% were related to Chinese herbal drugs,[10] and a smaller study in Singapore found more than half of DILI cases were associated with traditional Chinese medicines.[11] New data should start emerging from Latin America with the formation of the Latin DILI Network, which encompasses most South American countries along with Mexico.[12]

Pattern of Injury

Based on the ratio of serum ALT to alkaline phosphatase (expressed as multiples of upper limit of normal), the R ratio is used to classify DILI into

- Hepatocellular (R >5)
- Cholestatic (R <2)
- Mixed (R of 2–5)

Using the R ratio, it is apparent that most DILI cases in the large national registries are hepatocellular (**Fig. 2**). The pattern of injury will depend on the type of drug as demonstrated when examining the breakdown of the same figures in Asia where DILI from HDS is the predominant injury seen. More than 75% of cases in the Korean series were hepatocellular with very few cholestatic cases.[4]

The pattern of injury will depend on the type of drug but also influences the outcome because hepatocellular injury is more than twice as likely to lead to a worse outcome, such as death or liver transplantation, in both the US and the Spanish Registries.[8,9]

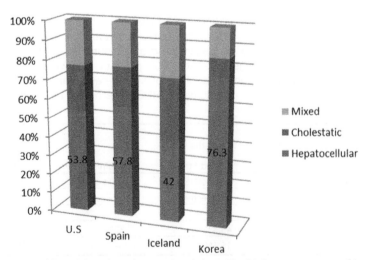

Fig. 2. Pattern of liver injury based on national data. The higher percentage of hepatocellular injury in Korea reflects the implicated drugs as the vast majority of cases there are related to HDS. (*Data from* Refs.[2,4,8,9])

Specific Drugs

The risk of DILI with any drug is difficult to ascertain using registry data where there is no information on the population at risk, but overall it is a rare event. However, the registry studies are similar to population-based studies in identifying antimicrobials as the leading cause of DILI at least in the United States and Europe.

In the US DILIN, the largest category of drugs causing DILI was antibiotics, and as shown in **Table 3**, of the top 10 implicated drugs, 9 were antibiotics, headed by amoxicillin-clavulanate,[8] which was also the leading agent in the Spanish DILI Registry.[9] In addition, the population-based study using the UK General Practice Research Database identified amoxicillin-clavulanate as second only to chlorpromazine in terms of the odds ratio in developing acute DILI.[5]

Antituberculosis (TB) medications are very commonly prescribed, particularly in the developing world. The risk of DILI is difficult to ascertain, but 5.3% of all the cases in the US DILIN were due to isoniazid (second only to amoxicillin-clavulanate) and 7% of the cases in the Spanish DILI Registry were due to isoniazid alone or in combination with other drugs.[8,9]

Similarly, statins are one of the most commonly prescribed medications, and liver enzyme monitoring is recommended. However, their actual risk of DILI is rare.[13,14] In the US DILIN, there were 29 cases of statin-related DILI of a total of 899 cases, much less than seen with several antimicrobials.[8]

Other than antimicrobials, nonsteroidal anti-inflammatory agents (NSAIDs) are another group that is commonly associated with DILI, particularly ibuprofen and diclofenac, accounting for up to 6% to 7% of cases in Iceland and Spain,[2,9] and to a lesser extent in the United States.[8]

Herbal and Dietary Supplements

The association between HDS use and DILI is being increasingly recognized, but studying this area is complicated by several issues:

- First, there is a complete lack of any population data.
- Second, assessing causality is problematic because patients often take a combination of HDS products, which often consist of multiple ingredients, and take them haphazardly.

Table 3
Top 10 individual agents causing drug-induced liver injury in the US drug-induced liver injury Network (total N = 899)

Rank	Individual Drug	N = 899
1	Amoxicillin-clavulanate	91
2	Isoniazid	48
3	Nitrofurantoin	42
4	Sulfamethoxazole/trimethoprim	31
5	Minocycline	28
6	Cefazolin	20
7	Azithromycin	18
8	Ciprofloxacin	16
9	Levofloxacin	13
10	Diclofenac	12

It is notable that of the 10 agents, 9 are antimicrobials.

- Third, HDS are not subject to the same federal regulations as prescription medicines so that actual content of each product is not always certain.

Despite these limitations, some interesting data have recently emerged. In the United States, the DILIN found 130 of 839 (15.5%) DILI cases were caused by HDS, and the incidence appeared to be increasing.[15] The 130 cases were divided into 45 cases due to body-building supplements (predominantly anabolic steroids) and 85 non-body-building HDS. The striking differences were the prolonged jaundice in the body-building cases, but they all resolved, whereas the remaining non-body-building cases were predominantly in middle-aged women and were more likely to result in a severe outcome such as death or transplant, even compared with DILI related to medications. Spanish and Latin American investigators also noted the pronounced jaundice and favorable outcome in young men taking body-building anabolic steroids.[16] The Korean experience with non-body-building HDS demonstrated that 4 of 371 patients with DILI died or needed liver transplant and ranged in age from 40 to 48 years.[4]

Demographic Factors

Age
The large national DILI registries indicate that the average age of patients presenting with DILI is between 49 and 53 years.[8,9] This age span is similar to the average age in Korea where HDS is much more prevalent and is likely a reflection of increased prescription medication and HDS use in middle-aged and older people.[4] Whether older age is a risk factor for DILI has been examined in the Spanish Registry. There was no effect on age in the overall cohort of 603 DILI cases, but when the cases were broken down into cholestatic and hepatocellular injury, older age was independently associated with the former and younger age was independently associated with the latter,[17] confirming an earlier finding.[18]

Recent data from the World Health Organization Safety Report Database examining 236 drugs known to be associated with DILI using data-mining methods also suggested that elderly patients (65 years or older) were much more likely to develop cholestatic injury, whereas acute liver injury was more common in children.[19] The effect in children may have been related to mitochondrial dysfunction, whereas the cholestatic DILI seen in the elderly may have reflected the higher lipophilicity and biliary excretion in the drugs they were more commonly taking.

In the US DILIN, children are included, and there are some interesting differences with adults.[20] Although antimicrobials were common causes, amoxicillin-clavulanate was not one of the agents. Most cases had hepatocellular injury, with some very severe or fatal; chronic DILI was less common (7%), but 64% of all the cases had autoantibodies with a much higher incidence of eosinophilia compared with adult counterparts.

Children also appear to be at increased risk of DILI from certain drugs, particularly valproate and other antiepileptic medications.[21]

Gender
Most of the large registry studies suggest a female preponderance of idiosyncratic DILI[2–4,8] with the exception of the Spain registry studies, where there was a slight increase in male patients.[9] Although female gender is not independently associated with DILI, it was associated with worse outcome, such as acute liver failure or the need for liver transplantation[17] in the Spanish Registry but was not seen in the US DILIN.[22] In addition, women were more likely to develop chronic injury (defined as >3 months) in an older Spanish cohort.[18]

Although gender does not appear to increase the risk for DILI overall, for individual drugs such as macrolide antibiotics and diclofenac, there may be an increased risk in women.[5]

Race/ethnicity

The effect of race/ethnicity on DILI is unclear because the European Registries almost universally comprise Caucasians. There is limited information in the US DILIN with a more heterogeneous population. The natural history study from the US DILIN demonstrated that almost 10% of patients died within 6 months of DILI onset and 19% had evidence of chronic injury (persisting beyond 6 months).[22] Asian race was an independent predictor of reduced time to liver-related death or liver transplantation, and African American race was an independent risk factor for chronic DILI.

Daily Dose and Polypharmacy

An interesting observation is that almost all drugs that have been withdrawn from the market or have black-box warnings due to hepatotoxicity were given in doses of greater than 50 mg. This phenomenon was examined using pharmaceutical databases in the United States and Sweden, and it did appear that there was a statistically significant relationship between the daily dose of medication and the risk of a severe outcome due to hepatotoxicity such as liver failure, transplantation, or death. In addition, 77% of DILI cases occurred in medications given at a dose of 50 mg or more.[23]

The US DILIN failed to show an association between daily dose and outcome in 383 DILI cases but did note that a daily dosage of greater than or equal to 50 mg was associated with a shorter latency and a different pattern of injury, with less cholestasis.[24] If a drug has significant hepatic metabolism and is given in a daily dose greater than 50 mg, the risk of DILI is also increased.[25]

The UK General Practice Research Database found that, when 2 or more hepatotoxic drugs were given concurrently, the risk of DILI increased 6-fold.[5]

Hospitalization

The referral bias of the large DILI registries is reflected in the overrepresentation of severe cases, meaning many are hospitalized, for instance, more than half in the US DILIN.[8] However, DILI, defined as elevation of liver enzymes, is typically seen in the outpatient setting, but several studies indicate that the incidence of DILI in the inpatient setting is as high as 1.4%[26] and is even higher when examining patients with jaundice or non-acetaminophen-related acute liver failure.[27] Again, the commonly associated agents are antimicrobials, anti-TB, and some cancer drugs.

Underlying Liver Disease

The suggestion that DILI superimposed on chronic underlying liver disease should be more severe or associated with a worse outcome is controversial. The long-term follow-up from the US DILIN noted that 24% of patients who died or were transplanted had underlying liver disease compared with 11% of patients who survived ($P<.02$).[22] However, underlying liver disease was self-reported, and the severity was unclear. Azithromycin DILI appears to be particularly more common in patients with underlying liver disease.[8] Statins are frequently used in patients with underlying fatty liver disease without an increase in the risk of DILI,[28,29] and it is unclear whether chronic viral hepatitis increases the risk of DILI from anti-TB medications[30,31] but may do so with anti-HIV medications.[32–34]

GENETIC ASSOCIATIONS WITH DRUG-INDUCED LIVER INJURY
Background

Epidemiologic studies indicate that the prevalence of DILI varies geographically, which likely reflects differing environmental and genetic risk factors for DILI. It is currently unknown the extent to which this variation is environmental versus genetic. No studies of immigrants have been published to determine if their prevalence of DILI reflects that of their host or mother country. Genetic studies have clearly shown that a genetic component does exist at least for select drugs based on candidate gene studies and genome-wide association studies. Certain HLA haplotypes have been proposed to increase the risk of DILI. Whether a genetic component exists for general susceptibility to DILI remains uncertain.

The liver plays a key role in metabolizing toxins and drugs via enzyme-mediated oxidative metabolism and conjugation reactions followed by biliary transport and secretion (**Fig. 3**). The genes encoding the enzymes and transporters involved in this process are highly redundant and polymorphic,[35] which may have protected early human populations from catastrophic exposure to environmental toxins as new areas were settled. Because of natural selection, the frequency of these polymorphisms varies widely among different populations. Unfortunately, the polymorphic nature of these genes may also lead to rare idiosyncratic reactions to toxin or drug exposure that actually cause liver injury or may in some individuals accentuate formation of dose-dependent hepatotoxins, such as acetaldehyde from ethanol. Not every alcoholic develops cirrhosis. The immune environment of the liver is normally a highly tolerant one in part due to its constant exposure to foreign antigen. Some drugs, however, are well known potentially to induce immune-mediated liver damage infrequently (eg, halothane) that may even mimic autoimmune hepatitis. Consequently, immuno-modulatory gene polymorphisms and mutations may also contribute to induction of DILI.

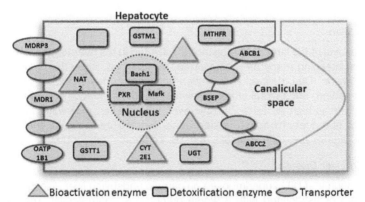

Fig. 3. Candidate gene approach to DILI genetics discovery. The large number of hepatic proteins involved in drug metabolism can be placed in 3 broad categories: bioactivation and detoxification enzymes and transporters. Drug hepatotoxicity may be dose dependent and may be due to the parent drug or its metabolites. Therefore, the relative activity levels of proteins involved in drug metabolism are likely important determinants of susceptibility to DILI. The redox state of hepatocytes is also known to affect the activity of these proteins. The genes encoding hepatocyte bioactivation and detoxification enzymes as well as transporters involved in drug metabolism are highly polymorphic, which may lead to uncommon or rare idiosyncratic reactions that only cause liver injury in select individuals.

Not surprisingly, given these 2 potential mechanisms of DILI, early candidate gene studies in DILI focused mainly on genes encoding hepatic enzymes and transporters involved in drug metabolism as well as immunomodulatory genes. More recently, large collaborative efforts have spawned a few genome-wide association studies (GWAS) and whole-genome sequencing (WGS) studies to confirm prior observations and to identify genes that may unexpectedly be associated with DILI. Results are available from only a handful of GWAS currently. More than 90% of published DILI genetic studies are small case control candidate gene studies, and only 1 WGS study has been published to date (**Fig. 4**). More than half of the case control studies focus on anti-TB treatment (AT).

Goals of Genetic Studies

There are several potential benefits in pursuing genetic analysis of DILI, including those listed:

- Identify those most susceptible to DILI in order to make genetic prescreening cost-effective
- Determine genetic risk factors for specific drugs or populations
- Identify genetic factors that predict DILI susceptibility regardless of drug or ethnic group
- Use genetic information to prevent exposure to drugs to which one is susceptible (ie, personalized medicine) or to indicate closer monitoring during treatment
- To increase the mechanistic understanding of DILI, which may suggest novel treatments for DILI

Candidate Gene Studies

The drug association that has been most often studied is DILI during AT given the high prevalence of TB in certain regions and the high frequency of AT-associated DILI, which lends itself to case-control studies. Isoniazid is thought to be responsible for most of the liver injury associated with AT. In some cases, contradictory results have been obtained within the same country, such as India, which may reflect local ethnic variation or small case numbers (**Fig. 5**). The genetic polymorphisms most frequently associated with AT-induced liver injury are found in *N*-acetyltransferase 2 (NAT2), glutathione S-transferase M1 (GSTM1), glutathione S-transferase T1

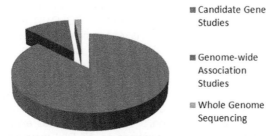

■ Candidate Gene Studies

■ Genome-wide Association Studies

▨ Whole Genome Sequencing

Fig. 4. DILI genetic study alternatives. Abundant candidate gene studies have been performed to uncover genes and polymorphisms responsible for DILI, but the scope of these studies is necessarily limited by preconceptions as to the cause of DILI. GWAS and WGS represent unbiased approaches to improving the understanding of DILI. To date, few of the latter approaches have been applied to those with DILI, but there have been some preliminary results that show promise.

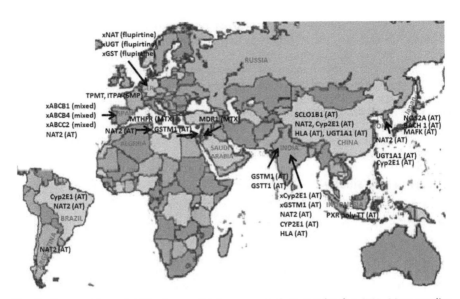

Fig. 5. Geographic variability in candidate gene analysis results for DILI. Most studies focused on AT-induced liver injury because it is very common. NAT2 polymorphisms, which lead to slow acetylation of AT drugs, were the most commonly associated with AT. Most of the other polymorphisms or mutations associated with DILI were population specific. An "x" before a gene name indicates no association was found. Some negative association results may have been due to the limited power of a smaller study to detect a weak or moderate association.

(GSTT1), Cytochrome P450 2E1 (Cyp2E1), and HLA genes.[36–43] NAT2 polymorphisms causing slow acetylation are associated with AT-DILI, and certain Cyp2E1 polymorphisms may increase the severity of AT-DILI.[41] Null mutations in GSTM1 and GSTT1 have often been associated with AT-DILI, but not always.[38] Not all studies have shown an association between AT-DILI and NAT2 polymorphisms, either. However, a meta-analysis of results from AT-DILI studies confirmed this association across different ethnic groups.[44]

Some other drug metabolism–related genes associated with AT-DILI by case control studies include SCLO1B1, NOS2A, BACH 1, MAFK, UDP-glucuronosyltransferase 1A1 (UGT1A1), and pregnane X receptor (PXR).[45–48] SCLO181 encodes the organic anion transporting polypeptide 1B1, which is responsible for the hepatic uptake of xenobiotics and conjugated bile acids.[45] The inducible isoform of nitric oxide synthase (coded by NOS2A) regulates the redox state of the cell, which may affect the activity of drug-metabolizing enzymes. BTB and CNC homology 1 protein (coded by BACH1) and Mafk (coded by MAFK) are transcription factors that regulate expression of antioxidant enzymes such as glutathione S-transferase.[46] UGT1A1 is a detoxification enzyme responsible for glucuronidation.[47] The PXR regulates expression of several detoxification enzymes.[48] These associations to AT-DILI were not very strong in most studies and have not led to pretesting of individuals before AT to prevent DILI.

HLA associations have been identified in case control studies for DILI related to other drugs as well, including nevirapine,[49–51] lapatinib,[52–54] and ticlopidine.[55] Meta-analysis has been useful in confirming the association of nevirapine with HLA haplotypes.[56] Conversely, DILI due to 2 immunomodulatory drugs (methotrexate and 6-mercaptopurine) has been associated with genetic polymorphisms in multi-drug resistance gene, methylenetetrahydrofolate reductase, thiopurine methyltrans-ferase, and inosine triphosphate pyrophosphatase.[57–60] NSAIDs also frequently induce hepatotoxicity; however, checking candidate gene polymorphisms as risk factors for NSAID-induced hepatotoxicity was unrevealing in a Spanish population.[61] The former results suggested that immune responses play a general role in DILI regardless of the drug in question. Unfortunately, the associated HLA haplotypes or alleles were typically population specific and drug specific and not useful for general DILI prevention.

Two case control studies have identified associations that were not drug specific. In Spain, a mixed group of DILI cases was associated with GSTM1/GSTT1 null mutations.[62] A Chinese study found that UGT1A9 polymorphisms were associated with DILI, regardless of cause.[63] These general associations were intriguing, but did not have a high positive predictive value and have not been replicated. In contrast, a Spanish DILI study of 141 individuals with DILI from varied causes suggested that ABCB1, ABCB4, and ABCC2 polymorphisms do not enhance the risk of drug-induced hepatotoxicity.[64] Much larger populations likely need to be studied to identify genetic risk factors common to liver injury due to different drugs. To that end, several international collaborations have been formed to increase the power of DILI studies to identify genetic risk factors. A uniform definition of DILI across studies may also help diminish discrepancies between studies.

Genome-wide Association Studies and Whole-Genome Sequencing Studies

In order to identify genetic polymorphisms that would be clinically useful, assumptions about the mechanism of DILI may need to be disregarded. Hence, GWAS and WGS studies have been published by large consortiums, and studies are ongoing. The quality and size of the GWAS have increased over time and have produced useful results, particularly for individual drugs with a high frequency of DILI (**Table 4**). The definition of DILI, the methodology used, and statistical analysis in the different GWAS have been variable. Replication groups were not used in all studies to confirm results. A small GWAS study showed an association between rho GTPase, a signaling molecule, and methotrexate-induced liver injury.[65] All of the highly significant genetic associations thus far are restricted to HLA alleles or haplotypes, emphasizing the importance perhaps of T-cell responses in DILI in general.[66–71] The HLA associations identified by GWAS do overlap between certain drugs, but none is universal for all the drugs. Some associations as with Lumiracoxib do cross ethnic groups.[70] The HLA association with flucloxacillin-induced DILI was surprisingly strong, but given the frequency of HLA-B*5701, only 0.1% of individuals with that genotype are predicted to develop liver injury if exposed to flucloxacillin.[69] Only one WGS study has been reported, and the results confirmed a prior GWAS result.[67]

A GWAS of 783 individuals of European ancestry who experienced DILI due to more than 200 different implicated drugs was published by international collaborators in 2012.[72] No significant associations were identified after accounting for the known HLA associations with DILI due to flucloxacillin and amoxicillin/clavulanate. A trend toward an association for hepatocellular DILI was seen for STAT4, an immunomodulatory gene. No general HLA associations were confirmed. The lack of reproducible findings for mixed cases of DILI supports the idea that only weak to moderate determinants of DILI may be present in mixed cases and/or that strong associations reflect rare genetic variations. By increasing the number of cases in GWAS or WGS studies, such risk factors for DILI may be soon identified.

Table 4
Genome-wide association studies for drug-induced liver injury

Drug Name	Class	Gene Association	OR	P Value	Cohort	N	Reference
Methotrexate	Immunomodulator	ARHGAP24 (rhoGTPase)	NA	9.0×10^{-3}	Japanese	8	65
Flupirtine	Analgesic	HLA DRB1*16:01-DQB1*05:02	18.7	6.7×10^{-5}	German	10	66
Lapatinib	Tyrosine kinase inhibitor	HLA-DRB1*07:01	—	2.0×10^{-18}	International	34	67
Amoxicillin-clavulanate	Antimicrobial	HLA-A*0201	2.2	2.0×10^{-6}	NW European & Spanish	177	68
		HLA-DQB1*0602	3.3	1.4×10^{-6}	NW European & Spanish	177	69
Flucloxacillin	Antimicrobial	HLA-B*5701	80.6	9.0×10^{-19}	United Kingdcm	51	70
Lumiracoxib	Cyclo-oxygenase inhibitor	HLA-DRB1*1501-DQA1*0102	5.0	6.8×10^{-25}	International	98	71
Ximelagatran	Thrombin inhibitor	HLA-DRB1*07:01	4.4	4×10^{-5}	European	74	72
		HLA-DQA1*02	4.4	2×10^{-6}	European	74	73

All of the highly significant genetic associations thus far are associated with HLA alleles or haplotypes. Some HLA alleles (eg, HLA-DRB1*07:01) associate with multiple drugs. Certain HLA associations as with Lumiracoxib do cross ethnic groups. A small number of cases appear to be sufficient to identify strong associations as with Flucloxacillin and HLA-B*5701. Odds ratios (OR) and P values are given for secondary fine gene mapping where available rather than single-nucleotide polymorphism screening.

Key Genetic Findings

Genetic analysis of DILI is limited to date, and several large studies are ongoing. The key findings thus far are listed as follows:

- Polymorphisms of genes involved in drug metabolism and transport are risk factors for DILI
- HLA polymorphisms are also associated with DILI
- Most genetic risk factors for DILI identified so far are drug and population specific
- Genetic pretesting of individuals is not yet possible

Future Directions for Genetic Analysis of Drug-Induced Liver Injury

Of course, there are many directions in which to follow up on the above key findings. The following are some suggested avenues:

- Expanded GWAS and WGS studies—both drug specific and nonspecific analyses
- Microbiome analysis—Are the wrong genome being studied? The microbiome clearly affects drug metabolism and immune responses
- Environment influence and epigenetic factors—Gene expression is modified by other factors besides one's gene sequence
- Proteomics and metabolomics—Likewise, protein activity is not simply a function of gene expression. Genetic analysis should be integrated with proteomics and metabolomics analyses
- DILI treatment trials—Is enough known yet? Genetic study results to date suggest modulation of drug metabolism, antioxidant levels, and immune responses may ameliorate DILI

SUMMARY

The epidemiology of idiosyncratic DILI suggests that overall it is an uncommon event. In the United States and Europe, prescription antimicrobials are the most common cause, but HDS are increasingly associated with DILI, particularly in Korea and Japan. The pattern of injury differs according to the implicated drug. Several differences are apparent in the risk of DILI with regards to demographic factors, and some of these factors influence the severity of the injury and its outcome. Genetic analysis of DILI is limited, although several large studies are ongoing. Multiple polymorphisms of HLA genes and genes involved in drug metabolism and transport have been identified as risk factors for DILI.

REFERENCES

1. Zhang W, Roederer MW, Chen WQ, et al. Pharmacogenetics of drugs withdrawn from the market. Pharmacogenomics 2012;13:223–31.
2. Björnsson ES, Bergmann OM, Björnsson HK, et al. Incidence, presentation, and outcomes in patients with drug-induced liver injury in the general population of Iceland. Gastroenterology 2013;144:1419–25.
3. Sgro C, Clinard F, Ouazir K, et al. Incidence of drug-induced hepatic injuries: a French population-based study. Hepatology 2002;36:451–5.
4. Suk KT, Kim DJ, Kim CH, et al. A prospective nationwide study of drug-induced liver injury in Korea. Am J Gastroenterol 2012;107:1380–7.
5. de Abajo FJ, Montero D, Madurga M, et al. Acute and clinically relevant drug-induced liver injury: a population based case-control study. Br J Clin Pharmacol 2004;58:71–80.

6. Ruigómez A, Brauer R, Rodríguez LA, et al. Ascertainment of acute liver injury in two European primary care databases. Eur J Clin Pharmacol 2014;70:1227–35.

7. De Valle MB, Av Klinteberg V, Alem N, et al. Drug-induced liver injury in a Swedish University hospital out-patient hepatology clinic. Aliment Pharmacol Ther 2006; 24:1187–95.

8. Chalasani N, Bonkovsky HL, Fontana R, et al, United States drug induced liver injury Network. Features and outcomes of 899 patients with drug-induced liver injury: the DILIN prospective study. Gastroenterology 2015;148:1340–52.

9. Andrade RJ, Lucena MI, Fernández MC, et al, Spanish Group for the Study of Drug-Induced Liver Disease. Drug-induced liver injury: an analysis of 461 incidences submitted to the Spanish registry over a 10-year period. Gastroenterology 2005;129:512–21.

10. Takikawa H, Murata Y, Horiike N, et al. Drug-induced liver injury in Japan: an analysis of 1676 cases between 1997 and 2006. Hepatol Res 2009;39:427–31.

11. Wai CT. Presentation of drug-induced liver injury in Singapore. Singapore Med J 2006;47:116–20.

12. Bessone F, Hernandez N, Lucena MI, et al, Latin Dili Network Latindilin And Spanish Dili Registry. The Latin American DILI registry experience: a successful ongoing collaborative strategic initiative. Int J Mol Sci 2016;17:313.

13. Björnsson E, Jacobsen EI, Kalaitzakis E. Hepatotoxicity associated with statins: reports of idiosyncratic liver injury post-marketing. J Hepatol 2012;56:374–80.

14. Charles EC, Olson KL, Sandhoff BG, et al. Evaluation of cases of severe statin-related transaminitis within a large health maintenance organization. Am J Med 2005;118:618–24.

15. Navarro VJ, Barnhart H, Bonkovsky HL, et al. Liver injury from herbals and dietary supplements in the U.S. Drug-Induced Liver Injury Network. Hepatology 2014;60: 1399–408.

16. Robles-Diaz M, Gonzalez-Jimenez A, Medina-Caliz I, et al, Spanish DILI Registry, SLatinDILI Network. Distinct phenotype of hepatotoxicity associated with illicit use of anabolic androgenic steroids. Aliment Pharmacol Ther 2015;41:116–25.

17. Lucena MI, Andrade RJ, Kaplowitz N, et al, Spanish Group for the Study of Drug-Induced Liver Disease. Phenotypic characterization of idiosyncratic drug-induced liver injury: the influence of age and sex. Hepatology 2009;49:2001–9.

18. Andrade RJ, Lucena MI, Kaplowitz N, et al. Outcome of acute idiosyncratic drug-induced liver injury: long-term follow-up in a hepatotoxicity registry. Hepatology 2006;44:1581–8.

19. Hunt CM, Yuen NA, Stirnadel-Farrant HA, et al. Age-related differences in reporting of drug-associated liver injury: data-mining of WHO safety report database. Regul Toxicol Pharmacol 2014;70:519–26.

20. Molleston JP, Fontana RJ, Lopez MJ, et al, Drug-Induced Liver Injury Network. Characteristics of idiosyncratic drug-induced liver injury in children: results from the DILIN prospective study. J Pediatr Gastroenterol Nutr 2011;53:182–9.

21. Murray KF, Hadzic N, Wirth S, et al. Drug-related hepatotoxicity and acute liver failure. J Pediatr Gastroenterol Nutr 2008;47:395–405.

22. Fontana RJ, Hayashi PH, Gu J, et al, DILIN Network. Idiosyncratic drug-induced liver injury is associated with substantial morbidity and mortality within 6 months from onset. Gastroenterology 2014;147:96–108.

23. Lammert C, Einarsson S, Saha C, et al. Relationship between daily dose of oral medications and idiosyncratic drug-induced liver injury: search for signals. Hepatology 2008;47:2003–9.

24. Vuppalanchi R, Gotur R, Reddy KR, et al. Relationship between characteristics of medications and drug-induced liver disease phenotype and outcome. Clin Gastroenterol Hepatol 2014;12:1550–5.

25. Lammert C, Bjornsson E, Niklasson A, et al. Oral medications with significant hepatic metabolism at higher risk for hepatic adverse events. Hepatology 2010;51: 615–20.

26. Meier Y, Cavallaro M, Roos M, et al. Incidence of drug-induced liver injury in medical inpatients. Eur J Clin Pharmacol 2005;61:135–43.

27. Reuben A, Koch DG, Lee WM, Acute Liver Failure Study Group. Drug-induced acute liver failure: results of a U.S. multicenter, prospective study. Hepatology 2010;52:2065–76.

28. Chalasani N, Aljadhey H, Kesterson J, et al. Patients with elevated liver enzymes are not at higher risk for statin hepatotoxicity. Gastroenterology 2004;126: 1287–92.

29. Lewis JH, Mortensen ME, Zweig S, et al, Pravastatin in Chronic Liver Disease Study Investigators. Efficacy and safety of high-dose pravastatin in hypercholesterolemic patients with well-compensated chronic liver disease: results of a prospective, randomized, double-blind, placebo-controlled, multicenter trial. Hepatology 2007;46:1453–63.

30. Wong WM, Wu PC, Yuen MF, et al. Antituberculosis drug-related liver dysfunction in chronic hepatitis B infection. Hepatology 2000;31:201–6.

31. Lee BH, Koh WJ, Choi MS, et al. Inactive hepatitis B surface antigen carrier state and hepatotoxicity during antituberculosis chemotherapy. Chest 2005;127: 1304–11.

32. den Brinker M, Wit FW, Wertheim-van Dillen PM, et al. Hepatitis B and C virus coinfection and the risk for hepatotoxicity of highly active antiretroviral therapy in HIV-1 infection. AIDS 2000;14:2895–902.

33. Sulkowski MS, Thomas DL, Mehta SH, et al. Hepatotoxicity associated with nevirapine or efavirenz-containing antiretroviral therapy: role of hepatitis C and B infections. Hepatology 2002;35:182–9.

34. Kramer JR, Giordano TP, Souchek J, et al. Hepatitis C coinfection increases the risk of fulminant hepatic failure in patients with HIV in the HAART era. J Hepatol 2005;42:309–14.

35. Kalow W. Genetic variation in the human hepatic cytochrome P-450 system [review]. Eur J Clin Pharmacol 1987;31(6):633–41.

36. Huang YS, Chern HD, Su WJ, et al. Polymorphism of the N-acetyltransferase 2 gene as a susceptibility risk factor for antituberculosis drug-induced hepatitis. Hepatology 2002;35(4):883–9.

37. Sharma SK, Jha BK, Sharma A, et al. Genetic polymorphisms of CYP2E1 and GSTM1 loci and susceptibility to anti-tuberculosis drug-induced hepatotoxicity. Int J Tuberc Lung Dis 2014;18(5):588–93.

38. Gupta VH, Singh M, Amarapurkar DN, et al. Association of GST null genotypes with anti-tuberculosis drug induced hepatotoxicity in Western Indian population. Ann Hepatol 2013;12(6):959–65.

39. Chatterjee S, Lyle N, Mandal A, et al. GSTT1 and GSTM1 gene deletions are not associated with hepatotoxicity caused by antitubercular drugs. J Clin Pharm Ther 2010;35(4):465–70.

40. Huang YS, Chern HD, Su WJ, et al. Cytochrome P450 2E1 genotype and the susceptibility to antituberculosis drug-induced hepatitis. Hepatology 2003;37(4): 924–30.

41. Bose PD, Sarma MP, Medhi S, et al. Role of polymorphic N-acetyl transferase2 and cytochrome P4502E1 gene in antituberculosis treatment-induced hepatitis. J Gastroenterol Hepatol 2011;26(2):312–8.
42. An HR, Wu XQ, Wang ZY, et al. NAT2 and CYP2E1 polymorphisms associated with antituberculosis drug-induced hepatotoxicity in Chinese patients. Clin Exp Pharmacol Physiol 2012;39(6):535–43.
43. Lee SW, Chung LS, Huang HH, et al. NAT2 and CYP2E1 polymorphisms and susceptibility to first-line anti-tuberculosis drug-induced hepatitis. Int J Tuberc Lung Dis 2010;14(5):622–6.
44. Wang PY, Xie SY, Hao Q, et al. NAT2 polymorphisms and susceptibility to anti-tuberculosis drug-induced liver injury: a meta-analysis. Int J Tuberc Lung Dis 2012;16(5):589–95.
45. Chen R, Wang J, Tang S, et al. Association of polymorphisms in drug transporter genes (SLCO1B1 and SLC10A1) and anti-tuberculosis drug-induced hepatotoxicity in a Chinese cohort. Tuberculosis (Edinb) 2015;95(1):68–74.
46. Nanashima K, Mawatari T, Tahara N, et al. Genetic variants in antioxidant pathway: risk factors for hepatotoxicity in tuberculosis patients. Tuberculosis (Edinb) 2012;92(3):253–9.
47. Chang JC, Liu EH, Lee CN, et al. UGT1A1 polymorphisms associated with risk of induced liver disorders by anti-tuberculosis medications. Int J Tuberc Lung Dis 2012;16(3):376–8.
48. Zazuli Z, Barliana MI, Mulyani UA, et al. Polymorphism of PXR gene associated with the increased risk of drug-induced liver injury in Indonesian pulmonary tuberculosis patients. J Clin Pharm Ther 2015;40(6):680–4.
49. Gao S, Gui XE, Liang K, et al. HLA-dependent hypersensitivity reaction to nevirapine in Chinese Han HIV-infected patients. AIDS Res Hum Retroviruses 2012; 28(6):540–3.
50. Phillips E, Bartlett JA, Sanne I, et al. Associations between HLA-DRB1*0102, HLA-B*5801, and hepatotoxicity during initiation of nevirapine-containing regimens in South Africa. J Acquir Immune Defic Syndr 2013;62(2):e55–7.
51. Carr DF, Chaponda M, Jorgensen AL, et al. Association of human leukocyte antigen alleles and nevirapine hypersensitivity in a Malawian HIV-infected population. Clin Infect Dis 2013;56(9):1330–9.
52. Spraggs CF, Budde LR, Briley LP, et al. HLA-DQA1*02:01 is a major risk factor for lapatinib-induced hepatotoxicity in women with advanced breast cancer. J Clin Oncol 2011;29(6):667–73.
53. Spraggs CF, Parham LR, Hunt CM, et al. Lapatinib-induced liver injury characterized by class II HLA and Gilbert's syndrome genotypes. Clin Pharmacol Ther 2012;91(4):647–52.
54. Schaid DJ, Spraggs CF, McDonnell SK, et al. Prospective validation of HLA-DRB1*07:01 allele carriage as a predictive risk factor for lapatinib-induced liver injury. J Clin Oncol 2014;32(22):2296–303.
55. Hirata K, Takagi H, Yamamoto M, et al. Ticlopidine-induced hepatotoxicity is associated with specific human leukocyte antigen genomic subtypes in Japanese patients: a preliminary case-control study. Pharmacogenomics J 2008; 8(1):29–33.
56. Cornejo Castro EM, Carr DF, Jorgensen AL, et al. HLA-allelotype associations with nevirapine-induced hypersensitivity reactions and hepatotoxicity: a systematic review of the literature and meta-analysis [review]. Pharmacogenet Genomics 2015;25(4):186–98.

57. Samara SA, Irshaid YM, Mustafa KN. Association of MDR1 C3435T and RFC1 G80A polymorphisms with methotrexate toxicity and response in Jordanian rheumatoid arthritis patients. Int J Clin Pharmacol Ther 2014;52(9):746–55.

58. Adam de Beaumais T, Fakhoury M, Medard Y, et al. Determinants of mercaptopurine toxicity in paediatric acute lymphoblastic leukemia maintenance therapy. Br J Clin Pharmacol 2011;71(4):575–84.

59. Karathanasis NV, Stiakaki E, Goulielmos GN, et al. The role of the methylenetetrahydrofolate reductase 677 and 1298 polymorphisms in Cretan children with acute lymphoblastic leukemia. Genet Test Mol Biomarkers 2011;15(1–2):5–10.

60. Mazor Y, Koifman E, Elkin H, et al. Risk factors for serious adverse effects of thiopurines in patients with Crohn's disease. Curr Drug Saf 2013;8(3):181–5.

61. Agúndez JA, Lucena MI, Martínez C, et al. Assessment of nonsteroidal anti-inflammatory drug-induced hepatotoxicity [review]. Expert Opin Drug Metab Toxicol 2011;7(7):817–28.

62. Lucena MI, Andrade RJ, Martínez C, et al, Spanish Group for the Study of Drug-Induced Liver Disease. Glutathione S-transferase m1 and t1 null genotypes increase susceptibility to idiosyncratic drug-induced liver injury. Hepatology 2008;48(2):588–96 [Erratum appears in: Hepatology 2009;49(3):1058].

63. Jiang J, Zhang X, Huo R, et al. Association study of UGT1A9 promoter polymorphisms with DILI based on systematically regional variation screen in Chinese population. Pharmacogenomics J 2015;15(4):326–31.

64. Ulzurrun E, Stephens C, Ruiz-Cabello F, et al. Selected ABCB1, ABCB4 and ABCC2 polymorphisms do not enhance the risk of drug-induced hepatotoxicity in a Spanish cohort. PLoS One 2014;9(4):e94675 [Erratum appears in PLoS One 2015;10(10):e0141400].

65. Horinouchi M, Yagi M, Imanishi H, et al. Association of genetic polymorphisms with hepatotoxicity in patients with childhood acute lymphoblastic leukemia or lymphoma. Pediatr Hematol Oncol 2010;27(5):344–54.

66. Nicoletti P, Werk AN, Sawle A, et al, International Drug-induced Liver Injury Consortium (iDILIC). HLA-DRB1*16: 01-DQB1*05: 02 is a novel genetic risk factor for flupirtine-induced liver injury. Pharmacogenet Genomics 2016;26(5): 218–24.

67. Parham LR, Briley LP, Li L, et al. Comprehensive genome-wide evaluation of lapatinib-induced liver injury yields a single genetic signal centered on known risk allele HLA-DRB1*07:01. Pharmacogenomics J 2016;16(2):180–5.

68. Lucena MI, Molokhia M, Shen Y, et al, Spanish DILI Registry, EUDRAGENE, DILIN, DILIGEN, International SAEC. Susceptibility to amoxicillin-clavulanate-induced liver injury is influenced by multiple HLA class I and II alleles. Gastroenterology 2011;141(1):338–47.

69. Daly AK, Donaldson PT, Bhatnagar P, et al, DILIGEN Study, International SAE Consortium. HLA-B*5701 genotype is a major determinant of drug-induced liver injury due to flucloxacillin. Nat Genet 2009;41(7):816–9.

70. Singer JB, Lewitzky S, Leroy E, et al. A genome-wide study identifies HLA alleles associated with lumiracoxib-related liver injury. Nat Genet 2010;42(8):711–4.

71. Kindmark A, Jawaid A, Harbron CG, et al. Genome-wide pharmacogenetic investigation of a hepatic adverse event without clinical signs of immunopathology suggests an underlying immune pathogenesis. Pharmacogenomics J 2008; 8(3):186–95.

72. Urban TJ, Shen Y, Stolz A, et al, Drug-Induced Liver Injury Network, DILIGEN, EUDRAGENE, Spanish DILI Registry, International Serious Adverse Events

Consortium. Limited contribution of common genetic variants to risk for liver injury due to a variety of drugs. Pharmacogenet Genomics 2012;22(11):784–95.

73. Yip VL, Alfirevic A, Pirmohamed M. Genetics of immune-mediated adverse drug reactions: a comprehensive and clinical review. Clin Rev Allergy Immunol 2015; 48:165–75.

Adverse Drug Reactions

Type A (Intrinsic) or Type B (Idiosyncratic)

Carlo J. Iasella, PharmD[a],*, Heather J. Johnson, PharmD[a], Michael A. Dunn, MD[b]

KEYWORDS

- Hepatotoxicity • Drug-induced liver injury • Adverse drug reaction
- Type A adverse drug reaction • Type B adverse drug reaction • Intrinsic
- Idiosyncratic • LiverTox

KEY POINTS

- Type A, or intrinsic, adverse drug reactions are dose-related, predictable toxic effects of medications, such as acute liver failure resulting from acetaminophen overdose.
- Type B or idiosyncratic adverse drug reactions are less related to dose and are associated with drug, patient, and environmental risk factors, which can be difficult to predict.
- Resources such as LiverTox assist with earlier detection of idiosyncratic adverse reactions in postmarketing use and can help guide diagnosis and management.

INTRODUCTION

In the United States today, drug-induced liver injury is the leading cause of acute liver failure (ALF), ahead of viral hepatitis and other causes.[1,2] More than1000 agents have been identified as causes of hepatic injury and, as reporting increases and new agents come to market, this number will continue to rise.[3] The adverse drug reactions experienced from these substances have typically been divided into Type A intrinsic reactions or Type B idiosyncratic reactions. Type A adverse drug reactions are dose-dependent, predictable toxicities. Type B adverse reactions are not easily explained by dose or expected pharmacologic response, rather they involve less predictable responses in susceptible individuals. Both types of adverse drug reactions are responsible for significant morbidity and mortality in many Western countries.

Most cases of drug-induced liver injury are the result of Type A adverse events; however, many more medications have been reported as causing Type B events. From 1990 to 2002, drug-induced liver injury from acetaminophen, isoniazid,

Disclosure Statement: The authors have nothing to disclose.
[a] Department of Pharmacy and Therapeutics, University of Pittsburgh School of Pharmacy, 3501 Terrace Street, Pittsburgh, PA 15261, USA; [b] Division of Gastroenterology, Hepatology and Nutrition, Center for Liver Diseases, University of Pittsburgh, 200 Lothrop Street, PUH, M2, C-wing, Pittsburgh, PA 15213, USA
* Corresponding author.
E-mail address: carlo.iasella@pitt.edu

Clin Liver Dis 21 (2017) 73–87
http://dx.doi.org/10.1016/j.cld.2016.08.005
1089-3261/17/© 2016 Elsevier Inc. All rights reserved.

valproate, phenytoin, and propylthiouracil was responsible for 15% of all liver transplantations in the United States.[4] More than half of these cases involved therapeutic use of the medications rather than intentional overdose. Although acetaminophen, which causes a Type A adverse event, accounts for most drug-induced ALF, Type B adverse drug events are implicated in more than 10% of ALF cases.[5]

Although understanding of Type A adverse events is relatively well established, new information about Type B responses and their risk factors continue to shape how clinicians diagnose and manage these responses. Drug-induced liver injury identified in postmarketing experience is the leading cause of withdrawal or new warnings for medications that have already been approved.[5,6] Most medications that require postmarketing action cause Type B responses. These reactions are difficult to detect in clinical trials because they often do not occur in animal models and occur rarely in the general population. This means that idiosyncratic reactions may not be observed in premarketing studies in which the number of participants is limited and duration of exposure is short, and are only seen in postmarketing surveillance, as depicted in **Fig. 1**. Fortunately, resources such as LiverTox, an online database maintained by the National Institutes of Health, exist to assist clinicians with identifying, managing, and reporting drug-induced liver injury.

TYPE A (INTRINSIC) ADVERSE DRUG REACTIONS

Adverse drug reactions classified as Type A, or intrinsic, are defined as predictable adverse effects associated with an agent and are related to dose.[7] As the dose of the administered agent increases, the risk of adverse event increases with it, in accordance with the pharmacologic profile of the agent.[7,8] Type A adverse effects are predictable side effects and may also be characterized as drug toxicities. Because of their predictable nature, Type A adverse effects generally have relatively low mortality because responses can be monitored and managed.[7] Because intrinsic adverse effects are usually identified in animal models or clinical trials in humans, medications that demonstrate these effects at therapeutic doses often never come to market.

Common examples of medications causing Type A adverse effects leading to liver injury are listed in **Table 1**. The classic example of a dose-dependent hepatotoxic response is acetaminophen. Acetaminophen is associated with fulminant hepatic failure when administered at toxic doses; however, hepatic dysfunction is rarely seen at doses below 4 g per day in healthy patients. As long as the drug is administered at the therapeutically appropriate dose, hepatic adverse effects are very rare.

Chronic exposure to certain medications can increase the risk of developing Type A adverse reactions. In a mouse model, chronic exposure to acetaminophen in combination with subacute high-dose exposures resulted in severe hepatotoxicity, ALF, and death.[9] Additionally, chronic exposure alone, without the acute overdose, led to ALF in some older mice. Finally, N-acetylcysteine (NAC), which is normally an effective antidote for acetaminophen hepatotoxicity, did not significantly improve ALF prevention or recovery compared with placebo. These findings suggest that exposure to hepatotoxic medications over time may be important in the development of intrinsic hepatotoxic reactions.

TYPE B (IDIOSYNCRATIC) ADVERSE DRUG REACTIONS

Type B adverse drug reactions, or idiosyncratic drug reactions, are unanticipated adverse effects associated with an agent.[7] They result from a combination of factors unique to the individual.[5,8,10–12] Differences between Type A and Type B adverse drug

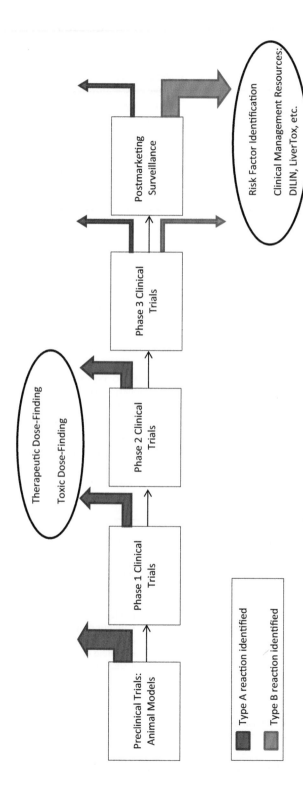

Fig. 1. Identification of drug-induced injury in drug development and surveillance process. Adverse drug reactions are identified at different parts of the drug discovery and Food and Drug Administration (FDA)-approval process. Type A reactions are typically observed in animal studies with subsequent phase 1 and phase 2 studies identifying toxic doses. Type B reactions rarely present in preclinical or clinical trials due to the limited number of subjects in these studies. These effects are seen in postmarketing experience in which resources such as LiverTox and the Drug-Induced Liver Injury Network (DILIN) can assist with timely identification and clinical management. The arrows represent discovery of Type A or Type B adverse effects in the drug development process. The thickness of the arrows signifies the relative frequency with which each type of adverse effect is discovered in the process.

Table 1
Drugs associated with Type A (intrinsic) adverse drug events involving the liver

Drug	Class
Acetaminophen	Analgesic, antipyretic
Amiodarone	Antiarrhythmic
Bromfenac[a]	Nonsteroidal antiinflammatory drugs
Cyclophosphamide	Antineoplastic
Cyclosporine	Immunosuppressant
Methotrexate	Antineoplastic, immunosuppressant
Niacin	Antilipemic
Tetracycline	Antibiotic

[a] Systemic formulations withdrawn from market.

reactions are summarized in **Table 2**. Although it is difficult to estimate the true incidence of idiosyncratic drug-induced liver injury due to incomplete recognition and reporting, it is thought to range from 1 in 1000 to 1 in 200,000, depending on the agent.[13] Common classes of agents causing idiosyncratic drug-induced liver injury include antibiotics, nonsteroidal antiinflammatory drugs, and anticonvulsants. Idiosyncratic reactions have highly variable presentations. They can be further subdivided into immunologic (immunoallergic and autoimmune) and nonimmunologic adverse reactions.[5,8,14]

Idiosyncratic adverse reactions have been considered to be dose-independent; however, several reports suggest specific situations in which dose predicts response to some extent. One retrospective database review examined medications most commonly prescribed in the United States and stratified their reported hepatotoxicity based on the average prescribed dose. Three times as many medications with reports of drug-induced liver failure resulting in death had average prescribed doses greater than or equal to 50 mg, compared with medications with average doses less than or equal to 10 mg (odds ratio [OR] 3.10, 95% CI 1.19–8.12, $P = .021$).[15] Overall, a

Table 2
Type A versus Type B drug-induced liver injury

	Type A Drug-Induced Liver Injury	Type B Drug-Induced Liver Injury
Patient characteristics increasing risk	• High-dose exposure • Chronic exposure • Pre-existing hepatic dysfunction	• Concomitant medications or polypharmacy • Infection • Immunosuppression • Extremes of age • Female gender • Genetic variations
Clinical manifestations	Toxic or overdose reactions	• Immunoallergic reactions • Autoimmune reactions • Nonimmunologic reactions
Diagnostic methods	• Physical examination • Liver function tests	• Diagnosis of exclusion • Hy's Law • Immunoglobulin levels • Biopsy

significantly higher incidence of liver failure as a reported adverse effect was seen for higher dose medications (OR 2.38, 95% CI 1.03–5.50, P = .042). An analysis of Swedish drug-induced liver injury cases found that 76.9% (n = 460) of reported events were associated with medications administered at doses of 50 mg per day or greater, whereas only 8.9% (n = 53) were associated with medication doses of 10 mg per day or less.[15] These findings indicate that there is a probable threshold of exposure below which idiosyncratic reactions are unlikely to occur. Although increasing dose will not necessarily increase the risk of idiosyncratic reaction for a particular medication, doses less than 10 mg seem unlikely to elicit a response.

Risk Factors

Several medication, environmental, and patient-specific risk factors have been associated with Type B adverse drug reactions.[8] Broadly, drug-specific risk factors include metabolic pathways, presence of toxic metabolites, and potency.[8,15] Patient-specific risk factors might include concomitant use of other medications or herbals, age, nutritional status, immune system function, gender, genetics, and physical activity.[8] Diet, chemical exposure, antioxidants, and probiotics are all considered environmental factors.[6] Type B adverse reactions are thought to arise only when multiple risk factors are present in a given individual.

Drug metabolism and potency are important for the development of idiosyncratic drug reactions. As discussed previously, although dose does not correlate with Type B adverse drug reactions, these events are far less likely for medications that are administered at low doses.[15] Medications that adversely affect mitochondrial function, including tetracycline, valproate, and oncologic chemotherapy agents, can predispose individuals to idiosyncratic reactions through deposition and accumulation of lipid droplets in hepatocytes.[8,11] For most idiosyncratic reactions, the administered agent is not responsible for the observed adverse effect but, instead, a toxic or reactive metabolite is generated.[8] Although idiosyncratic drug reactions can occur in many different organ systems, the liver tends to be an especially common site of toxicity as the organ where most toxic metabolites are generated.[8,12]

Patient-associated risk factors are not yet well understood; however, a few factors have been shown to increase risk for Type B reactions. Pre-existing diseases can increase an individual's susceptibility for an idiosyncratic reaction. Viral infections may sensitize the innate immune system via activation of cytokine and chemokine pathways. In rat models, drug-induced activation of inflammatory pathways followed by administration of nontoxic doses of ranitidine resulted in liver failure, whereas rats administered famotidine, a medication of the same class but with a much lower reported rate of idiosyncratic hepatotoxicity, did not develop liver failure.[16]

Immunosuppression may also predispose individuals to idiosyncratic drug reactions. Type B drug-induced liver injury is more common in human immunodeficiency virus (HIV)-positive patients, as well as liver transplant recipients, although other factors, such as medication burden and pre-existing liver dysfunction, may contribute as well.[17,18] The combination of a patient-specific factor, inflammation, along with a drug-specific factor, such as ranitidine's versus famotidine's potential for toxicity, may predispose to an idiosyncratic reaction. Besides infection, pre-existing disease, such as baseline hepatic impairment, can increase the risk for Type B reactions.[8] Concomitant use of other medications, herbals, or dietary supplements can also increase the likelihood of these types of reactions. Medications that alter metabolic pathways, such as cytochrome P450, can either both increase production of and impair clearance of toxic metabolites.[8] Age is another important risk factor for the development of adverse drug reactions. Specifically, the very young and very old seem to be at an increased risk for Type B reactions from particular agents.[8,10] Children have an increased risk for hepatotoxicity resulting from antimicrobials and antiepileptics, such as valproate, which has been attributed to differences in metabolic enzyme activity.[8,10] The risk of liver injury from medications, such as isoniazid, amoxicillin-clavulanate, and nitrofurantoin, increases with age. It is unclear if these differences are due to an inherent change with age itself or to coexistence of other medical conditions, malnutrition, or polypharmacy, which are often observed in this population.[8,10,11] Women tend to be at higher risk for idiosyncratic reactions than men, especially immunologic adverse reactions.[10] Finally, genetic variations that affect metabolism or mitochondrial activity can alter the chance that Type B reactions occur.[0,10]

Presentation and Diagnosis

Diagnosis of idiosyncratic drug-induced liver injury is challenging. Laboratory findings, hepatobiliary imaging, and liver biopsy, in addition to a comprehensive patient history, can support a working diagnosis of Type B adverse drug reaction hepatotoxicity.[10] Acute hepatitis C virus (HCV) and hepatitis E can present a clinical picture that is indistinguishable from drug-induced liver injury, especially when initial antibody tests remain negative. HCV RNA testing should be performed in cases of suspected drug-induced liver injury to rule out HCV.[10] Wilson disease and Budd-Chiari syndrome can also be mistaken for drug-induced liver injury. Autoimmune hepatitis can be either an alternative diagnosis to drug-induced liver injury or an idiosyncratic reaction to a medication, such as minocycline, α-methyldopa, or nitrofurantoin.[10,20,21] In cases in which these medications are the cause, latency periods may be as long as a year or more. Liver biopsy may be useful in the diagnosis of idiosyncratic drug-induced liver injury; however, it is not required. It can be difficult to distinguish drug-induced injury from nondrug autoimmune hepatitis on biopsy by any single pathologic finding; however, combinations of individual factors can help to differentiate them.[22] In a systematic histologic evaluation of 63 biopsies, features such as severe portal inflammation, prominent intra-acinar eosinophils, prominent portal plasma cells, rosette formation, fibrosis, and severe focal necrosis favored nondrug autoimmune hepatitis, whereas prominent intra-acinar lymphocytes, cholestasis canalicular, prominent portal neutrophils, and hepatocellular cholestasis favored drug-induced injury.[22] Diagnostic algorithms for assessing drug-induced liver injury based on serum aminotransferases and alkaline phosphatase were published in a 2014 guideline from the American College of Gastroenterology.[10]

Because of the myriad of presentations of liver injury resulting from Type B adverse drug reactions, severity of injury and prognosis varies greatly based on individual drugs and patients. Fortunately, recovery from drug-induced liver injury is as high as 90% overall.[10] However, patients experiencing drug-induced ALF from idiosyncratic adverse drug reactions seem to be at an increased risk for death or need for transplant than those suffering ALF due to intrinsic adverse drug reactions. Patients with ALF due to acetaminophen had higher transplant-free survival than those with ALF associated with idiosyncratic drug reactions (63% vs 23%).[10,23] Liver injury patterns with high degrees of necrosis, fibrosis, microvesicular steatosis, or ductular involvement are associated with poorer outcomes compared with those with intra-hepatic eosinophils or granulomas.[24] Although rechallenging patients with prior drug-induced liver injury can help establish a medication as the cause of liver injury, rechallenge is a high-risk course of action that should generally be avoided except in life-threatening situations in which no alternative agent would be appropriate.[10]

Management

The primary treatment of idiosyncratic drug-induced liver injury is removal of the suspected causal agent.[10] In the case of immunologic idiosyncratic reactions, antihistamines and corticosteroids have been used, although there are no controlled trials that support these therapies in the acute setting or for chronic injury.[10] For acetaminophen overdose resulting in ALF, NAC has established efficacy, and there are some data to support its use in idiosyncratic drug-induced liver injury. A randomized, double-blind, prospective trial compared NAC with placebo in subjects with nonacetaminophen ALF and found that transplant-free survival at 3 weeks was improved in the NAC group (40%) compared with the placebo group (27%, $P = .043$).[25] This effect seems to be applicable only to adults. Another study found that 1-year survival was lower in children receiving NAC for nonacetaminophen ALF versus placebo.[26]

Idiosyncratic Reaction Classifications

Idiosyncratic drug-induced liver injury can be divided broadly into immunologic and nonimmunological reactions. Immunologic Type B adverse drug reactions include hypersensitivity or allergic reactions, as well as autoimmune reactions.[5,14] Distinctions have been made between liver injury that is immunoallergic in nature versus drug-induced liver injury with autoimmune features. Symptoms of immunoallergic-type reactions include jaundice that is accompanied by fever, rash, itching, arthralgias, facial edema, and lymphadenopathy.[14] These tend to develop after latency periods of less than 1 month.[5,14] Other characteristics of this type of reaction include eosinophilia, the presence of antibodies, lymphocytosis, and elevated inflammatory markers such as C-reactive protein and erythrocyte sedimentation rate. Additionally, there is rapid recurrence of hepatotoxicity when rechallenged with the offending agent.[5] Immunoallergic liver injury usually improves gradually when the offending agent is removed, although rarely chronic injury, including vanishing bile duct syndrome, has been reported.[14]

Autoimmune drug-induced liver injury is less predictable than immunoallergic reactions. Clinical manifestations can vary greatly. Findings will often include abdominal pain, nausea, jaundice, with elevations in immunoglobulin levels, antinuclear antibodies, antimitochondrial antibodies, or other signs of autoimmunity.[10,27] Latency periods also range widely from 3 months to years after initially beginning the causal agent. If biopsy is performed, lobular and portal inflammation with interface hepatitis and lymphohistiocytic and plasma cell infiltrates can be observed.[14] Hepatocellular injury occurs more often than cholestatic or mixed patterns of disease. ALF is rare in autoimmune-type reactions. Instead, a prolonged syndrome results in a chronic autoimmune hepatitis.[14] Slow improvement is usually seen after the offending agent is withdrawn. Corticosteroids are commonly used in the same manner as for nondrug-induced autoimmune hepatitis and are generally considered to be beneficial, with biochemical and symptomatic improvement; however, controlled trials confirming this benefit are lacking. Unlike the need for years long therapy with nondrug autoimmune hepatitis, steroid therapy can often be withdrawn after no more than 6 months without recurrence.[14]

Nonimmunologic idiosyncratic reactions typically have a much longer latency period of up to 6 months.[5] These reactions are often a result of alterations in metabolic pathways leading to the formation of a toxic compound. An example of this phenomenon is isoniazid, which is metabolized differently in certain ethnic groups based on genetic variations responsible for fast versus slow acetylation.[13,28] Metabolic processes can also lead to autoimmune-like responses. Substances may be metabolized by cytochrome P450 enzymes to highly reactive intermediate compounds. These compounds may covalently bond to the enzyme, creating a drug-hapten adduct that inactivates the enzyme, directly damages the cell, and evokes an immune response against the adduct.[13,14] Genetic alterations in metabolism alone are not solely responsible for idiosyncratic reactions of this type. Most individuals with a given enzyme variant will develop an adaptive response after mild aminotransferase elevations that eventually subside, although a few will develop drug-induced liver injury, as is commonly demonstrated with 3-hydroxy-3-methylglutaryl coenzyme A (HMG-CoA) reductase inhibitors (see later discussion).[13] This adaptation supports the notion that other factors are important for the development of Type D reactions. Subsequent exposures to the offending agent may or may not cause recurrence of hepatic injury, depending on environmental factors.[5]

PREDICTING DRUG-INDUCED LIVER INJURY

Several methods have been used to predict the occurrence of and severity of drug-induced liver injury. The most well-known and frequently cited of these is Hy's Law. Named for the late Dr Hyman Zimmerman, whose research and clinical insight formed much of the basis for current thinking on hepatotoxicity, Hy's Law helps to evaluate the risk of drug-induced injury developing into ALF. Briefly, Hy's Law is based on observations that when jaundice becomes evident in combination with drug-induced hepatocellular injury, the mortality rate due to liver failure ranges between 10% and 50%.[29] When ALT levels exceed 3 times the upper limit of normal and total bilirubin exceeds twice normal in the setting of drug-induced injury, Hy's law predicts severe toxicity. Hy's Law is useful for predicting hepatotoxicity in clinical drug development, for example, as an important monitoring parameter in investigational clinical drug trials, as well as predicting risk in clinical scenarios. Recently, other approaches for predicting drug-induced ALF have been proposed to improve on the relatively low specificity of Hy's Law; however, it remains a well-established, validated predictor in hepatotoxicity.[29,30]

RESOURCES FOR CLINICIANS

Initially launched in 2012, LiverTox (available at: www.livertox.nih.gov) is a free online resource that allows clinicians to access current, comprehensive information about hepatotoxicity caused by medications and to assist with diagnosis and management of drug-induced liver injury.[3] The LiverTox Web site was created as a collaborative effort between the Liver Disease Research Branch of the National Institute of Diabetes and Digestive and Kidney Diseases (NIDDK) and the Division of Specialized Information Services of the National Library of Medicine (NLM), National Institutes of Health, and is regularly maintained and improved. Content is authored primarily by members of the Liver Disease Research Branch of the NIDDK, while members of the NLM developed the Web site. All sections of LiverTox are reviewed for accuracy and completeness by at least 1 independent reviewer, including many of the investigators of the Drug-induced Liver Injury Network.

LiverTox is divided into 3 primary sections: (1) introduction and overview of drug-induced liver injury, (2) specific drug records, and (3) a case submission registry.[3] The introduction component is a general review of drug-induced liver injury, including criteria for diagnosis, determination of severity and cause, clinical pathologic findings, treatment and management information, and standardized nomenclature. The specific drug records comprise the bulk of the Web site. Records exist only for medications currently approved in the United States, as well as commercially available herbals and dietary supplements. Each individual record contains the same basic information: Introduction, describing the agent and its uses; Background, containing basic information on the agents class, mechanism of action, and efficacy; Hepatotoxicity, describing type of liver injury, rates of serum enzyme elevations, time to onset, pattern of biomarker elevations, immunoallergic or autoimmune features (if any), severity, and prognosis; Mechanism of Liver Injury; Outcome and Management, discussing severity of injury and corresponding management or treatment, as well as recommendations for rechallenging or use of a related agent; Case Reports; Chemical and Product Information; and References. Finally, LiverTox contains a Case Submission Registry that encourages users to submit case reports in a standardized format. Information submitted by users is maintained in a secure database, which will allow for analysis of trends in drug-induced liver injury and patterns of liver injury associated with various agents. Cases that represent verified instances of drug-induced liver injury can be deidentified and made publically available for other users.

LiverTox is a useful tool for clinicians because it represents the largest publically available database specifically focused on hepatotoxicity. For most of the listed agents, the drug record and each of the sections are complete. Some medications are missing sections in which information is limited or there is little evidence of hepatotoxicity. Other agents lack individual records and are instead listed by class. Although the site currently has a large number of entries, including herbal and dietary supplements, it lacks a comprehensive listing of these nonprescription agents. There are plans to add more in the future. For clinicians, LiverTox is an authoritative, useful tool for quickly accessing information about drugs with established reports of hepatotoxicity.

Another resource that is available for clinicians is the Liver Toxicity Knowledge Base Benchmark Dataset (LTKB-BD). This data set was created by the National Center for Toxicologic Research and is housed on the Food and Drug Administration (FDA) Web site.[31] Prescription labeling was used to classify medications as "most drug-induced liver injury-concern drugs," "less drug-induced liver injury-concern drugs," and "no drug-induced liver injury-concern drugs." So far, 287 prescription drug labels have been examined with plans to continue to update the set in the future.

The LTKB-BD could be helpful for identifying medications with known risk for drug-induced liver injury and stratifying risk based on multiple potential causative agents. At this point, the number of included agents is far fewer than LiverTox and, compared to LiverTox, it lacks case report information in addition to the material included on medication labeling. Additionally, LTKB-BD focuses solely on classifying concern of drug-induced liver injury and does not provide guidance for diagnosis or management.

EVOLUTION OF DRUG-INDUCED INJURY RECOGNITION AND MANAGEMENT
Isoniazid

The ways in which idiosyncratic drug-induced injury is identified have evolved over time. The current architecture drug-induced liver injury monitoring in the United States is depicted in **Fig. 2**. Electronic resources have allowed for much quicker identification of these uncommon adverse events. The isoniazid experience demonstrates the challenges posed in identifying idiosyncratic injury in the past. Isoniazid is an antituberculosis antibiotic that causes aminotransferase elevations in about 10% of patients, with 1% of patients going on to develop severe hepatitis.[32] Isoniazid-induced hepatitis is characterized by anorexia, nausea, vomiting, abdominal pain, and jaundice, in addition to aminotransferase elevations usually exceeding 10 times the upper limit of

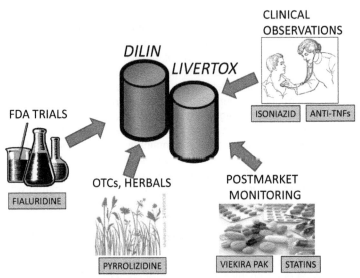

Fig. 2. Current architecture of United States drug-induced liver injury monitoring. DILIN is a National Institutes of Health-funded network of 8 academic centers begun in 2004. It collaborates with the online Livertox.nih.gov Web-based resource begun in 2012 by the NIDDK in collaboration with the NLM. Major inputs for LiverTox include (1) data from FDA clinical trials, for example, severe hepatotoxicity caused by fialuridine during its phase 2 evaluation as a hepatitis B antiviral; (2) reports of hepatotoxicity resulting from nonprescription and herbal compounds, for example, pyrrolizidine alkaloids; (3) postmarketing surveillance reports of approved drugs, for example, severe toxicity of Viekira Pak, a hepatitis C antiviral combination, in decompensated cirrhosis, and data showing that prolonged statin use is safe when low-grade aminotransferase elevations occur; and (4) clinical observations such as the large body of publications on isoniazid toxicity and reports of hepatotoxicity in patients treated with anti-TNF-α agents. OTCs, over-the-counter drugs.

normal. Morbidity and mortality from isoniazid hepatitis are significant, with fulminant liver failure requiring urgent liver transplantation, and occur in 5% to 10% of patients with clinical hepatitis but only 0.02% of patients taking isoniazid overall.[32–34]

Isoniazid was first used for the treatment of tuberculosis (TB) in 1954, before widespread electronic dissemination of information.[35] Initial studies indicated that isoniazid had few side effects and it was used as a cornerstone of multidrug regimens for TB. Reports of hepatotoxicity were rare and initially attributed to other antimicrobials taken concomitantly with isoniazid. However, in 1963 when isoniazid was recommended as monotherapy for prevention of active TB, case reports of hepatotoxicity in patients taking isoniazid alone led to identification of isoniazid itself as producing idiosyncratic hepatotoxicity.

Tumor Necrosis Factor-α Antagonists

One class of medications with emerging evidence of idiosyncratic drug-induced liver injury is the tumor necrosis factor-α (TNF-α) antagonists. A review of existing case reports from 2013 identified 6 published reports of autoimmune hepatotoxicity that were considered likely to have been caused by exposure to a TNF-α antagonist.[36] Multiple agents from the class were identified, including infliximab, adalimumab, and etanercept. Subjects were primarily female (5 out of 6) with average peak ALT of 914 units/L, alkaline phosphatase of 202 units/L, and total bilirubin of 9.8 mg/dL. The average latency period was 16 weeks. Of the 6 identified cases, 5 were treated with corticosteroids, which were able to eventually be withdrawn without further liver injury.

Two of the subjects who had adverse reactions to infliximab were then given etanercept after resolution of their symptoms without recurrence.[36] Infliximab is a chimeric human-murine monoclonal antibody that targets TNF-α, whereas etanercept is a DNA-derived protein composed of a TNF-α receptor linked to a fragment of human IgG.[37] Both prevent TNF-α interaction with cell surface receptors; however, etanercept is unlikely to lead to the development of an antidrug antibody response. Though the occurrence rate of TNF-α–induced drug-induced injury is low, electronic resources such as LiverTox can help clinicians diagnose and manage this adverse drug event based on current understanding of the response.

Viral Hepatitis Treatments

Several medications have been studied and used to treat viral hepatitis; however, some of those medications have resulted in hepatotoxic drug-induced injury. One important agent in the timeline of drug-induced injury is fialuridine. In 1993, fialuridine was studied in 15 subjects for the treatment of chronic hepatitis B after successfully completing animal studies.[38] Despite a favorable adverse effect profile in animal models, 5 of the 15 subjects participating in its initial human evaluation died as a result of lactic acidosis and ALF attributed to mitochondrial toxicity, whereas another 2 subjects required urgent liver transplantation. A more recent antiviral combination medication, ombitasvir, paritaprevir, ritonavir, plus dasabuvir (packaged as Viekera) used to treat HCV was associated with drug-induced injury. In postmarketing surveillance, this combination was shown to cause decompensated cirrhosis in patients with existing moderate to severe hepatic impairment, Child class B or C, in at least 26 patients at 1 to 4 weeks postinitiation of treatment.[39] The Web site HCVguidelines.org is a joint effort between the American Association for the Study of Liver Disease and the Infectious Disease Society of America.[40] It is a living document that is regularly updated as new agents and literature become available for the management of HCV. To help clinicians avoid potentially dangerous worsening liver failure, the current version recommends against the use of products containing ombitasvir and dasabuvir for the treatment of patients with decompensated cirrhosis. The adaptability and responsiveness of electronic resources, such as HCVguidelines.org and LiverTox, are changing the way clinicians make decisions about drug-induced injury and other treatment hazards by allowing information to be collected and processed in an expeditious manner that reaches practitioners quickly.

OTHER EXAMPLES AND MANAGEMENT STRATEGIES FOR IDIOSYNCRATIC DRUG-INDUCED INJURY
3-Hydroxy-3-Methylglutaryl Coenzyme A Reductase Inhibitors

A class of medications often linked to idiosyncratic drug-induced injury is the HMG-CoA reductase inhibitors. Commonly referred to as statins, these medications have been known to cause transient transaminitis; however, several large, randomized, prospective studies have shown that persistent aminotransferase elevations are not significantly different when compared with placebo.[41–43] A retrospective review of Scandinavian patients treated with statin therapy estimated the rate of statin-induced drug-induced injury to be 1.6 per 100,000 patients treated, with a small proportion of cases being associated with liver transplantation or death.[44] When statin-induced drug-induced injury does occur, it usually manifests 3 to 4 months after initiation. Experts have pointed out that the rare occurrence of serious drug-induced injury events while on statins does not vary greatly from the overall rate of liver failure in the general population, and avoidance of statins can put patients at a much higher risk of cardiovascular events.[45,46] Additionally, there is no evidence demonstrating that patients with pre-existing liver disease are at an increased risk for severe idiosyncratic drug-induced injury resulting from statin use.[45,46]

Herbal and Alternative Medicine

Herbal and dietary supplements present additional challenges to understanding drug-induced injury. These products can result in unanticipated direct hepatotoxicity because there is no requirement to demonstrate their safety or efficacy by the FDA. Additionally, many herbal and dietary supplements can interact with medication metabolism, leading to an increased risk for the development of drug-induced injury from those medications. Because of the limited regulation on the manufacturing processes of these substances, they carry the additional risks of misbranding and adulteration. Products with substandard manufacturing processes could contain substances not listed on their labels that are hepatotoxic and could potentiate idiosyncratic reactions to other agents.[8,10]

SUMMARY

Drug-induced liver injury is a problem associated with significant clinical impact in the United States. Classifying adverse drug events as intrinsic or idiosyncratic can help clinicians better understand the underlying mechanisms behind the response. Although intrinsic Type A response are reasonably well understood due to their predictable occurrence with increased exposure, the mechanisms and risk factors associated with Type B idiosyncratic responses are less clear. With the emergence of electronic resources, such as LiverTox, the ability to translate identification and assessment of drug-induced injury into clinically useful information is progressing to a more real-time model. As practice moves toward personalized medicine and finding the right drug for each individual patient, identifying patient-specific and environmental risk factors will be important in supporting appropriate clinical decisions.

REFERENCES

1. Ostapowicz G, Fontana RJ, Schiødt FV, et al. Results of a prospective study of acute liver failure at 17 tertiary care centers in the United States. Ann Intern Med 2002;137(12):947–55.
2. Fontana RJ, Seeff LB, Andrade RJ, et al. Standardization of nomenclature and causality assessment in drug-induced liver injury: summary of a clinical research workshop. Hepatology 2010;52(2):730–42.
3. LiverTox database. Bethesda (MD): US National Library of Medicine, National Institutes of Health, US Department of Health & Human Services; 2016. Available at: http://livertox.nih.gov. Accessed April 13, 2016.
4. Russo MW, Galanko JA, Shrestha R, et al. Liver transplantation for acute liver failure from drug induced liver injury in the United States. Liver Transpl 2004;10(8): 1018–23.
5. Kaplowitz N. Idiosyncratic drug hepatotoxicity. Nat Rev Drug Discov 2005;4(6): 489–99.
6. Bonkovsky HL, Jones DP, Russo MW, et al. Drug-induced liver injury. In: Boyer TD, Manns MP, Sanyal AJ, editors. Zakim and Boyer's hepatology. 6th edition. Philadelphia: WB Saunders; 2012. p. 417–61.

7. Edwards IR, Aronson JK. Adverse drug reactions: definitions, diagnosis, and management. Lancet 2000;356(9237):1255–9.

8. Ulrich RG. Idiosyncratic toxicity: a convergence of risk factors. Annu Rev Med 2007;58:17–34.

9. Kane AE, Huizer-Pajkos A, Mach J, et al. N-Acetyl cysteine does not prevent liver toxicity from chronic low dose plus sub-acute high dose paracetamol exposure in young or old mice. Fundam Clin Pharmacol 2016;30(3):263–75.

10. Chalasani N, Marrero JA, Ahn J, et al. ACG clinical guideline: the diagnosis and management of focal liver lesions. Am J Gastroenterol 2014;109(9):1–20.

11. Fontana RJ. Pathogenesis of idiosyncratic drug-induced liver injury and clinical perspectives. Gastroenterology 2014;146(4):914–28.

12. Uetrecht J, Naisbitt DJ. Idiosyncratic adverse drug reactions: current concepts. Pharmacol Rev 2013;65(2):779–808.

13. Lee WM. 152-Toxin- and drug-induced liver disease. In: Goldman L, Schafer AI, editors. Goldman-Cecil medicine, twenty-fifth edition. 25th edition. Philadelphia: Elsevier Inc; 2012. p. 979–84.

14. Delemos AS, Foureau DM, Jacobs C, et al. Drug-induced liver injury with autoimmune features. Semin Liver Dis 2014;34(2):194–204.

15. Lammert C, Einarsson S, Saha C, et al. Relationship between daily dose of oral medications and idiosyncratic drug-induced liver injury: search for signals. Hepatology 2008;47(6):2003–9.

16. Luyendyk JP. Ranitidine treatment during a modest inflammatory response precipitates idiosyncrasy-like liver injury in rats. J Pharmacol Exp Ther 2003; 307(1):9–16.

17. Sembera S, Lammert C, Talwalkar JA, et al. Frequency, clinical presentation, and outcomes of drug-induced liver injury after liver transplantation. Liver Transpl 2012;18(7):803–10.

18. Levy M. Role of viral infections in the induction of adverse drug reactions. Drug Saf 1997;16(1):1–8.

19. Stewart JD, Horvath R, Baruffini E, et al. Polymerase γ gene POLG determines the risk of sodium valproate-induced liver toxicity. Hepatology 2010;52(5): 1791–6.

20. Björnsson E, Talwalkar J, Treeprasertsuk S, et al. Drug-induced autoimmune hepatitis: clinical characteristics and prognosis. Hepatology 2010;51(6):2040–8.

21. Czaja AJ. Drug-induced autoimmune-like hepatitis. Dig Dis Sci 2011;56(4): 958–76.

22. Suzuki A, Brunt EM, Kleiner DE, et al. The use of liver biopsy evaluation in discrimination of idiopathic autoimmune hepatitis versus drug-induced liver injury. Hepatology 2011;54(3):931–9.

23. Reuben A, Koch DG, Lee WM. Drug-induced acute liver failure: results of a U.S. multicenter, prospective study. Hepatology 2010;52(6):2065–76.

24. Kleiner DE, Chalasani NP, Lee WM, et al. Hepatic histological findings in suspected drug-induced liver injury: systematic evaluation and clinical associations. Hepatology 2014;59(2):661–70.

25. Lee WM, Hynan LS, Rossaro L, et al. Intravenous N-Acetylcysteine improves transplant-free survival in early stage non-acetaminophen acute liver failure. Gastroenterology 2009;137(3):856–64, 864.e1.

26. Squires RH, Dhawan A, Alonso E, et al. Intravenous N-acetylcysteine in pediatric patients with nonacetaminophen acute liver failure: a placebo-controlled clinical trial. Hepatology 2013;57(4):1542–9.

27. Devarbhavi H. An update on drug-induced liver injury. J Clin Exp Hepatol 2012; 2(3):247–59.

28. Huang YS. Genetic polymorphisms of drug-metabolizing enzymes and the susceptibility to antituberculosis drug-induced liver injury. Expert Opin Drug Metab Toxicol 2007;3(1):1–8.

29. Robles-Diaz M, Isabel Lucena M, Kaplowitz N, et al. Use of Hy's law and a new composite algorithm to predict acute liver failure in patients with drug-induced liver injury. Gastroenterology 2014;147(1):109–18.e5.

30. Lo Re V, Haynes K, Forde KA, et al. Risk of acute liver failure in patients with drug-induced liver injury: evaluation of Hy's law and a new prognostic model. Clin Gastroenterol Hepatol 2015;13(13):2360–8.

31. Liver Toxicity Knowledge Base (LTKB) - LTKB Benchmark Dataset. National Center for Toxicological Research. FDA.gov. Available at: http://www.fda.gov/ScienceResearch/BioinformaticsTools/LiverToxicityKnowledgeBase/ucm2268 11.htm. Accessed May 11, 2016.

32. Verma S, Kaplowitz N. Hepatology of antituberculosis drugs. In: Kaplowitz N, DeLeve LD, editors. Drug-induced liver disease. 2nd edition. New York: Informa Healthcare; 2007. p. 547–66.

33. Ben Mahmoud L, Ghozzi H, Kamoun A, et al. Polymorphism of the N-acetyltransferase 2 gene as a susceptibility risk factor for antituberculosis drug-induced hepatotoxicity in Tunisian patients with tuberculosis. Pathol Biol 2012;60(5): 324–30.

34. Brunton LL, Lazo JS, Parker KL. Chemotherapy of tuberculosis, mycobacterium avium complex disease, and leprosy. In: Brunton LL, Chabner B, Knollmann B, editors. Goodman & Gilman's the pharmacological basis of therapeutics. 12th edition. New York: McGraw-Hill; 2006. p. 1–36.

35. Isoniazid. Bethesda (MD): US National Library of Medicine, National Institutes of Health, US Department of Health & Human Services; 2016. Available at: http://livertox.nih.gov/Isoniazid.htm#reference. Accessed April 13, 2016.

36. Ghabril M, Bonkovsky HL, Kum C, et al. Liver injury from tumor necrosis factor-α antagonists: analysis of thirty-four cases. Clin Gastroenterol Hepatol 2013;11(5): 558–64.e3.

37. Breedveld F. New tumor necrosis factor-alpha biologic therapies for rheumatoid arthritis. Eur Cytokine Netw 1998;9(3):233–8.

38. McKenzie R, Fried MW, Sallie R, et al. Hepatic failure and lactic acidosis due to fialuridine (FIAU), an investigational nucleoside analogue for chronic hepatitis B. N Engl J Med 1995;333(17):1099–105.

39. U.S. Food and Drug Administration. Hepatitis C treatments Viekira Pak and Technivie: drug safety communication - risk of serious liver injury. Safety alerts for human medical products. Silver Springs (MD): US Food and Drug Administration; 2015. Available at: http://www.fda.gov/Safety/MedWatch/SafetyInformation/SafetyAlertsforHumanMedicalProducts/ucm468757.htm?source=govdelivery&utm_medium=email&utm_source=govdelivery. Accessed April 14, 2016.

40. Unique Patient Populations: Patients with decompensated cirrhosis. Recommendations for Testing, Managing, and Treating Hepatitis C; HCVGuidelines.org. 2016. Available at: http://www.hcvguidelines.org/full-report/unique-patient-populations-patients-decompensated-cirrhosis. Accessed April 14, 2016.

41. Collins GS, Altman DG. Predicting the adverse risk of statin treatment: an independent and external validation of Qstatin risk scores in the UK. Heart 2012; 98(14):1091–7.

42. Scandinavian Simvastatin Survival Study Group. Randomised trial of cholesterol lowering in 4444 patients with coronary heart disease: the Scandinavian Simvastatin Survival Study (4S). Lancet 1994;344(8934):1383–9.
43. Downs JR, Clearfield M, Weis S, et al. Primary prevention of acute coronary events with lovastatin in men and women with average cholesterol levels. J Am Med Assoc 1998;279(20):1615–22.
44. Björnsson E, Jacobsen EI, Kalaitzakis E. Hepatotoxicity associated with statins: reports of idiosyncratic liver injury post-marketing. J Hepatol 2012;56(2):374–80.
45. Bader T. Yes! Statins can be given to liver patients. J Hepatol 2012;56(2):305–7.
46. Cohen DE, Anania FA, Chalasani N. An assessment of statin safety by hepatologists. Am J Cardiol 2006;97(8A):77C–81C.

Phenotypes and Pathology of Drug-Induced Liver Disease

Zachary D. Goodman, MD, PhD

KEYWORDS

- Liver biopsy • Histopathology • Hepatotoxicity • Drug-induced liver injury

KEY POINTS

- Liver tissue has a limited number of morphologic patterns that occur in response to various forms of injury.
- Drug hepatotoxicity can mimic virtually all forms of naturally occurring liver disease.
- Drugs with hepatotoxic potential generally cause recurring patterns of injury that are characteristic for each drug.
- Liver biopsy is often useful in determining whether histologic features characteristic of a particular drug-induced injury are present.

Chemical hepatotoxicity is a well-recognized phenomenon, whereas hepatic injury caused by medications available for therapeutic use is an uncommon but still far from rare occurrence in medical practice.[1–6] The drug approval process in developed countries keeps most highly toxic agents from reaching the market, so that the frequency of hepatotoxicity from any particular drug is generally less than 1% (usually much less). Nevertheless, there are so many different drugs in use that the aggregate number of cases is appreciable. Furthermore, as discussed elsewhere in this issue, the widespread use of herbal remedies and dietary supplements that are generally not regulated has resulted in numerous instances of toxic hepatic injury for which firm statistical documentation is not available.

CLINICAL SYNDROMES AND HISTOLOGIC CORRELATES

The diagnosis of hepatotoxicity is complicated because drug-induced liver injury is a great imitator, capable of mimicking all types of liver disease from other causes, in

The author has nothing to disclose.
Liver Pathology Research and Consultation, Center for Liver Diseases, Inova Fairfax Hospital, 3300 Gallows Road, Falls Church, VA 22042, USA
E-mail address: zachary.goodman@inova.org

clinical presentation and pathologic features (**Table 1**). Frequent presentations that bring patients to clinical attention and prompt liver biopsy include the following:

- Asymptomatic liver test abnormalities: routine screening tests detect many cases of mild liver injury in asymptomatic patients who only have liver test abnormalities, usually mildly elevated aspartate aminotransferase, alanine aminotransferase, or alkaline phosphatase.
- Acute seronegative viral hepatitis-like illness with anorexia, malaise, elevated transaminases with or without jaundice.
- Cholestatic hepatitis: viral hepatitis-like but with jaundice greater than one would expect from the degree of liver injury.
- Fulminant liver failure: jaundice and very high transaminases followed by hepatic coma over a period of a few days to a few weeks.
- Venous outflow obstruction: usually an acute process with features of fulminant liver failure and with rapidly accumulating ascites.
- Autoimmune hepatitis-like, which may have acute or fulminant presentation or may have an insidious onset with minimum symptoms.

Table 1
Clinical syndromes that can be mimicked by drug-induced liver injury and their pathologic counterparts

Clinical Syndrome	Pathologic Phenotypes
Asymptomatic liver test abnormalities	Adaptive changes Steatosis Phospholipidosis Mild necroinflammatory changes
Acute viral hepatitis-like ± jaundice	Acute panlobular hepatitis Mononucleosis-like hepatitis Hepatitis with confluent necrosis
Autoimmune hepatitis-like	Autoimmune hepatitis-like with severe injury, plasma cells ± confluent necrosis and/or fibrosis
Acute liver failure	Submassive or massive lytic necrosis Submassive or massive coagulative necrosis Microvesicular steatosis
Venous outflow obstruction	Hepatic vein thrombosis with severe congestion and necrosis Veno-occlusive disease (sinusoidal obstruction syndrome) Nodular regenerative hyperplasia
Obstructive jaundice-like	Bland cholestasis Cholestasis with mild hepatocellular injury Cholestasis with acute cholangitis
Cholestatic hepatitis	Combined hepatocellular and cholestatic injury ± cholangitis
Chronic cholestasis	Chronic cholestasis and ductopenia following acute cholestatic injury
Fibrosis and cirrhosis	Cirrhosis ± hepatitis, steatohepatitis or other liver disease
Noncirrhotic portal hypertension	Nodular regenerative hyperplasia Hepatoportal sclerosis
Liver disease with signs of hypersensitivity and/or disease in other organs	Acute or cholestatic hepatitis ± confluent necrosis
Primary hepatic neoplasms	Hepatocellular adenoma Hepatocellular carcinoma Hepatic angiosarcoma

- Obstructive jaundice-like: high bilirubin and alkaline phosphatase with normal or only mildly elevated transaminases.
- Chronic cholestasis when an initial obstructive jaundice-like injury fails to resolve with time.
- Liver disease accompanied by signs of hypersensitivity: any of the previously listed presentations but also with fever, skin rash, and/or eosinophilia DRESS syndrome (drug rash with eosinophilia and systemic symptoms)[1] should raise the suspicion of a hypersensitivity-type drug reaction.
- Fibrosis, cirrhosis, or noncirrhotic portal hypertension may follow an acute injury or may have a clinically silent insidious onset.
- Hepatic masses attributable to drugs and toxins include several types of primary liver tumors and tumor-like lesions.

DIAGNOSIS OF DRUG-INDUCED LIVER DISEASE

Because drug hepatotoxicity can simulate nearly any clinical syndrome or pathologic lesion that may occur in the liver, the diagnosis cannot be made on morphologic grounds alone or based on any specific laboratory test or biomarker. Because injury from any individual agent is uncommon, and because so many drug exposures occur for every actual instance of drug-related injury, every case requires careful analysis before attributing the cause to a specific drug. The difficulty of establishing a diagnosis whether by expert opinion or assessment tools, such as the Roussel-Uclaf Causality Assessment Method, is discussed elsewhere in this issue and in several reviews.[1-3,7-9] Histologic features are rarely considered because of a perceived lack of specificity, although this is not entirely true. An older method for evaluating suspected adverse drug reactions developed by Irey[10,11] uses criteria similar to those of expert opinion and Roussel-Uclaf Causality Assessment Method but also includes histologic pattern of injury as a critical feature. Key points in the evaluation are temporal eligibility with proper time sequence and appropriate latent period; exclusion of other drugs, drug interactions, and complications of the underlying disease being treated or an intercurrent primary liver disease; precedent for this type of injury by the suspected drug in the medical literature; pattern of injury and whether it is characteristic of reactions to the suspected drug; and dechallenge, because if the patient recovers after the drug is stopped, the likelihood that the drug was the cause is increased. After gathering the information and weighing the relative positive and negative findings, then one arrives at an expert opinion on the likelihood that a suspect drug was responsible for the liver injury.

A key element of this type of analysis is knowledge about previous experience with the drug, its likelihood of causing hepatotoxicity, and the features that have been documented. Most hepatotoxic drug reactions are idiosyncratic, and many drugs are known to cause more than one type of injury. Nevertheless, most drugs that are capable of hepatotoxicity tend to cause the same type or types of injury in susceptible individuals. There are several excellent books and reviews about drug hepatotoxicity, but until recently, accurate and timely information about many drugs was difficult to obtain. This changed dramatically in 2012 with the release of the LiverTox Web site (http//livertox.nih.gov), a joint product of the Liver Disease Research Branch of National Institute of Diabetes and Digestive and Kidney Diseases and the National Library of Medicine. This continually updated database contains accurate and up to date information on nearly all drugs currently used in the United States with summaries of known hepatotoxicity and an exhaustive annotated reference list for each agent.

Table 2
Morphologic Patterns Associated with Drug and Chemical Induced Hepatotoxicity

Morphologic Patterns	Examples
Adaptive changes, reflecting morphologic adaptation to drug metabolism	
Ground-glass cytoplasm is uniform pale eosinophilia of liver cells due to proliferation of smooth endoplasmic reticulum, reflecting induction of drug metabolizing enzymes	Phenobarbital (**Fig. 1**), diphenylhydantoin
Lipofuscin pigment granular and golden brown, accumulates in zone 3 liver cells.	Phenothiazines, cascara
Phospholipidosis by light microscopy is characterized by enlargement of foamy hepatocytes and Kupffer cells. By electron microscopy they can be seen to be due to characteristic lamellar lysosomal inclusions.	Amiodarone
Acute hepatotoxicity	
Hepatitis-like injury involves all zones of the acinus, with ballooning and acidophilic degeneration of hepatocytes, apopto-tic bodies, and small foci of necrosis. Minimal portal inflammation.	Isoniazid, rifampin sulfonamides, sulfasalazine (**Fig. 2**), methyldopa halothane, phenylbutazone, indomethacin, disulfiram
Mononucleosis-like hepatitis - increased cellularity of sinusoids in a so-called "beading arrangement", marked infiltration of portal spaces with lymphocytes, eosinophils, scattered acidophilic bodies and foci of necrosis, and multiple mitotic figures in liver cells.	Diphenylhydantoin (**Fig. 3**), sulfonamides, dapsone.
Submassive necrosis usually affects zone 3 ("centrilobular"), but may occur in zone 1 (periportal). It consists of confluent necrosis and loss of liver cells from an entire microcirculatory zone with collapse of supporting stroma but no fibrosis (or at most only early fibrosis). Inflammatory cells are seen in the stroma, and the portal areas might show inflammation as well. When the necrosis affects zone 1, there is often considerable cholestasis.	Zone 3 - Halothane, acetaminophen (**Fig. 4**), troglitazone (**Fig. 4**) ketoconazole, toxic mushrooms, black cohosh. Zone 1 - Halothane
Massive necrosis shows total loss of hepatocytes with collapse of the residual stroma, prominent ductular proliferation, and infiltration by neutrophils.	Any that cause submassive necrosis (see above)
Acute intrahepatic cholestasis	
• Cholestasis without hepatocellular injury ("Bland" cholestasis)	Anabolic and contraceptive steroids
• Cholestasis with minimal hepatocellular injury	Chlorpromazine, prochlorperazine (**Fig. 5**), erythromycin, amoxicillin-clavulanate, tolbutamide, mercaptopurine

(continued on next page)

Table 2 (continued)	
Morphologic Patterns	**Examples**
• Cholestasis + bile duct degeneration • Cholestasis with acute cholangitis	Paraquat poisoning Erythromycin (**Fig. 6**), chlorpromazine, amoxicillin-clavulanate, allopurinol, hydralazine
Acute cholestatic hepatitis (combined hepatocellular-cholestatic injury) leads to hepatocellular degeneration and/or necrosis along with a significant degree of intrahepatic cholestasis.	Carbamazepine (**Fig. 7**), diphenylhydantoin isoniazid, phenylbutazone,
Microvesicular steatosis in which the hepatocytes become enlarged and have one or two centrally placed nuclei. The cytoplasm is finely vacuolated with vacuoles varying from less than one up to eight microns in diameter.	Tetracycline, valproate (**Fig. 8**), salicylate intoxication, zidovudine, didanosine.
Vascular lesions include necrotizing angiitis with inflammation, edema and fibrinoid necrosis of the vessel wall; and lesser degrees of vasculitis of both veins and arteries.	Diphenylhydantoin, allopurinol, penicillin, sulfonamides, chlorothiazide
Chronic hepatotoxicity	
Chronic autoimmune-like hepatitis with considerable chronic portal and periportal inflammation, plasma cells, interface hepatitis and sometimes portal-periportal and bridging fibrosis.	Nitrofurantoin, minocycline (**Fig. 9**), methyldopa
Steatohepatitis, with fat, hepatocellular ballooning, Mallory-Denk bodies and fibrosis.	Alcohol (the prototype), amiodarone, tamoxifen (**Fig. 10**)
Chronic intrahepatic cholestasis with periportal bile pigment, cholate stasis and copper accumulation.	Chlorpromazine, prochlorperazine, methyltestosterone, imipramine, tolbutamide, haloperidol, thiabendazole
Macrovesicular steatosis can be recognized when most of the liver cells contain one large droplet of fat that pushes the nucleus to the periphery.	Alcohol, corticosteroids, methotrexate
Granulomatous reactions	
• Simple or "bland" granulomas • Granulomatous hepatitis, accompanied by hepatitis-like hepatocellular injury • Granulomas with vasculitis.	Sulfonamides, sulfonylureas, diltiazem (**Fig. 11**), quinidine, carbamazepine, phenylbutazone, allopurinol
Fibrosis accompanies many injuries as the result of chronicity. With a few drugs and chemicals, fibrosis (portal, periportal, bridging, etc) is the principal finding.	Methotrexate (**Fig. 12**), hyperalimentation
Cirrhosis with bridging fibrosis, loss of acinar architecture, and the formation of structurally abnormal nodules.	Methotrexate, amiodarone, total parenteral nutrition, chlorpromazine

(continued on next page)

Morphologic Patterns	Examples

Table 2
(continued)

Morphologic Patterns	Examples
Vascular lesions	
• Sinusoidal dilatation	Oral contraceptive steroids
• Peliosis hepatis, varying-sized cysts that contain blood and usually do not have an endothelial lining.	Androgenic/anabolic steroids, danazol, tamoxifen
• Veno-occlusive disease (also called sinusoidal obstruction syndrome) with occlusion of the terminal hepatic venules and severe congestion and necrosis.	Radiation, busulfan (**Fig. 13**), comfrey, hypervitaminosis A, azathioprine,
• Hepatic vein thrombosis	Oral contraceptive steroids
Neoplasms	
• Benign - Hepatocellular adenoma	Oral contraceptive steroids (**Fig. 14**)
• Malignant Hepatocellular carcinoma	Alcohol (?), anabolic steroids, contraceptive steroids (?)
Angiosarcoma	Anabolic steroids, arsenicals

Based on the information in LiverTox, Björnsson and Hoofnagle[12] recently published a listing of 671 drugs, grouped by the number of reported cases of convincing hepatotoxicity caused by those agents. Cases of hepatotoxicity are vastly underreported in the literature, primarily because of the reluctance of journal editors to publish individual case reports. Nevertheless, the number of reported cases caused by each drug can be taken as a reflection of the likelihood of its hepatotoxicity. Category A has 48 drugs with more than 50 reported cases; category B has 76 drugs with 12 to 49 cases; category C has 96 drugs with 4 to 11 cases; category D has 126 drugs with one to three convincing cases; and category E has 318 drugs with no convincing cases of hepatotoxicity. There is also a category T with seven drugs (acetaminophen, aspitin, niacin, vitamin A, buprenonphine, methylprednisolone, and tetracycline) that are directly toxic in very high disease or intravenous administration. The complete list is published[12] and is scheduled but has not yet been posted on LiverTox. Even so, the listing is extremely valuable when assessing an individual case of suspected drug-induced liver injury. If the

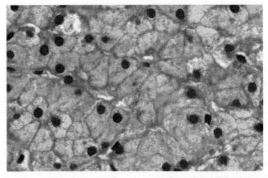

Fig. 1. Adaptive change characterized by drug-induced proliferation of smooth endoplasmic produces uniformly pale ground-glass cytoplasm in the hepatocytes of this patient on long-term phenobarbital (H&E, original magnification ×400).

drugs the patient was taking are not in categories A or B (ie, at least 12 reported cases), then it is still possible that the suspect drug is responsible, but more stringent evidence is needed than for a drug with more than 100 documented cases. Exceptions may be made for newly marketed drugs and for unregulated herbal products and dietary supplements, which are discussed elsewhere in this issue.

MORPHOLOGIC FEATURES THAT SUGGEST DRUG-INDUCED LIVER INJURY

Drug-induced injury can cause virtually any type of injury that occurs in the liver (**Table 2**), and so one cannot make an absolute diagnosis based on morphology alone. Some patterns, however, and unusual combinations of features should make one especially suspicious that a drug is the cause of the injury. In the setting of a hospital or medical practice in the developed world, all are more likely caused by drug-induced liver injury than by natural occurrence (ie, viral or autoimmune liver disease). These histologic patterns include:

- Severe acute hepatitis
  - Submassive or massive necrosis
  - Zonal necrosis
  - Coagulative necrosis
- Cholestatic hepatitis
- Hepatitis with eosinophils
- Granulomatous hepatitis
- Microvesicular steatosis
- Veno-occlusive disease or sinusoidal obstruction syndrome

Patients who are evaluated by expert hepatologists, especially hepatologists with expertise in drug-induced liver disease, would not be likely to have a liver biopsy in this circumstance, because a careful drug history would have revealed the likely underlying cause. Most patients, however, are initially evaluated by physicians who are not experts in this area, so when the initial laboratory tests and imaging studies do not reveal an obvious cause, the patient is often sent to an interventional radiologist for a liver biopsy. In such circumstances, the pathologist may be the first to suggest drug-induce liver injury. The pathologist may also be able to exclude drug-induced

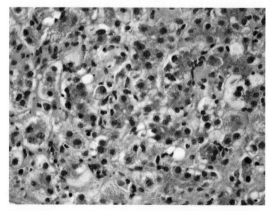

Fig. 2. Acute hepatitis, similar to typical acute viral hepatitis, caused by sulfasalazine. The biopsy shows lobular disarray with apoptotic bodies, hepatocellular ballooning and focal necrosis, Kupffer cell hypertrophy, and sinusoidal inflammation (H&E, original magnification ×400).

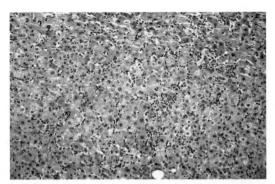

Fig. 3. Mononucleosis-like hepatitis, similar to Epstein-Barr virus infection, caused by diphenylhydantoin. The biopsy shows a marked sinusoidal mononuclear inflammatory cell infiltrate that is out of proportion to the degree of hepatocellular injury (H&E, original magnification ×400).

injury. For example, if the patient has a biopsy that shows severe steatohepatitis but he or she is not taking a drug, such as amiodarone or tamoxifen, then the steatohepatitis is presumed to be caused by alcohol or metabolic syndrome related nonalcoholic steatohepatitis, and the drug exposure is considered coincidental.

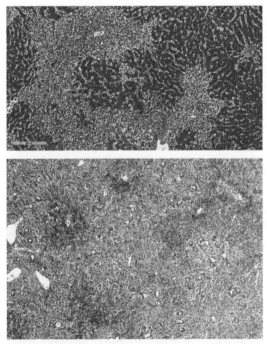

Fig. 4. Submassive and massive hepatic necrosis, with drug-induced acute liver failure. (*Top*) Submassive necrosis caused by acetaminophen overdose produces coagulative necrosis in the centrilobular (zone 3) regions of the liver. Necrotic liver cells and macrophages remain in areas that have lost viable hepatocytes. (*Bottom*) Massive necrosis caused by idiosyncratic reaction to troglitazone produced lytic necrosis of all hepatocytes with stromal collapse. There are only inflammatory cells and proliferating ductules in place of missing hepatocytes (H&E, original magnification ×200).

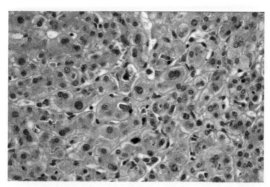

Fig. 5. Cholestasis with mild hepatocellular injury caused by prochlorperazine. There is marked canalicular and hepatocellular bile stasis, and there is variability in the hepatocyte size with many binucleate hepatocytes, indicating regenerative activity (H&E, original magnification ×400).

Acute liver injury may take the form of panacinar degeneration (hepatitis-like), sub-massive or massive necrosis, mononucleosis-like hepatitis, acute combined hepato-cellular/cholestatic injury, acute intrahepatic cholestasis, microvesicular steatosis, vasculitis of the hypersensitivity type, and necrotizing angiitis. Several chronic hepatic lesions can also result, including chronic active hepatitis, chronic intrahepatic cholestasis, macrovesicular steatosis, phospholipidosis, steatohepatitis, granulomatous reactions, fibrosis, cirrhosis, sinusoidal dilatation, peliosis hepatis, veno-occlusive disease, hepatic vein thrombosis, and benign and malignant neoplasms. For any

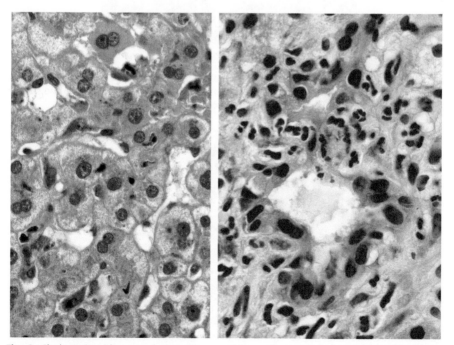

Fig. 6. Cholestasis with acute cholangitis caused by erythromycin hepatotoxicity. The biopsy shows severe canalicular and hepatocellular bile stasis (*left*) with bile duct damage and infiltration by neutrophils (*right*), indicating acute cholangitis (H&E, original magnification ×1000).

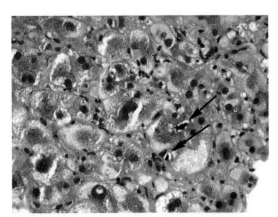

Fig. 7. Combined hepatocellular-cholestatic injury (acute cholestatic hepatitis) caused by carbamazepine. The biopsy shows hepatocellular ballooning and dropout along with prominent intracellular and canalicular bile stasis (*arrows*) (H&E, original magnification ×400).

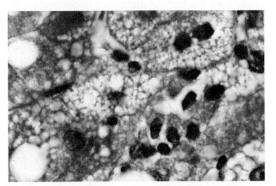

Fig. 8. Microvesicular steatosis caused by valproate hepatotoxicity. The hepatocytes contain numerous, predominantly small, fat vacuoles ranging from barely visible up to the size of the nucleus or larger (H&E, original magnification ×1000).

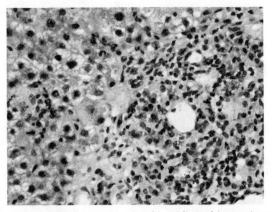

Fig. 9. Chronic autoimmune-like hepatitis, mimicking idiopathic autoimmune hepatitis in a patient on chronic minocycline therapy. The portal tracts have chronic inflammation that contains numerous plasma cells (*right*), and there is periportal interface hepatitis (*center*) (H&E, original magnification ×400).

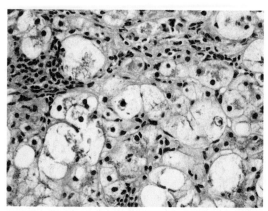

Fig. 10. Steatohepatitis in a patient on chronic tamoxifen therapy to prevent recurrence of breast cancer. There is steatosis with prominent hepatocellular ballooning, Mallory-Denk bodies, mixed lobular inflammation, and pericellular fibrosis, identical to alcoholic hepatitis or metabolic syndrome associated nonalcoholic steatohepatitis. Repeat biopsy 6 months after stopping tamoxifen showed almost complete resolution of the steatohepatitis (H&E, original magnification ×400).

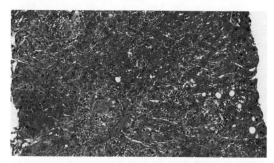

Fig. 11. Granulomatous hepatitis in a patient taking diltiazem. The biopsy shows multiple granulomas composed of epithelioid histiocytes and lymphocytes with a prominent giant cell in the granuloma in the center of the field. Smaller clusters of inflammatory cells are scattered throughout the parenchyma (H&E, original magnification ×200).

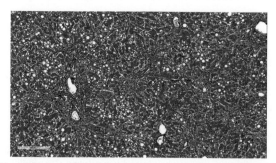

Fig. 12. Hepatic fibrosis associated with long-term methotrexate therapy. In this wedge biopsy, the Masson trichrome stain shows fibrous expansion of the portal tracts with sinusoidal and bridging fibrosis but not yet cirrhosis. The hepatocytes have a mild degree of macrovesicular steatosis, which is also typical of methotrexate (Masson trichrome, ×200).

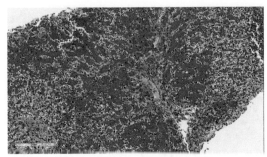

Fig. 13. Sinusoidal obstruction syndrome (veno-occlusive disease) in a patient following chemotherapy and radiation in preparation for bone marrow transplant. This Masson trichrome stain shows a patent central vein in the center of the field; the hepatic sinusoids are massively congested; and there is dropout of centrilobular hepatocytes with replacement by hypertrophied, lipofuscin-laden macrophages (Masson trichrome, ×200).

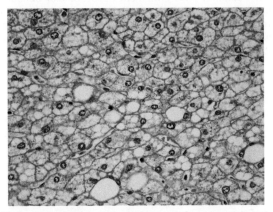

Fig. 14. Hepatocellular adenoma in a long-time user of contraceptive steroids. The tumor consists of a solid growth of large, pale, benign hepatocytes without portal areas or other lobular architecture (H&E, original magnification ×400).

individual drug, one type of injury may be characteristic, but it is almost invariable that other types of injury are seen, frequently for some agents, rarely for others.

REFERENCES

1. Zimmerman HJ. Hepatotoxicity. 2nd edition. Philadelphia: Lippincott Williams & Wilkins; 1999.
2. Lee WM, Senior JR. Recognizing drug-induced liver injury: current problems, possible solutions. Toxicol Pathol 2005;33:155–64.
3. Verma S, Kaplowitz N. Diagnosis, management and prevention of drug-induced liver injury. Gut 2009;58:1555–64.
4. Lewis JH, Kleiner DE. Hepatic injury due to drugs, herbal compounds, chemicals and toxins. In: Burt AD, Portmann BC, Ferrell LD, editors. MacSween's pathology of the liver. 6th edition. Edinburgh (United Kingdom): Churchill Livingstone Elsevier; 2012. p. 645–760.
5. Hoofnagle JH, Serrano J, Knoben JE, et al. LiverTox: a website on drug-induced liver injury. Hepatology 2013;57:873–4.

6. LiverTox Website. Available at: http//www.livertox.nih.gov. Accessed September 25, 2016.
7. Rockey DC, Seeff LB, Rochon J, et al. Causality assessment in drug-induced liver injury using a structured expert opinion process: comparison to the Roussel-Uclaf causality method. Hepatology 2010;51:2117–26.
8. Fontana RJ. Pathogenesis of idiosyncratic drug-induced liver injury and clinical perspectives. Gastroenterology 2014;146:914–28.
9. Lewis JH. Causality assessment: which is best – expert opinion of RUCAM? Clin Liver Dis 2014;4:4–8.
10. Irey NB. Tissue reactions to drugs. Am J Pathol 1976;82:617–48.
11. Irey NB. When is a disease drug-induced?. In: Riddell RH, editor. Pathology of drug-induced and toxic diseases. New York: Churchill-Livingstone; 1982. p. 1–18.
12. Bjönsson ES, Hoofnagle JH. Categorization of drugs implicate in causing liver injury: critical assessment based on published case reports. Hepatology 2016; 63:590–603.

Drug Hepatotoxicity
Environmental Factors

Jonathan G. Stine, MD, MSc[a], Naga P. Chalasani, MD[b],*

KEYWORDS

- Drug-induced liver injury • Liver toxicity • Cirrhosis • Acute liver failure • Alcohol
- Smoking

KEY POINTS

- In general, human data on the environment and drug-induced liver injury (DILI) are sparse and the majority of understanding is derived from animal studies of both intrinsic and idiosyncratic injury.
- Smoking can induce cytochrome P450 (CYP) enzymes but this does not necessarily translate into DILI.
- Alcohol consumption is a clear risk factor for hepatotoxicity from acetaminophen (APAP) and may predispose to injury from antituberculosis (anti-TB) medications but large international registries have not found an association between excessive alcohol consumption and DILI in general.
- Understanding of the role of infection, proinflammatory states, the hepatic clock, environmental pollutants, and the microbiome in predisposing an individual to DILI is still evolving.

INTRODUCTION

It is estimated that more than 1100 drugs or herbal agents are associated with DILI.[1] DILI can present as various forms of both acute and chronic liver disease and, although self-limited in the majority of cases, can have more severe consequences,

Research reported in this publication was supported by the National Institute of Diabetes and Digestive and Kidney Diseases of the National Institutes of Health under award number T32DK007769.
The content is solely the responsibility of the authors and does not necessarily represent the official views of the National Institutes of Health.
Disclosure: Dr N.P. Chalasani serves as a consultant to many pharmaceutical companies for both nonalcoholic steatohepatitis and drug hepatotoxicity, but none of them represents significant and direct conflict with this review article. Dr J.G. Stine has nothing to disclose.
^a Division of Gastroenterology & Hepatology, Department of Medicine, University of Virginia, 1215 Lee Street, PO Box 800708, MSB 2145, Charlottesville, VA 22908, USA; ^b Division of Gastroenterology and Hepatology, Department of Medicine, Indiana University School of Medicine, 702 Rotary Building, Suite 225, Indianapolis, IN 46202, USA
* Corresponding author.
E-mail address: nchalasa@iu.edu

Clin Liver Dis 21 (2017) 103–113
http://dx.doi.org/10.1016/j.cld.2016.08.008
liver.theclinics.com

with approximately a 10% case fatality or transplantation rate within the first 6 months of DILI onset and a 20% rate of progression to chronic liver injury.[2–8] DILI remains the leading cause of acute liver failure (ALF) both in the United States and internationally.[1–3,5,9,10] Geographic variation is common in the most frequently implicated agents[1,9,11] for a variety of reasons, including host and environmental factors, such as xcessive alcohol and tobacco consumption, infection, pro-inflammatory states, and variations in circadian rhythm. Although host factors are much more robustly described across the body of literature, the environment promoting hepatotoxicity is an ever-expanding and in some instances unexplored field. Environmental factors are important considerations for both intrinsic, or dose-dependent DILI, and idiosyncratic DILI (iDILI). Intrinsic DILI, although more rare, occurs in individuals at the same toxic dose threshold.[12,13] iDILI remains more problematic, less understood, and much more dependent on both environmental and genetic covariates to produce a milieu of susceptibility at the individual level. Currently available testing to both predict and diagnose iDILI in premarketing and postmarketing trials is largely ineffective[14] and most cases of iDILI are discovered when medications are prescribed in much greater volume after regulatory approval.[15] This review focuses on the available evidence supporting specific environmental factors (**Box 1**) and their influence on the likelihood and outcomes of DILI.

GEOGRAPHIC VARIATION

The World Health Organization (WHO) initially began the Programme for International Drug Monitoring (PDIM) in 1968 involving 10 countries, a majority of which were in the regions of Europe or North America (including the United States), in a collaborative effort to pool national data from spontaneous adverse event reporting systems.[16] Ultimately, this collaboration led to the creation of VigiBase in the mid-1990s, a database system comprised of more than 7 million individual case safety reports that became accessible for medical research in 2012 and publically searchable in a limited fashion in 2015 (http://www.vigisearch.org).[16] This collaboration has expanded to more than 80 nations and currently includes the regions of Africa, Asia, and Latin America.[16]

In an analysis of VigiBase that spanned data from 2000 to 2009, Agaard and colleagues[17] found geographic variation in both frequency of adverse drug reaction (ADR) reporting as well as the type of medication associated with the ADR. Low-income countries, as defined by the World Bank, were less likely to report ADRs.[17]

Box 1
Environmental risk factors for drug-induced liver injury

Intrinsic
   Circadian rhythm
   Hepatic clock
   Infection
   Inflammation
   Intestinal microbiome

Extrinsic
   Alcohol consumption
   Regional geographic variation
   Smoking
   Socioeconomic status
   Environmental pollution

Low-income countries reported a greater frequency of ADRs with antibiotics and anti-fungal and antiviral medications whereas ADRs were more common for immunomod-ulatory and antineoplastic drugs in high-income nations.[17] The investigators postulated that ADR reporting was more a feature of income rather than actual geog-raphy and highlighted the need to improve ADR reporting rates in low-income nations, in particular African nations that contribute less than 1% of the total individual case safety report volume.[18] Despite this, several important differences between African nations and all other countries in the WHO-PDIM are worth noting. African nations report DILI occurring on average in a younger population (18–44 years of age) compared with 45 to 64 years of age in the rest of the world, and 28% of all ADRs re-ported were attributable to antiviral medications used to treat HIV.[18] Further high-lighting geographic differences in DILI, an analysis of VigiBase by Suzuki and colleagues,[19] limited to the United States, England, and Sweden, found that of the 385 unique medications reported, only 9.7% appeared in all 3 registries. Of the 47 drugs subjected to regulatory action, only 6 were found in all 3 regions.[19] Reports from European centers were also more homogenous compared with reports from the United States.[19] A recent report from a single center in India that does not perform liver transplantation incorporating 303 cases of hepatotoxicity from 1997 to 2008 found that 58% were attributable to tuberculosis agents[10]; strikingly, no cases of APAP toxicity were reported. Despite this, a 17.3% case-fatality rate was reported, owing largely to ALF from anti-TB drugs.[10]

EXCESSIVE ALCOHOL CONSUMPTION

Although excessive alcohol consumption has historically been incorporated into cau-sality assessment, namely that put forth by the Council for International Organizations of Medical Sciences,[12] only a handful of medications have been demonstrated to have increased hepatotoxic potential in the setting of excessive alcohol use, namely APAP, highly active antiretroviral therapy (HAART), halothane, and anti-TB therapy with isoni-azid or methotrexate.[12]

Coined *alcohol-APAP syndrome (AAS)*, the risk of APAP toxicity in the setting of alcohol use has been well described since the 1980s.[20–24] AAS is related to CYP2E1 induction as well as glutathione depletion directly attributable to the toxic ef-fects of alcohol.[22] Concurrent malnutrition can predispose a patient to liver injury in this setting through impaired glucuronidation.[22,25,26]

The chronicity of consumption of alcohol may also a role in hepatotoxicity. In a se-ries of 645 patients with singe-dose APAP toxicity, Schmidt and colleagues[20] found that chronic alcohol abuse was an independent predictor for mortality while controlling for other confounding factors (odds ratio [OR] 3.52; 95% CI, 1.78–6.97), including renal failure, which has previously been implicated in the increased mortality in this patient population.[27] When APAP overdose superimposed on chronic alcohol consumption (defined as >21 drinks per week for men and >14 drinks per week for women) presents with acute renal failure with creatinine greater than 3.0 mg/dL, prothrombin time greater than 100 seconds, and grades III–IV portosystemic encephalopathy, the prog-nosis is uniformly fatal.[27] In a prospective nested case-control study of 150 patients with anti-TB drugs, associated DILI drawn from an overall cohort of 3900 patients exposed to anti-TB drugs, Gaude and colleagues[28] found that 42.2% of DILI cases had significant chronic alcohol consumption and that alcohol abuse was predictive of DILI risk on adjusted multivariable analysis.

On the other hand, acute alcohol ingestion may be protective against hepatotoxic-ity. In animal models, acute alcohol ingestion inhibits CYP2E1 oxidation of APAP, ultimately resulting in a lower level of N-acetyl-p-benzoquinone imine, the reactive metabolite responsible for the known hepatotoxic potential.[29] This has been corroborated in human observational study because acute ingestion of alcohol in alcoholic patients was associated with a profound reduction in risk (OR 0.08; 95% CI, 0.01–0.66) of APAP hepatotoxicity.[20]

Alcohol is also thought to play a role in hepatotoxicity attributed to HAART when used for the treatment of HIV (namely protease inhibitors and non-nucleoside reverse transcriptase inhibitors).[30] Excessive alcohol use may also lead to decreased treatment efficacy and acceleration of HIV to AIDS through changes in CYP2E1 and CYP3A4 activity.[31] This is important to recognize given that approximately one-fourth of patients with newly diagnosed HIV are alcohol dependent.[30] With the widespread use of similar classes of medications to treat chronic hepatitis C virus (HCV) as a part of the new all-oral direct-acting antiviral regimens and the overlap with comorbid polysubstance abuse, including alcohol, it will be interesting to see if alcohol consumption with the direct-acting antivirals predisposes to either hepatotoxicity or loss of treatment effect, because reports of the hepatotoxic potential of these medications have already surfaced.[32] There have been several reports of increased hepatotoxicity with HAART in patients with HIV/HCV coinfection who abuse alcohol.[33,34]

Alcohol abuse in heavy quantities is associated with accelerated fibrosis in patients who are prescribed chronic immunosuppressive therapy with the antimetabolite methotrexate.[35,36] In a meta-analysis of 15 studies, including 636 patients, Whiting-O'Keefe and colleagues[36] found the pooled risk of advanced fibrosis was 17.8% versus 4.5% ($P = .003$) in heavy drinkers, which was defined as greater than or equal to 100 g of alcohol per week. This population also had histologic progression more frequently (73% vs 26%, $P = .002$).[36] In accordance with expert opinion, pretreatment liver biopsy is often considered on an individual basis in patients with a history of heavy alcohol consumption to assess for advanced fibrosis prior to initiation of methotrexate.

Despite the evidence put forth from the aforementioned studies, several large registries have not validated the risk of excessive alcohol consumption and any association with DILI.[5,11,37] A majority of patients in a Spanish registry of 461 subjects with DILI had alcohol consumption less than 40 g/d.

SMOKING

In contrast to the available body of evidence for excessive alcohol and its role in hepatotoxicity development, the literature describing tobacco smoking is much less prevalent and is based solely on observational studies. A Brazilian series of 131 subjects treated with anti-TB drugs found a decreased risk of developing anti-TB DILI in active smokers compared with lifelong nonsmokers (OR 0.28; 95 CI, 0.11–0.64; $P<.01$).[38] Additionally, the investigators found that CYP2E1, despite known to be induced by smoking, was not associated with hepatotoxicity, confirming previous reports.[39,40] CYP1A2 may also be up-regulated by smoking without known clinically relevant hepaotoxicity.[40] A single-center experience in Denmark of 602 patients with APAP toxicity found that 70% were daily tobacco users and this was predictive of severity of injury (diagnosed by significantly higher peak aminotransferase and international normalized ratio levels) as well as all-cause mortality (OR 3.64; 95% CI, 1.23–10.75).[41] On the other hand, Wada and colleagues[42] found that, of the 33 patients in a series of 123 patients with prostate cancer treated with the antiandrogenic drug flutamide, which is metabolized by both CYP1A2 and CYP3A enzymes, smoking was associated with significantly lower odds of hepatotoxicity.

INFECTION AND INFLAMMATION

Infection and inflammation, through innate immune responses to the invasion of the body by foreign agents, including bacteria, viruses, and fungus, may predispose a patient to either intrinsic DILI or iDILI. The risk of intrinsic, or dose-dependent, DILI is due largely to a left shift in the dose-response curve, thereby sensitizing hepatocytes to injury,[43–45] through a complex proinflammatory cascade involving pathogen-associated molecular patterns, damage-associated molecular patterns, Toll-like receptors, Kupffer cells, tumor necrosis factor (TNF)-α, natural killer cells, interferon gamma, polymorphonuclear neutrophils, endothelial cells, prostaglandins, dendritic and stellate cells, and both the coagulation[46] and complement systems, the specifics of which are beyond the scope of this review but have been described in detail by other investigators.[13]

Animal models using both lipopolysaccharide (LPS) and TNF-α exposed mice have found that these models of inflammation predispose to intrinsic DILI from both APAP and trovafloxacin.[43,45] The timing of LPS administration varied in hepatotoxicity risk in APAP animal models, where LPS given 2 hours before APAP had significantly greater risk compared with LPS administration 24 hours prior to APAP.[47] Animal models investigating the exogenous stress of cocaine administration have found that LPS augments the injury from cocaine.[48] Because both TNF-α and LPS are surrogates for circulating endotoxemia, it is surprising that advanced fibrosis and cirrhosis have not been[49] documented to significantly increase the risk of DILI for a large number of medications; however, most medications have not been largely studied in patients with cirrhosis and dose adjustment for cirrhosis is often lacking in the prescribing information, despite changes in both pharmacokinetics and pharmacodynamics in this special population.[49]

Inflammation and infection also seem to play a greater role in iDILI and ultimately hepatic necrosis. Similar to intrinsic DILI, a majority of evidence is afforded from animal models. In the setting of LPS-induced endotoxemia, various medications, such as amiodarone, diclofenac, halothane, ranitidine, sulindac, and trovafloxacin, have been implicated in iDILI.[13,44,50–53] Proinflammatory TNF-α also plays a role in iDILI because blocking TNF-α with pentoxifylline in several of these animal models proved effective in decreasing the severity of liver injury.[44,50] The coagulation system is also activated in periods of acute inflammation and the balance between procoagulation and anticoagulation shifts toward thrombotic risk. LPS administration in animal models has led to increased levels of circulating plasminogen activator inhibitor 1 (PAI-1) and ultimately increased fibrin deposition in experimentally induced iDILI.[54] PAI-1 may also play a role in the mechanism of intrinsic DILI form APAP[46] and has been implicated in other inflammatory processes in the liver (namely nonalcoholic steatohepatitis).[55] Furthermore, anticoagulation with heparin-reduced fibrin deposition and thrombin generation has been shown to lead to an attenuation of the hepatotoxic response,[54] and treatment with tissue plasminogen activator (streptokinase) has been shown to reduce hepatotoxicity through a similar mechanism.[56] Collectively, these animal models suggest that activation of the coagulation cascade leads to fibrin deposition and ultimately tissue hypoxia and worsening cellular death and necrosis, findings that warrant validation in human models where to date, the majority of serum testing has focused on drug-induced ALF and the role of microparticles.[57] These membrane fragments of 0.1 µm to 1.0 µm are derived from systemic inflammation and seem predictive of worse clinical outcomes in ALF, including those cases that are drug-induced.

CIRCADIAN RHYTHM AND THE HEPATIC CLOCK

Circadian time is an important process affecting both the pharmacokinetic as well as the pharmacodynamic properties of drugs across a 24-hour span.[58] This so-called hepatic clock is driven by the central suprachiasmatic nucleus of the hypothalamus, which organizes the majority of circadian change at the cellular level.[59] Fasting-feeding cycles in association with rest-activity rhythms help synchronize the hepatic clock, including the control of xenobiotic detoxification, in effect allowing for the temporal coordination of metabolism.[59,60]

Although the available data are mostly from animal models investigating anti-TB medications and APAP,[58,61–66] there have been extensions in the human population.[67] Through lipid peroxidation inducing mitochondrial toxicity, Souayed and colleagues[58] found that toxic doses of isoniazid in mice at 1 and 9 zeitgeber time produced severe hepatic necrosis whereas dosing at 17 zeitgeber time did not. Deletion of circadian gene Per1 has been shown to change the hepatotoxic risk from alcohol,[62] whereas mPer2 has a role in the diurnal variation of APAP toxicity, both in mice.[64]

Patients taking APAP may also be predisposed due to hepatotoxicity due to 24-hour circadian variation.[59,68] This may be due in part to the normal pattern of intermittent fasting states over a 24-hour period because during times of fasting,[68] glutathione levels are known to drop,[69,70] thus potentially decreasing a protective mechanism that normally prevents toxicity from APAP. Fasting states are also known to disrupt detoxification of anti-TB drugs leading to change in the CYP system, predisposing to liver toxicity.[71,72]

Although recommendations for timing of medication administration or dose reduction based on circadian rhythm and resultant drug metabolism effects is a long way off, these results are nonetheless collectively intriguing. APAP is generally taken during times of illness, namely fever or pain, both of which are associated with fasting states. More prospective study in human based populations is needed.

GUT MICROBIOME

The role of the gut microbiome is also being explored for its potential as a means to protect against APAP-induced and antimicrobial DILI.[73–75] Possamai and colleagues[73] found that when given an intravenous dose of hepatotoxic APAP, the urinary ratio of APAP-sulphate:glucuronide was significantly different when comparing the conventionally housed mice to the germ-free mice because the germ-free mice were found to have higher concentrations; however, interruption of Toll-like receptor 4 signaling was also protective, leading the investigators to conclude that the microbiome itself may play a role but not offer the complete explanation for the observed differences. Xue and colleagues[74] recently published their experience with 3,4-dihydroxyphenylacetic acid, a microbiota-derived metabolite, and its protective role through nuclear factor–erythroid 2–related factor when exposed to toxic levels of APAP, also in mice. Using urinary bile acids as a surrogate for antimicrobial hepatoxicity, Bhowmik and colleagues[75] demonstrated that gut microbiota may play a significant role in bile acid homeostasis and metabolism because germ-free mice had elevated levels of cholic acid and α-muricholic acid/β-muricholic acid, which could predispose to hepatotoxicity in this sterile environment. The authors are unaware of any studies in human models investigated the role of the gut microbiome in predisposing or preventing DILI.

ENVIRONMENTAL POLLUTION

Exposure through an environment rich with pollution can place an individual at risk for hepatotoxicity and although the majority of liver injury is fairly benign with a modest elevation in liver-associated enzymes,[76] rare instances of fatal hepatitis have been reported.[77] In a retrospective case-control study of 247 subjects, D'Andrea and Reddy[76] found significantly elevated liver-associated enzymes in cases of oil spill clean-up workers exposed to potential toxins from the Gulf oil spill along the coast of Louisiana, perhaps directly attributable to benzenes and paraphenols. Exposure to organic pesticides, such as chlorpyrifos, endosulfan, and pyrethroids,[78,79] often through wastewater exposure,[80] has also been associated with hepatotoxicity. The importance of this cannot be understated, because a prospective study by Cecchi and colleagues[81] of 97 women living in the rural Rio Negro province of Argentina found a predominant increase in alanine aminotransferase (ALT) values in the second trimester of pregnancy, with ALT greater than aspartate aminotransferase (AST). These laboratory abnormalities were not predictive, however, of worse maternal-fetal outcomes in the immediate postpartum period as measured by incidence rates of premature birth and miscarriage, and no cases of fatal hepatitis or nonfatal ALF were reported.[81]

SUMMARY

The role of environmental factors in predisposing a patient to both intrinsic DILI and iDILI remains a work in progress. Through the evolution of animal models, the complicated interaction between modifiable risk factors, such as tobacco smoking, excessive alcohol consumption, intestinal microbiome, environmental pollutants, and proinflammatory and/or hypercoagulable states, is only beginning to be understood. Although much research attention remains focused to identifying specific individual risk factors with genome-wide association studies, perhaps more attention should be focused on confirming the environmental observations from these animal models in human-based studies, both on observational and interventional levels. Understanding the environmental risk factors with a goal toward modification and prevention may be fruitful in light of medical treatment of both acute and chronic DILI limited by a lack of specific therapies and antidotes currently available; judicious use of a potentially hepatotoxic drug in a patient with underlying risk factors remains the mainstay of DILI management.

REFERENCES

1. Reuben A, Koch DG, Lee WM. Drug-induced acute liver failure: results of a U.S. multicenter, prospective study. Hepatology 2010;52(6):2065–76.
2. Bjornsson E, Jerlstad P, Bergqvist A, et al. Fulminant drug-induced hepatic failure leading to death or liver transplantation in Sweden. Scand J Gastroenterol 2005; 40(9):1095–101.
3. Chalasani N, Fontana RJ, Bonkovsky HL, et al. Causes, clinical features, and outcomes from a prospective study of drug-induced liver injury in the United States. Gastroenterology 2008;135(6):1924–34.e1921–24.
4. Stine JG, Lewis JH. Drug-induced liver injury: a summary of recent advances. Expert Opin Drug Metab Toxicol 2011;7(7):875–90.
5. Andrade RJ, Lucena MI, Fernandez MC, et al. Drug-induced liver injury: an analysis of 461 incidences submitted to the Spanish registry over a 10-year period. Gastroenterology 2005;129(2):512–21.
6. Chalasani NP, Hayashi PH, Bonkovsky HL, et al. ACG Clinical Guideline: the diagnosis and management of idiosyncratic drug-induced liver injury. Am J Gastroenterol 2014;109(7):950–66 [quiz: 967].
7. Stine JG, Chalasani N. Chronic liver injury induced by drugs: a systematic review. Liver Int 2015;35(11):2343–53.

8. Fontana RJ, Hayashi PH, Gu J, et al. Idiosyncratic drug-induced liver injury is associated with substantial morbidity and mortality within 6 months from onset. Gastroenterology 2014;147(1):96–108.e104.

9. Devarbhavi H, Singh R, Patil M, et al. Outcome and determinants of mortality in 269 patients with combination anti-tuberculosis drug-induced liver injury. J Gastroenterol Hepatol 2013;28(1):161–7.

10. Devarbhavi H, Dierkhising R, Kremers WK, et al. Single-center experience with drug-induced liver injury from India: causes, outcome, prognosis, and predictors of mortality. Am J Gastroenterol 2010;105(11):2396–404.

11. Chalasani N, Bonkovsky HL, Fontana R, et al. Features and outcomes of 889 patients with drug-induced liver injury: the DILIN prospective study. Gastroenterology 2015;48(7):1340–52.e7.

12. Zimmerman HJ. Hepatotoxicity: the adverse effects of drugs and other chemicals on the liver. 2nd edition. Philadelphia: Lippincott-Williams & Wilkins; 1999.

13. Kaplowitz N, DeLeve LD, editors. Drug-induced liver disease. 3rd edition. London: Elsevier/Academic Press; 2013. p. 746.

14. FDA drug stopping rules 2009. Available at: http://www.fda.gov/downloads/Drugs/.../Guidances/UCM174090.pdf. Accessed April 11, 2016.

15. Lewis JH. The art and science of diagnosing and managing drug-induced liver injury in 2015 and beyond. Clin Gastroenterol Hepatol 2015;13(12):2173–89.e8.

16. Lindquist M. VigiBase, the WHO global ICSR database system: basic facts. Drug Inform J 2007;42:409–19.

17. Aagaard L, Strandell J, Melskens L, et al. Global patterns of adverse drug reactions over a decade: analyses of spontaneous reports to VigiBase. Drug Saf 2012;35(12):1171–82.

18. Ampadu HH, Hoekman J, de Bruin ML, et al. Adverse drug reaction reporting in Africa and a comparison of individual case safety report characteristics between Africa and the rest of the world: analyses of spontaneous reports in vigiBase((R)). Drug Saf 2016;39(4):335–45.

19. Suzuki A, Andrade RJ, Bjornsson E, et al. Drugs associated with hepatotoxicity and their reporting frequency of liver adverse events in VigiBase: unified list based on international collaborative work. Drug Saf 2010;33(6):503–22.

20. Schmidt LE, Dalhoff K, Poulsen HE. Acute versus chronic alcohol consumption in acetaminophen-induced hepatotoxicity. Hepatology 2002;35(4):876–82.

21. Maddrey WC. Hepatic effects of acetaminophen. Enhanced toxicity in alcoholics. J Clin Gastroenterol 1987;9(2):180–5.

22. Zimmerman HJ, Maddrey WC. Acetaminophen (paracetamol) hepatotoxicity with regular intake of alcohol: analysis of instances of therapeutic misadventure. Hepatology 1995;22(3):767–73.

23. Draganov P, Durrence H, Cox C, et al. Alcohol-acetaminophen syndrome. Even moderate social drinkers are at risk. Postgrad Med 2000;107(1):189–95.

24. Seeff LB, Cuccherini BA, Zimmerman HJ, et al. Acetaminophen hepatotoxicity in alcoholics. A therapeutic misadventure. Ann Intern Med 1986;104(3):399–404.

25. Lauterburg BH, Davies S, Mitchell JR. Ethanol suppresses hepatic glutathione synthesis in rats in vivo. J Pharmacol Exp Ther 1984;230(1):7–11.

26. Lauterburg BH, Velez ME. Glutathione deficiency in alcoholics: risk factor for paracetamol hepatotoxicity. Gut 1988;29(9):1153–7.

27. Bray GP, Mowat C, Muir DF, et al. The effect of chronic alcohol intake on prognosis and outcome in paracetamol overdose. Hum Exp Toxicol 1991;10(6):435–8.

28. Gaude GS, Chaudhury A, Hattiholi J. Drug-induced hepatitis and the risk factors for liver injury in pulmonary tuberculosis patients. J Family Med Prim Care 2015; 4(2):238–43.

29. Altomare E, Leo MA, Lieber CS. Interaction of acute ethanol administration with acetaminophen metabolism and toxicity in rats fed alcohol chronically. Alcohol Clin Exp Res 1984;8(4):405–8.

30. Barve S, Kapoor R, Moghe A, et al. Focus on the liver: alcohol use, highly active antiretroviral therapy, and liver disease in HIV-infected patients. Alcohol Res Health 2010;33(3):229–36.

31. Kumar S, Jin M, Ande A, et al. Alcohol consumption effect on antiretroviral therapy and HIV-1 pathogenesis: role of cytochrome P450 isozymes. Expert Opin Drug Metab Toxicol 2012;8(11):1363–75.

32. Stine JG, Intagliata N, Shah NL, et al. Hepatic decompensation likely attributable to simeprevir in patients with advanced cirrhosis. Dig Dis Sci 2015;60(4):1031–5.

33. Pol S, Lamorthe B, Thi NT, et al. Retrospective analysis of the impact of HIV infection and alcohol use on chronic hepatitis C in a large cohort of drug users. J Hepatol 1998;28(6):945–50.

34. Wit FW, Weverling GJ, Weel J, et al. Incidence of and risk factors for severe hepatotoxicity associated with antiretroviral combination therapy. J Infect Dis 2002; 186(1):23–31.

35. Malatjalian DA, Ross JB, Williams CN, et al. Methotrexate hepatotoxicity in psoriatics: report of 104 patients from Nova Scotia, with analysis of risks from obesity, diabetes and alcohol consumption during long term follow-up. Can J Gastroenterol 1996;10(6):369–75.

36. Whiting-O'Keefe QE, Fye KH, Sack KD. Methotrexate and histologic hepatic abnormalities: a meta-analysis. Am J Med 1991;90(6):711–6.

37. Andrade RJ, Lucena MI, Kaplowitz N, et al. Outcome of acute idiosyncratic drug-induced liver injury: long-term follow-up in a hepatotoxicity registry. Hepatology 2006;44(6):1581–8.

38. Zaverucha-do-Valle C, Monteiro SP, El-Jaick KB, et al. The role of cigarette smoking and liver enzymes polymorphisms in anti-tuberculosis drug-induced hepatotoxicity in Brazilian patients. Tuberculosis (Edinb) 2014;94(3):299–305.

39. Czekaj P, Wiaderkiewicz A, Florek E, et al. Tobacco smoke-dependent changes in cytochrome P450 1A1, 1A2, and 2E1 protein expressions in fetuses, newborns, pregnant rats, and human placenta. Arch Toxicol 2005;79(1):13–24.

40. Hoofnagle JH. Drug-induced liver injury network (DILIN). Hepatology 2004;40(4): 773.

41. Schmidt LE, Dalhoff K. The impact of current tobacco use on the outcome of paracetamol poisoning. Aliment Pharmacol Ther 2003;18(10):979–85.

42. Wada T, Ueda M, Abe K, et al. Risk factor of liver disorders caused by flutamide–statistical analysis using multivariate logistic regression analysis. Hinyokika Kiyo 1999;45(8):521–6 [in Japanese].

43. Liguori MJ, Ditewig AC, Maddox JF, et al. Comparison of TNFalpha to lipopolysaccharide as an inflammagen to characterize the idiosyncratic hepatotoxicity potential of drugs: trovafloxacin as an example. Int J Mol Sci 2010;11(11): 4697–714.

44. Shaw PJ, Ganey PE, Roth RA. Idiosyncratic drug-induced liver injury and the role of inflammatory stress with an emphasis on an animal model of trovafloxacin hepatotoxicity. Toxicol Sci 2010;118(1):7–18.

45. Maddox JF, Amuzie CJ, Li M, et al. Bacterial- and viral-induced inflammation increases sensitivity to acetaminophen hepatotoxicity. J Toxicol Environ Health A 2010;73(1):58–73.

46. Ganey PE, Luyendyk JP, Newport SW, et al. Role of the coagulation system in acetaminophen-induced hepatotoxicity in mice. Hepatology 2007;46(4):1177–86.

47. Liu J, Sendelbach LE, Parkinson A, et al. Endotoxin pretreatment protects against the hepatotoxicity of acetaminophen and carbon tetrachloride: role of cytochrome P450 suppression. Toxicology 2000;147(3):167–76.

48. Labib R, Turkall R, Abdel-Rahman MS. Endotoxin potentiates the hepatotoxicity of cocaine in male mice. J Toxicol Environ Health A 2002;65(14):977–93.

49. Lewis JH, Stine JG. Review article: prescribing medications in patients with cirrhosis - a practical guide. Aliment Pharmacol Ther 2013;37(12):1132–56.

50. Lu J, Jones AD, Harkema JR, et al. Amiodarone exposure during modest inflammation induces idiosyncrasy-like liver injury in rats: role of tumor necrosis factor-alpha. Toxicol Sci 2012;125(1):126–33.

51. Zou W, Beggs KM, Sparkenbaugh EM, et al. Sulindac metabolism and synergy with tumor necrosis factor-alpha in a drug-inflammation interaction model of idiosyncratic liver injury. J Pharmacol Exp Ther 2009;331(1):114–21.

52. Tukov FF, Luyendyk JP, Ganey PE, et al. The role of tumor necrosis factor alpha in lipopolysaccharide/ranitidine-induced inflammatory liver injury. Toxicol Sci 2007; 100(1):267–80.

53. Cheng L, You Q, Yin H, et al. Effect of polyI: C cotreatment on halothane-induced liver injury in mice. Hepatology 2009;49(1):215–26.

54. Shaw PJ, Fullerton AM, Scott MA, et al. The role of the hemostatic system in murine liver injury induced by coexposure to lipopolysaccharide and trovafloxacin, a drug with idiosyncratic liability. Toxicol Appl Pharmacol 2009;236(3):293–300.

55. Verrijken A, Francque S, Mertens I, et al. Prothrombotic factors in histologically proven NAFLD and NASH. Hepatology 2014;59(1):121–9.

56. Luyendyk JP, Maddox JF, Green CD, et al. Role of hepatic fibrin in idiosyncrasy-like liver injury from lipopolysaccharide-ranitidine coexposure in rats. Hepatology 2004;40(6):1342–51.

57. Stravitz RT, Bowling R, Bradford RL, et al. Role of procoagulant microparticles in mediating complications and outcome of acute liver injury/acute liver failure. Hepatology 2013;58(1):304–13.

58. Souayed N, Chennoufi M, Boughattas F, et al. Circadian variation in murine hepatotoxicity to the antituberculosis agent <<Isoniazide>>. Chronobiol Int 2015; 32(9):1201–10.

59. Levi F, Schibler U. Circadian rhythms: mechanisms and therapeutic implications. Annu Rev Pharmacol Toxicol 2007;47:593–628.

60. DeBruyne JP, Weaver DR, Dallmann R. The hepatic circadian clock modulates xenobiotic metabolism in mice. J Biol Rhythms 2014;29(4):277–87.

61. Johnson BP, Walisser JA, Liu Y, et al. Hepatocyte circadian clock controls acetaminophen bioactivation through NADPH-cytochrome P450 oxidoreductase. Proc Natl Acad Sci U S A 2014;111(52):18757–62.

62. Wang T, Yang P, Zhan Y, et al. Deletion of circadian gene Per1 alleviates acute ethanol-induced hepatotoxicity in mice. Toxicology 2013;314(2–3):193–201.

63. Xu YQ, Zhang D, Jin T, et al. Diurnal variation of hepatic antioxidant gene expression in mice. PLoS One 2012;7(8):e44237.

64. Kakan X, Chen P, Zhang J. Clock gene mPer2 functions in diurnal variation of acetaminophen induced hepatotoxicity in mice. Exp Toxicol Pathol 2011;63(6): 581–5.

65. Boorman GA, Blackshear PE, Parker JS, et al. Hepatic gene expression changes throughout the day in the Fischer rat: implications for toxicogenomic experiments. Toxicol Sci 2005;86(1):185–93.
66. Bruckner JV, Ramanathan R, Lee KM, et al. Mechanisms of circadian rhythmicity of carbon tetrachloride hepatotoxicity. J Pharmacol Exp Ther 2002;300(1): 273–81.
67. Ngong JM, Waring RH. Circadian rhythms of paracetamol metabolism in healthy subjects; a preliminary report. Drug Metabol Drug Interact 1994; 11(4):317–30.
68. Schnell RC, Bozigian HP, Davies MH, et al. Circadian rhythm in acetaminophen toxicity: role of nonprotein sulfhydryls. Toxicol Appl Pharmacol 1983;71(3): 353–61.
69. Howell SR, Klaassen C. Circadian variation of hepatic UDP-glucuronic acid and the glucuronidation of xenobiotics in mice. Toxicol Lett 1991;57(1):73–9.
70. Martensson J. The effect of fasting on leukocyte and plasma glutathione and sulfur amino acid concentrations. Metabolism 1986;35(2):118–21.
71. Walter-Sack I, Klotz U. Influence of diet and nutritional status on drug metabolism. Clin Pharmacokinet 1996;31(1):47–64.
72. Buchanan N, Eyberg C, Davis MD. Isoniazid pharmacokinetics in kwashiorkor. S Afr Med J 1979;56(8):299–300.
73. Possamai LA, McPhail MJ, Khamri W, et al. The role of intestinal microbiota in murine models of acetaminophen-induced hepatotoxicity. Liver Int 2015;35(3): 764–73.
74. Xue H, Xie W, Jiang Z, et al. 3,4-Dihydroxyphenylacetic acid, a microbiota-derived metabolite of quercetin, attenuates acetaminophen (APAP)-induced liver injury through activation of Nrf-2. Xenobiotica 2016;46(10):1–9.
75. Bhowmik SK, An JH, Lee SH, et al. Alteration of bile acid metabolism in pseudo germ-free rats [corrected]. Arch Pharm Res 2012;35(11):1969–77.
76. D'Andrea MA, Reddy GK. Health consequences among subjects involved in Gulf oil spill clean-up activities. Am J Med 2013;126(11):966–74.
77. Payan-Renteria R, Garibay-Chavez G, Rangel-Ascencio R, et al. Effect of chronic pesticide exposure in farm workers of a Mexico community. Arch Environ Occup Health 2012;67(1):22–30.
78. Hodgson E, Rose RL. Organophosphorus chemicals: potent inhibitors of the human metabolism of steroid hormones and xenobiotics. Drug Metab Rev 2006; 38(1–2):149–62.
79. Hodgson E, Rose RL. Human metabolic interactions of environmental chemicals. J Biochem Mol Toxicol 2007;21(4):182–6.
80. Gao H, Liu Y, Guan W, et al. Hepatotoxicity and nephrotoxicity of organic contaminants in wastewater-irrigated soil. Environ Sci Pollut Res Int 2015;22(5): 3748–55.
81. Cecchi A, Rovedatti MG, Sabino G, et al. Environmental exposure to organophosphate pesticides: assessment of endocrine disruption and hepatotoxicity in pregnant women. Ecotoxicol Environ Saf 2012;80:280–7.

Drug Hepatotoxicity
Newer Agents

Chalermrat Bunchorntavakul, MD[a,b], K. Rajender Reddy, MD[c],*

KEYWORDS

- Drug-induced liver injury • Hepatotoxicity • Antibiotics • Antiretrovirals
- Tyrosine kinase inhibitors • Monoclonal antibodies • Anticoagulants • Antiplatelet

KEY POINTS

- Idiosyncratic hepatotoxicity is one of the most common reasons for an already approved drug being restricted or withdrawn.
- The incidence of clinically relevant hepatotoxicity from newer agents seems lower than that from older agents.
- Cases of severe hepatotoxicity have been reported and attributable to some of these newer agents, such as trastuzumab, ipilimumab, infliximab, imatinib, bosutinib, dasatinib, gefitinib, erlotinib, sunitinib, pazopanib, ponatinib, regorafenib, lapatinib, vemurafenib, crizotinib, dabigatran, rivaroxaban, clopidogrel, felbamate, lamotrigine, levetiracetam, venlafaxine, duloxetine, sertraline, darunavir, and maraviroc.

INTRODUCTION

Over the past decade, the dramatic growth in the number of new prescriptions and over-the-counter drugs has greatly improved the therapeutic armamentarium but at the expense of an increased risk of adverse drug events, in particular hepatotoxicity. Although uncommon, drug hepatotoxicity is increasingly seen in clinical practice and carries significant morbidity and mortality; approximately 30% of drug hepatotoxicity exhibit jaundice and it is one of the leading causes of acute liver failure (ALF) in the United States.[1] In addition, idiosyncratic hepatotoxicity is one of the most common reasons for an investigational drug not coming into the market and is the most common reason for an already approved drug being restricted or withdrawn. If significant liver injury is recognized during drug development, the drug would never be released into

Conflict of Interest: The authors have nothing to disclose.
[a] Division of Gastroenterology and Hepatology, Department of Medicine, University of Pennsylvania, 2 Dulles, 3400 Spruce Street, HUP, Philadelphia, PA 19104, USA; [b] Division of Gastroenterology and Hepatology, Department of Medicine, Rajavithi Hospital, College of Medicine, Rangsit University, Rajavithi Road, Ratchathewi, Bangkok 10400, Thailand; [c] Liver Transplantation, Viral Hepatitis Center, University of Pennsylvania, 2 Dulles, 3400 Spruce Street, HUP, Liver Transplant Office, Philadelphia, PA 19104, USA
* Corresponding author.
E-mail address: rajender.reddy@uphs.upenn.edu

Clin Liver Dis 21 (2017) 115–134
http://dx.doi.org/10.1016/j.cld.2016.08.009
1089-3261/17/© 2016 Elsevier Inc. All rights reserved.

liver.theclinics.com

the market. For drugs with lower incidence of hepatotoxicity, however, liver injury is often first recognized after approval. Unfortunately, the systematic data on hepatotoxicity of newer agents are not often easily accessible, mainly due to a limited number of cases. By using available data on PubMed and the LiverTox Web site (http://livertox. nlm.nih.gov),[2] this article focuses on hepatotoxicity of select agents that have been recently introduced into the clinical arena, such as tyrosine kinase inhibitors (TKIs), monoclonal antibodies (MABs), novel or non–vitamin K oral anticoagulants (NOACs), newer antiplatelet agents, antidiabetic agents, antiepileptic drugs (AEDs), antidepressants, antipsychotics, and antiretrovirals (ARVs). In addition, hepatotoxicity due to select antibiotics commonly used in clinical practice, including amoxicillin/clavulanate, azithromycin, cefazolin, and quinolones, also is reviewed because they were frequently implicated in hepatotoxicity by the US Drug-Induced Liver Injury (DILI) Network.[1]

ANTIBIOTICS
Amoxicillin/Clavulanate

Amoxicillin/clavulanate is currently the most commonly documented cause of nonacetaminophen DILI in the United States (91 of 899 cases)[1] and Spain (59 of 461 cases).[3] The incidence of hepatotoxicity is estimated to be 1.7 to 4 of 10,000 prescriptions.[2,4–6] The mechanism of hepatotoxicity is unclear but is probably immunoallergic in origin. Certain HLA haplotypes, especially HLA class II SNP rs9274407, have been associated with amoxicillin/clavulanate hepatotoxicity, particularly in those patients who exhibit immunoallergic features.[7] The hepatotoxicity is idiosyncratic and thought primarily related to the clavulanate component, because the combination is more often associated with hepatotoxicity than amoxicillin alone.[4,6] Unlike many other DILIs, where women are at higher risk, risk factors of amoxicillin/clavulanate hepatotoxicity include older age, male gender, longer duration of exposure, and repeated courses of therapy.[4,8–10]

The mean onset of jaundice has been 16 to 37 days after the start of therapy, but a delay of up to 6 to 8 weeks has been reported (jaundice occurred after cessation of therapy in up to 50% of cases in some series).[8,11–13] Hypersensitivity features (eg, rash, fever, arthralgia, and eosinophilia) occurred in 40% to 60% of cases,[8,11] whereas interstitial nephritis and sialadenitis developed in some cases.[14] Patterns of hepatotoxicity can be either hepatocellular (approximately one-third), cholestatic (approximately one-third), or mixed injury (approximately one-third),[8,11] although case series from Belgium and France reported that cholestatic injury was the most common pattern (66%–74%).[12,13] A prospective series of amoxicillin/clavulanate hepatotoxicity from Spain reported that age was the most important determinant in the biochemical manifestation of hepatotoxicity; younger age was associated with hepatocellular injury and shorter treatment duration, whereas cholestatic/mixed injury was related to older age and prolonged amoxicillin/clavulanate therapy.[8] Typical histologic features were centrilobular cholestasis with a mixed portal inflammatory infiltrate, variable portal edema, and interlobular bile duct injury with bile duct proliferation.[6,14] In addition, granulomatous hepatitis has also been reported.[13,15] Recovery usually occurs within 1 to 4 months after cessation of therapy, although poor outcomes, including death, liver transplantation (LT), and chronic liver damage, have been reported in 9% of cases.[8]

Cephalosporins

Cephalosporins are rarely associated with DILI and cefazolin seemed the most common implicated agent in this group (ranking 6 among all drugs in the US DILI Network).[1,16]

Cefazolin hepatotoxicity can develop after a single intravenous dose. It is characterized by a latency period of 1 to 3 weeks after exposure, cholestatic or mixed biochemical patterns, hypersensitivity features in approximately 25%, and a self-limited moderate to severe clinical course.[16] Other cephalosporins can cause a similar pattern of hepatotoxicity but can be more severe; 2 deaths from liver failure were observed in the US DILI Network.[1,16] In addition, ceftriaxone can be associated with formation of biliary sludge and jaundice, which is mostly seen in children but also reported in adults.[6,17,18]

Azithromycin

Similar to other macrolides, azithromycin has been linked to hepatotoxicity. Transient and asymptomatic elevation in serum alanine aminotransferases (ALTs) occur in 1% to 2% of patients treated by azithromycin for short periods, with similar rates also in a comparator arm in a clinical trial.[19] Rarely, cholestatic injury has occurred and was often associated with longer duration of therapy.[20–22] A case series of azithromycin hepatotoxicity in the US DILI Network (18 of 899 cases) reported that the patterns of hepatotoxicity were hepatocellular in 10 patients, cholestatic in 6 patients, and mixed in 2 patients, with clinical onset 1 to 3 weeks after azithromycin initiation.[23] Hypersensitivity features were common whereas previously this was considered unusual with macrolides. Severe cutaneous reactions that included Stevens-Johnson syndrome (SJS) and toxic epidermal necrolysis developed in 2 young women who had azithromycin hepatotoxicity.[23] Most patients recovered fully, but vanishing bile duct syndrome developed in 4 patients, and death or LT occurred in 2 patients who had underlying chronic liver disease.[23]

Quinolones

Although hepatotoxicity from quinolones is rare, with an estimated incidence of 1:100,000 persons exposed,[24] cases of quinolone hepatotoxicity have been increasingly seen, probably due to their wide use in clinical practice. Ciprofloxacin and levofloxacin were the eighth and ninth most common causes of DILI, respectively, in the US DILI Network.[1] All available quinolones have been implicated in causing hepatotoxicity included the first-generation agent, nalidixic acid; the second-generation drugs, norfloxacin, ciprofloxacin, and ofloxacin; and the third-generation products, levofloxacin, moxifloxacin, and gatifloxacin.[1,6,25] Quinolone hepatotoxicity seems to be a class effect in which the clinical presentation and phenotype of injury are similar among the different agents. It is likely an immunoallergic reaction and the predominant feature is hepatocellular injury with a short latency period (median 2–9 days).[26] Hypersensitivity features were present in approximately 60% of cases.[26] A majority of cases resolved after treatment discontinuation, but liver failure developed in up to 25%. Patients with mixed injury tended to have mild reversible disease without jaundice.[26] Prolonged cholestasis leading to vanishing bile duct syndrome has been reported after toxicity from ciprofloxacin.[26,27] Granulomatous hepatitis has been described with norfloxacin.[28]

Newer Antiretrovirals

Hepatotoxicity is a well-known side effect of ARVs, which can be explained by several mechanisms, such as hypersensitivity reactions (eg, abacavir, nevirapine, and fosamprenavir), mitochondrial toxicity (eg, stavudine and didanosine), steatosis (almost all ritonavir-boosted protease inhibitors [PIs]), direct hepatotoxicity (eg, efavirenz, nevirapine, and tipranavir), and immune reconstitution (potentially all ARVs), with an increased risk in patients coinfected with viral hepatitis.[29,30] Since 2007, several ARVs with novel mechanisms of action (HIV integrase inhibitors and C-C chemokine receptor type 5

(CCR5) coreceptor inhibitors) and newer ARVs from previously recognized therapeutic classes have been released into the market and seem to be associated with a lower rate of hepatotoxicity (**Table 1**).[29] Nevertheless, 2 of the newer ARVs, darunavir and maraviroc, have a warning issued concerning hepatotoxicity after their release.

Etravirine and rilpivirine, non-nucleoside reverse transcriptase inhibitors (NNRTIs), have been noted to have low incidence of hepatotoxicity in clinical trials, with higher incidence in hepatitis B virus (HBV)/HIV, hepatitis C virus (HCV)/HIV coinfected patients compared with HIV monoinfected patients.[31–33] Nevertheless, a case of severe hepatitis with hypersensitivity reaction associated with rilpivirine has been reported.[34] This hepatic hypersensitivity reaction, including fatal ALF, is a known complication of nevirapine, the first-generation NNRTIs.[29] Darunavir, the latest PI on the market, has been associated with some degree of hepatotoxicity. In clinical trials, ALT elevations greater than 5 times upper limit of normal (ULN) were seen in 7% to 11% of patients, which were similar to the comparator group (lopinavir).[29,35] These elevations were often asymptomatic and self-limited and resolved even with continuation of the medication.[2,29,35] Several reports of severe to fatal hepatotoxicity in patients treated with darunavir, however, in conjunction with other ARVs, have been published. The pattern of darunavir hepatotoxicity was often hepatocellular, arising after 1 to 8 weeks of therapy, and hypersensitivity features were rare.[2,29,36] Maraviroc, the only agent in the class of CCR5 antagonists, is extensively metabolized in the liver via the cytochrome P450 (CYP) system and is a substrate for P-glycoprotein (P-gp), making it susceptible to multiple drug interactions.[29] It was associated with low incidence of significant hepatotoxicity in clinical trials.[37,38] Few cases of hepatotoxicity, however, including ALF, have been reported in patients receiving maraviroc while they were receiving other medications.[2,29,39] Raltegravir, the first-in-class integrase inhibitor, was associated with ALT elevations greater than 5 times the ULN in approximately 4% and 14% of HIV monoinfected and HBV/HIV, HCV/HIV coinfected patients, respectively, in clinical

Table 1
Hepatotoxicity of newer antiretrovirals

Agents	Drug Class	Incidence of Serum Alanine Aminotransferase Elevation Grade 3/4 in Randomized Controlled Trials	Pattern of Hepatotoxicity	Food and Drug Administration Warning Regarding Hepatotoxicity
Etravirine	NNRTI	4% (2% in controls)	Hepatitis	No
Rilpivirine	NNRTI	1%–2% (2%–4% in controls)	Hepatitis, hypersensitivity reaction	No
Darunavir	PI	7%–11% (9%–12% in controls)	Hepatitis, ALF	Yes
Maraviroc	CCR5 antagonist (entry inhibitor)	3%–4% (3%–4% in controls)	Hepatitis, ALF	Yes
Raltegravir	Integrase inhibitor	2%–4% (2%–3% in controls)	Hepatitis, hypersensitivity reaction	No
Elvitegravir	Integrase inhibitor	2%–15% (5%–34% in controls)	Hepatitis	No
Dolutegravir	Integrase inhibitor	2%–3% (2% in controls)	Hepatitis	No

trials.[40–42] To date, there have been no published reports of severe hepatotoxicity attributed to raltegravir.[2,29,42] Nevertheless, raltegravir has been linked to instances of SJS and drug rash with eosinophilia and systemic symptoms (DRESS) syndrome, which can be accompanied by liver involvement.[2,29] In clinical trials, ALT elevations greater than 5 times the ULN occurred in 2% to 15% of patients treated with cobicistat-boosted elvitegravir combined with emtricitabine and tenofovir, which were similar or slightly lower than what occurred in comparator groups (efavirenz, raltegravir, or ritonavir-boosted atazanavir).[2,29,43] There is no information on cross-sensitivity for hepatic injury between elvitegravir and raltegravir, although cross-reactivity is likely to occur.[2,29,43] Dolutegravir, the more recent once-daily integrase inhibitor without booster, has shown a very low incidence of significant ALT elevation (<1%) in a phase III study.[44]

MOLECULAR TARGETED THERAPY
Tyrosine Kinase Inhibitors

Hepatotoxicity was one of the serious class-related safety issues signaled in preapproval stages with TKIs and is now increasingly being reported after their broader use in clinical oncology. Many TKIs had adequate data on hepatotoxicity, such as with the use of lapatinib, pazopanib, ponatinib, regorafenib, and sunitinib, and as such necessitated a boxed label warning.[45] In clinical trials, hepatocellular injury, characterized by abnormal transaminases, during treatment with TKIs is common and occurred in 23% to 50% of patients, which were mostly transient, and mostly resolved without treatment discontinuation, whereas approximately 2% to 5% of patients developed high-grade ALT elevation with or without jaundice.[45,46] In addition, severe hepatotoxicity during TKIs treatment has been reported after the use of imatinib,[47] bosutinib,[48,49] nilotinib,[50] dasatinib,[51] gefitinib,[52,53] erlotinib,[54,55] sorafenib,[56,57] sunitinib,[58] pazopanib,[59,60] ponatinib,[61] regorafenib,[46] lapatinib,[62,63] vemurafenib,[64] crizotinib, cabozantinib, vandetanib, and axitinib (**Table 2**).[45,46] Latency period after starting therapy to onset of ALT elevation has been 2 to 8 weeks in most cases but may be delayed in some patients receiving imatinib, pazopanib, and sunitinib.[45]

Mechanisms of TKI hepatotoxicity involve the formation of a reactive intermediate through metabolism via CYP pathway, accompanied by immune-mediated injury, disruption of hepatic bile acid transport, and mitochondrial dysfunction.[45,65] Hepatocellular necrosis with or without lymphocyte infiltration is the most common histologic finding in TKI-induced hepatotoxicity.[45,65] In addition, certain TKIs, such as erlotinib, nilotinib, pazopanib, sorafenib, and regorafenib, can inhibit UDP glucuronosyltransferase isoform 1A1 (UGT1A1), causing mild unconjugated hyperbilirubinemia, which is often clinically irrelevant.[45,50] Furthermore, caution should be exercised when using acetaminophen in cancer patients receiving imatinib, sunatinib, and the aforementioned TKIs, because reduced activity of UGT1A1 pathway may potentiate acetaminophen hepatotoxicity by enhancing production of the toxic metabolite through the CYP2E1 pathway.[45,66] Treatment with TKIs requires periodic transaminase monitoring and with treatment interruption/discontinuation for specified threshold elevations of ALT. Reinitiation of treatment or switching TKIs (available evidence suggests that there is no cross-reactivity between different TKIs even with the same tyrosine kinase target) may be feasible when liver injury resolves.[45]

Monoclonal Antibodies

MABs comprise a class of therapeutic biologics that has been increasingly used over the past decades for various indications, mainly cancer and autoimmune disorders.

Table 2
Hepatotoxicity due to tyrosine kinase inhibitors

Agents	Main Indications	Rates of Serum Alanine Aminotransferase Elevation Grade 3/4 (All Grades), %	Latency Period	Cases of Severe Hepatotoxicity (Death)	On-Treatment Liver Functions Monitoring Recommended
Imatinib[47]	CML, ALL, MDS, HES, GIST	3–6 (6–12)	2–20 wk	Yes (yes)	Yes
Bosutinib[48,49]	CML	4–9 (20)	Median 4 wk	Yes (no)	Yes
Ponatinib[61]	CML, ALL	8 (56)	Median 6 wk (1–40)	Yes (yes)	Yes
Nilotinib[50]	CML	1–4 (35–62)	NA	Yes (no)	Yes
Dasatinib[51]	CML, ALL	4–7 (50)	Median 8–12 wk	No (no)	No
Gefitinib[52,53]	NSCLC	2–4 (10–24)	Within 8 wk	Yes (no)	Yes
Erlotinib[54,55]	NSCLC, pancreatic CA	10–14 (35–45)	Within 2–4 wk	Yes (no)	Yes
Crizotinib	NSCLC	6 (57)	Within 8 wk	Yes (yes)	Yes
Lapatinib[62,63]	Breast CA	2–6 (37–53)	Median 7 wk (1–12)	Yes (yes)	Yes
Sorafenib[56,57]	HCC, RCC	2 (21–25)	Median 2 wk	No (no)	No
Sunitinib[58]	GIST, RCC, PNET	3 (40–60)	4–9 wk	Yes (yes)	Yes
Axitinib	RCC	<1 (22)	NA	No (no)	Yes
Pazopanib[59,60]	RCC, soft tissue sarcoma	12 (46–53)	Median 4 wk (1–18)	Yes (yes)	Yes
Cabozantinib	Medullary thyroid CA	3–6 (86)	NA	No (no)	No
Vandetanib	Medullary thyroid CA	2 (51)	NA	No (no)	No
Regorafenib[46]	Colorectal CA	6 (45–65)	2–6 wk	Yes (yes)	Yes
Vemurafenib	Melanoma	3 (35–38)	Median 3–6 wk	Yes (no)	Yes

Abbreviations: ALL, acute myeloid leukemia; CA, cancer; CML, chronic myeloid leukemia; GIST, gastrointestinal stromal tumor; HCC, hepatocellular carcinoma; HES, hypereosinophilic syndrome; MDS, myelodysplastic syndrome; NSCLC, non–small cell lung cancer; PNET, pancreatic neuroendocrine tumor; RCC, renal cell carcinoma.

Adapted from Shah RR, Morganroth J, Shah DR. Hepatotoxicity of tyrosine kinase inhibitors: clinical and regulatory perspectives. Drug Saf 2013;36(7):495–6; with permission.

The nomenclature of MABs is based on how they are derived and it includes mouse (-omab), chimeric (-ximab), humanized (-zumab), or fully human (-umab) sources. Among more than 45 currently approved MABs, only a few have been linked to hepatotoxicity and, in many instances, the cause of hepatic event is unclear (**Table 3**).[2] Bevacizumab, a MAB targeted against vascular endothelial growth factor, has not been clearly associated with significant hepatotoxicity in clinical trials and postmarketing reports.[2,67] In contrast, several studies have suggested the protective effect (antiangiogenesis) of bevacizumab against sinusoidal damage induced by other chemotherapeutic agents.[67–69] Trastuzumab, a MAB targeted against epidermal growth factor receptor HER-2, has been implicated in hepatotoxicity in several isolated case reports.[2,70–72] The pattern of hepatotoxicity is often hepatocellular, occurring after 1 to 8 cycles of trastuzumab.[2,70–72] Trastuzumab emtansine, a HER-2 (human epidermal growth factor receptor 2) MAB with cytotoxic activity of the microtubule-inhibitory agent DM1, has more potential for hepatotoxicity (17%–22%) than trastuzumab (1%–12%) in clinical trials.[72–74] Fatal ALF and nodular regenerative hyperplasia have also been reported with trastuzumab emtansine.[74–76]

Ipilimumab, a MAB targeted against cytotoxic T lymphocyte–associated antigen 4 (CTLA-4), was associated with ALT elevation in 3% to 9% of patients (0.5%–1.5% grade 3/4) during treatment, but most were self-limited and resolved even with continuing cyclic therapy.[2,77,78] The incidence of hepatotoxicity was augmented (up to 30%–50%) when it was used in combination with dacarbazine or vemurafenib.[64,79] The pattern of hepatotoxicity is most commonly hepatocellular but can be mixed, occurring after 2 to 4 cycles of therapy.[2,77,79] The mechanism of ipilimumab hepatotoxicity is likely immune mediated, likely as part of the immune-related adverse events associated with blocking CTLA-4.[2,77–79] Histologically, it often demonstrates a panlobular active hepatitis that resembles autoimmune hepatitis.[80] Serum autoantibodies, however, are usually not present. Prominent sinusoidal histiocytic infiltrates and central venulitis may be helpful histologic clues to the diagnosis of ipilimumab hepatotoxicity.[80] A course of corticosteroids is recommended for patients receiving ipilimumab who develop elevation of ALT greater than 5 times the ULN. Hepatototoxicity usually resolves with prompt corticosteroid treatment; however, few deaths have been reported due to severe immune-related adverse events (eg, SJS and capillary leak syndrome).[2,78] Rituximab and ofatumumab, MABs targeted against CD20, lack convincing data for causing clinically apparent hepatotoxicity.[67] Their treatment can be associated, however, with reactivation of inactive chronic hepatitis B (hepatitis B surface antigen [HBsAg]+), resolved hepatitis B (HBsAg−/anti-HBc+/DNA−), and occult hepatitis B infection (HBsAg−/anti-HBc+/DNA+) that may cause ALF and death or lead to LT.[81] Therefore, HBsAg and anti-HBc should be screened in all candidates prior to anti-CD20 therapy and then appropriate immunoprophylaxis instituted.[81,82]

Anti–tumor necrosis factor (TNF)-α agents, including infliximab, etanercept, adalimumab, certolizumab, and golimumab, can be linked to rare instances of clinically apparent hepatotoxicity.[2,83] In a national database of 6861 patients with rheumatoid arthritis treated by anti–TNF-α agents, the incidence of ALT elevation greater than 3 times the ULN was less than 1% and was less likely with etanercept compared with infliximab or adalimumab.[84] In an analysis of 34 cases of anti–TNF-α hepatotoxicity, infliximab (n = 26) was the most common implicated agent and the most frequent pattern was hepatocellular injury (75% of cases).[85] Presence of autoimmune markers, including antibodies against antinuclear, smooth muscle, and double-stranded DNA, were common (65%), and some had classic histologic features of autoimmune hepatitis. The cases of autoimmune hepatitis phenotype seemed to have longer latency

Table 3
Hepatotoxicity due to monoclonal antibodies

Agents	Targets	Incidence of Serum Alanine Aminotransferase Elevation, %	Pattern of Hepatotoxicity	Latency Period	Reactivation of Hepatitis B	Benefits from Corticosteroids
Trastuzumab	HER-2	1–12	Hepatitis	1–8 cycles	No (possible with other CMT)	No
Trastuzumab emtansine	HER-2/DM1	17–22	Hepatitis, ALF, portal hypertension, NRH	1–8 cycles	No (possible with other CMT)	No
Ipilimumab	CTLA-4	3–9	Hepatitis, AIH-like (often with immune-mediated AEs), cholestasis, mixed	2–4 cycles	No (possible with other CMT)	Yes (++)
Rituximab	CD20	<1	Hepatitis	NA	Yes (++)	No
Infliximab, etanercept, adalimumab	TNF-α	<1	Hepatitis, AIH-like, cholestasis, mixed	Median 13 wk (2–104)	Yes (+)	Yes (+)

Abbreviations: ++, high; +=, low-moderate; AE, adverse events; AIH, autoimmune hepatitis; CMT, chemotherapy; NRH, nodular regenerative hyperplasia.

period (16 [2–104 days] versus 10 [2–52] weeks), higher peak ALT (784 [140–2250] versus 528 [175–2491] U/L) and higher R values (13 [4–40] versus 6 [1.8–20]), compared with nonimmune hepatotoxicity cases.[85] In addition, nonautoimmune mixed pattern and predominant cholestasis have been observed. The prognosis is usually good after drug discontinuation, although some patients (approximately 50%) may benefit from a course of corticosteroids.[83,85] Concomitant treatment with methotrexate seemed to have some protective effect against anti–TNF-α hepatotoxicity.[83] The mechanism and the question whether anti–TNF-α hepatotoxicity has a class effect remains unclear; however, treatment with an alternative anti–TNF-α after resolution of hepatotoxicity seems well tolerated without recurrence.[85] Anti–TNF-α, in particular infliximab, has been associated with hepatitis B reactivation, including ALF, so that prophylactic therapy before starting is suggested in patients who are HBsAg positive.[81,86]

CARDIOVASCULAR AGENTS
Novel or Non–Vitamin K Oral Anticoagulants

NOACs have significant pharmacologic advantages over vitamin K antagonists (eg, warfarin), that include rapid onset of action, rapid resolution of the anticoagulation effect on discontinuation, few drug-drug interactions, predictable pharmacokinetics, and also, importantly, eliminating the requirement for regular monitoring of prothrombin time.[87] Ximelagatran, a direct thrombin inhibitor, was the first NOAC on the market; however, it was subsequently withdrawn from the market in 2006 due to the risk of hepatotoxicity observed in long-term clinical trials (8% of treated patients have elevated ALT >3 times the ULN).[88,89] More recently, second-generation NOACs (direct thrombin inhibitors, dabigatran, and factor Xa inhibitors, including rivaroxaban, apixaban, and edoxaban) have been approved mainly for treatment and prevention of deep venous thrombosis/pulmonary embolism and systemic embolism from nonvalvular atrial fibrillation.[89] In a systematic review and meta-analysis of phase III studies (29 randomized controlled trials evaluating 152,116 patients), NOACs were not associated with an increased risk of hepatotoxicity. Similar rates of hepatotoxicity were obtained for individual NOACs (0.1%–1%), which were lower than in control groups (warfarin, low-molecular-weight heparin, and placebo).[90]

Nevertheless, a review of greater than 57,000 spontaneous reports in the World Health Organization (WHO) database revealed a small risk of hepatotoxicity attributed to rivaroxaban (3.8%), apixaban (2.1%), and dabigatran (1.8%), with 3% to 12% of these hepatotoxicity events being liver failure (**Table 4**).[89] Likewise, another analysis of spontaneous reports submitted through the US Food and Drug Administration adverse event reporting system noted that hepatotoxicity represented 3.7% (146/13,096 reports) and 1.7% (222/3985 reports) of all reports for rivaroxaban and dabigatran, respectively.[91] Concomitant use of potentially hepatotoxic and/or interacting drugs, especially statins, paracetamol, and amiodarone, were present in 37% to 42% of the hepatotoxicity cases. Among ALF reports (41 dabigatran and 25 rivaroxaban), fatal outcome occurred in 44% to 51% of cases, whereas rapid onset of the event (<1 week) was noted in 44% to 47% of patients.[91] A reliable estimate of the incidence and severity of hepatotoxicity from edoxaban is not possible due to alimited number of cases of hepatotoxicity in the available databases.[89,91] Rivaroxaban hepatotoxicity is mainly hepatocellular, but cholestatic and mixed injuries have also been described.[92–94] The latency period is often 2 to 8 weeks but can be as early as 2 days after initiation of treatment.[92–94] Although dose-dependent hepatotoxicity (centrilobular necrosis) was observed in animal models, histologic findings of

Table 4
Metabolism and hepatotoxicity of novel oral anticoagulants

Agents	Rivaroxaban	Apixaban	Edoxaban	Dabigatran
Liver metabolism	Yes; elimination by CYP3A4	Yes; elimination by CYP3A4	Minimal (<4% of elimination)	No
Half-life	5–13 h	8–15 h	10–14 h	12–17 h
Renal clearance	~40%	~40%	~50%	~80%
P-gp substrate	Yes	Yes	Yes	Yes
Potential interaction	CYP3A4/P-gp inhibitors	CYP3A4/P-gp inhibitors	P-gp inhibitors	P-gp inhibitors
Usage in patients with cirrhosis	Yes (Child A/B)	Yes (Child A/B)	Yes (Child A/B)	Not recommended (no available safety data)
Total spontaneous reports[a]	20,295	3710	63	33,369
Specific hepatic events	775 (3.8%)	73 (2.0%)	7 (11.1%)	546 (1.6%)
Liver failure[b]	60/775 (7.7%)	2/73 (2.7%)	0/7	67/546 (12.3%)
Liver death[b]	17/775 (2.2%)	0/73	NA	22/546 (4.0%)

[a] Total spontaneous reports from WHO database (up to February 6, 2015).
[b] Percentage of specific hepatic events.
Adapted from Liakoni E, Ratz Bravo AE, Krahenbuhl S. Hepatotoxicity of New Oral Anticoagulants (NOACs). Drug Saf 2015;38(8):711–20.

rivaroxaban hepatotoxicity in humans are often dominant portal lymphocytic and eosinophil infiltrates, with varying degree of bile duct damage, which are suggestive of an immunoallergic reaction.[89,92,93,95] Besides, rivaroxaban hepatotoxicity associated with DRESS syndrome has also been reported.[89,95]

Newer Antiplatelet Agents

ADP receptor inhibitors, including clopidogrel, prasugrel, and ticagrelor, are increasingly used, replacing ticlopidine, for treatment and prevention of myocardial infarction and stroke. Hepatotoxicity from ADP receptor inhibitors is generally rare. In large clinical trials, ALT elevations were no more frequent with clopidogrel as with comparator arms (1%–3%) and no instances of clinically apparent hepatotoxicity were reported.[96,97] There have been several case reports, however, of significant hepatotoxicity, including ALF and death, associated with clopidogrel since its approval in 1997.[2,98,99] The pattern of hepatotoxicity is typically hepatocellular, but mixed or cholestatic injury has also been described. The median onset of symptoms has been 6 (2–24) weeks after treatment and is often self-limited with recovery within 1 to 3 months.[2,98,99] Hypersensitivity features may occur but are generally not prominent. Clopidogrel hepatotoxicity does not seem to have cross-sensitivity within ticlopidine, dipyridamole, or other ADP receptor inhibitors.[2,98,99] Prasugrel has been noted to have similar rates compared with controls of ALT elevation in clinical trials.[100] Although it has been used in a limited number of patients, there has been at least

1 case report of liver injury attributed to prasugrel, in the context of severe systemic inflammatory response syndrome, and this led to death.[101] To date, there has been no report of severe hepatotoxicity from ticagrelor.[2]

NEWER ANTIDIABETIC AGENTS

Recently, roles of the incretin pathway in the pathogenesis of type 2 diabetes mellitus have been defined and this has provided several potential targets for therapy; the main 2 are dipeptidyl peptidase (DDP)-4 inhibitors (vildagliptin, linagliptin, alogliptin, saxagliptin, and sitagliptin) and glucagon-like peptide 1 (GLP-1) agonists. With the possible exception of vildagliptin, none of other DPP-4 inhibitors has been associated with hepatotoxicity in their phase II–III clinical trials.[102,103] Two large pooled safety analysis of data from greater than 14,000 patients with type 2 diabetes mellitus reported that treatment with sitagliptin was not associated with increased risk of ALT elevation or hepatic events relative to comparators.[104,105] Nevertheless, few cases of hepatotoxicity potentially attributed to sitagliptin,[106,107] vildagliptin,[108] alogliptin,[109] and linagliptin[110] have been reported, although there have been uncertainties in causality relationship. Patterns of hepatotoxicity are mostly hepatocellular without hypersensitivity features, but cholestatic injury has also been described (with vildagliptin).[106–110] Monitoring of hepatic biochemical tests is recommended before and during treatment with vildagliptin and alogliptin, and their use is not recommended in patients with significant liver impairment.[109,111,112]

The GLP-1 agonists are recombinant polypeptides given parenterally, and they do not have significant hepatic metabolism. To date, there have been no convincing data implicating hepatotoxicity with GLP-1 agonists.[103,113] Sodium glucose cotransporter (SGLT)-2 inhibitors, including canagliflozin, dapagliflozin, and empagliflozin, are another new class of antidiabetic agents. None of SGLT-2 inhibitors has been associated with hepatotoxicity in clinical trials and in postmarketing surveillance so far.[2,103,114]

CENTRAL NERVOUS SYSTEM AGENTS
Newer Antiepileptic Drugs

In general, the newer-generation AEDs are better tolerated, have fewer drug interactions, and carry lower risk of hepatotoxicity when compared with the older-generation AEDs.[115,116] Nevertheless, cases of severe hepatotoxicity and ALF have been linked with this group of agents that include felbamate,[117] lamotrigine,[118,119] levetiracetam,[120] gabapentin,[121] pregabalin,[122,123] and oxcarbazepine.[115,124] Felbamate has a boxed label warning due to the risk of aplastic anemia and ALF.[117] The earliest onset of hepatotoxicity was 3 weeks after initiation of treatment, with a reported incidence of ALF in the United States of approximately 6 per 75,000 patient years of use.[117] Lamotrigine hepatotoxicity is typically hepatocellular and occurs along with major hypersensitivity reactions.[115,118,119] The incidence of clinically apparent lamotrigine hepatotoxicity is estimated to be 1 to 5 of 10,000 treated patients.[2,125] Skin rash is described in 10% of patients, with some progressing to SJS and toxic epidermal necrolysis. Risk factors for severe adverse reactions include young age, rapid escalation of dose, and concomitant use of valproate (increases serum lamotrigine level by more than 200%).[115,116] Unlike most AEDs that are hepatically metabolized, levetiracetam is excreted renally. Rarely, treatment with levetiracetam can be associated with asymptomatic ALT elevation, with latency period ranging from 1 week to 5 months.[2,125] Furthermore, a case of ALF after treatment with levetiracetam and carbamazepine has been reported, where hepatotoxicity recurred after re-exposure to levetiracetam.[120]

Even though cases of hepatotoxicity linked to gabapentin, pregabalin, and oxcarbaze-pine have been reported, the causality relationship has been somewhat less clear.[115,121–124] Pregabalin has been related to a few reports of hepatitis, including ALF, with a latency period of 8 days to 4 months.[122,123]

Newer Antidepressants

All antidepressant drugs may potentially cause liver injury, with an estimated incidence of asymptomatic ALT elevation in 0.5% to 3% of patients in general.[126] Severe hepato-toxicity and ALF has been reported after the use of some antidepressants, including monoamine oxidase (MAO) inhibitors, tricyclic antidepressants, venlafaxine, duloxetine, sertraline, bupropion, nefazodone, trazodone, and agomelatine, whereas citalopram, escitalopram, paroxetine, and fluvoxamine seemed to have lower risk.[126] Recently, se-lective serotonin reuptake inhibitors (SSRIs) and serotonin-norepinephrine reuptake in-hibitors (SNRIs) have largely replaced the older-generation antidepressants, such as tricyclic antidepressants and MAO inhibitors, mainly due to their favorable side-effect profiles. Nevertheless, SSRIs/SNRIs, in particular duloxetine, have accounted for a considerable number of cases of hepatotoxicity in the US DILI Network and WHO DILI database (**Table 5**).[1,127]

Although the rates of ALT elevation were comparable between duloxetine and pla-cebo in clinical trials, cases of duloxetine hepatotoxicity, including ALF and death,

Table 5
Hepatotoxicity from selective serotonin reuptake inhibitors and serotonin-norepinephrine reuptake inhibitors

Agents	Incidence of Serum Alanine Aminotransferase Elevation Greater than 3 Times the Upper Limit of Normal, %	Pattern of Hepatotoxicity	Mechanism	Latency Period	Cases of Liver Failure
Sertraline	0.5–1.3	Hepatitis, cholestasis, mixed	Immune-allergic, metabolic,	2 wk–6 mo	Yes
Paroxitine	1	Acute and chronic hepatitis, cholestasis	Metabolic	1 d–10 mo	No
Fluoxetine	0.5	Acute and chronic hepatitis, cholestasis, mixed	Metabolic	2.5 mo–1 y	No
Citalopram, escitalopram	<1	Hepatitis	Metabolic	4 d–8 wk	No
Fluvoxamine	NA	Hepatitis	Metabolic	9 d	No
Venlafaxine	0.4	Hepatitis, cholestasis	Metabolic, immune-allergic	10 d–6 mo	Yes
Duloxetine	1.1	Hepatitis, cholestasis, mixed	Metabolic, immune-allergic	2 wk–3 mo	Yes

have been increasingly reported since its approval in 2004.[115,128–130] The estimated incidence of significant hepatotoxicity is 26/100,000 patient-years. Pattern of hepatotoxicity is often hepatocellular, but mixed and cholestatic injury has also been described.[115,128–130] Hypersensitivity features are uncommon. A risk factor for duloxetine hepatotoxicity is preexisting chronic liver disease and, therefore, it should not be used in patients with evidence of chronic liver disease or substantial alcohol abuse.[115,128–130]

Newer Antipsychotic Agents

The initial antipsychotic medications introduced into clinical practice were the phenothiazines, but they have been largely replaced in recent years by the atypical agents due to greater potency and fewer extrapyramidal side effects.[2] Several atypical antipsychotic agents have been released over the past decade and they include aripiprazole, asenapine, brexpiprazole, iloperidone, lurasidone, paliperidone, and ziprasidone. Many, but not all, of the newer antipsychotic agents have been linked to an ALT elevation during therapy; however, clinically apparent hepatotoxicity with jaundice from these agents is rare.[2] In rare instances, ziprasidone can be associated with hepatotoxicity in the context of hypersensitivity reactions or DRESS syndrome.[2,131] Long-term treatment with several antipsychotic agents may cause significant weight gain and thereby induce nonalcoholic fatty liver disease.[2,132]

REFERENCES

1. Chalasani N, Bonkovsky HL, Fontana R, et al. Features and outcomes of 899 patients with drug-induced liver injury: the DILIN Prospective Study. Gastroenterology 2015;148(7):1340–52.e7.
2. Farnsworth N, Fagan SP, Berger DH, et al. Child-Turcotte-Pugh versus MELD score as a predictor of outcome after elective and emergent surgery in cirrhotic patients. Am J Surg 2004;188(5):580–3.
3. Andrade RJ, Lucena MI, Fernandez MC, et al. Drug-induced liver injury: an analysis of 461 incidences submitted to the Spanish registry over a 10-year period. Gastroenterology 2005;129(2):512–21.
4. Garcia Rodriguez LA, Stricker BH, Zimmerman HJ. Risk of acute liver injury associated with the combination of amoxicillin and clavulanic acid. Arch Intern Med 1996;156(12):1327–32.
5. O'Donohue J, Oien KA, Donaldson P, et al. Co-amoxiclav jaundice: clinical and histological features and HLA class II association. Gut 2000;47(5):717–20.
6. Stine JG, Lewis JH. Hepatotoxicity of antibiotics: a review and update for the clinician. Clin Liver Dis 2013;17(4):609–42, ix.
7. Lucena MI, Molokhia M, Shen Y, et al. Susceptibility to amoxicillin-clavulanate-induced liver injury is influenced by multiple HLA class I and II alleles. Gastroenterology 2011;141(1):338–47.
8. Lucena MI, Andrade RJ, Fernandez MC, et al. Determinants of the clinical expression of amoxicillin-clavulanate hepatotoxicity: a prospective series from Spain. Hepatology 2006;44(4):850–6.
9. Thomson JA, Fairley CK, Ugoni AM, et al. Risk factors for the development of amoxycillin-clavulanic acid associated jaundice. Med J Aust 1995;162(12):638–40.
10. de Abajo FJ, Montero D, Madurga M, et al. Acute and clinically relevant drug-induced liver injury: a population based case-control study. Br J Clin Pharmacol 2004;58(1):71–80.

11. Reddy KR, Brillant P, Schiff ER. Amoxicillin-clavulanate potassium-associated cholestasis. Gastroenterology 1989;96(4):1135–41.

12. Hautekeete ML, Horsmans Y, Van Waeyenberge C, et al. HLA association of amoxicillin-clavulanate–induced hepatitis. Gastroenterology 1999;117(5): 1181–6.

13. Larrey D, Vial T, Micaleff A, et al. Hepatitis associated with amoxycillin-clavulanic acid combination report of 15 cases. Gut 1992;33(3):368–71.

14. Hautekeete ML, Brenard R, Horsmans Y, et al. Liver injury related to amoxycillin-clavulanic acid: interlobular bile-duct lesions and extrahepatic manifestations. J Hepatol 1995;22(1):71–7.

15. Silvain C, Fort E, Levillain P, et al. Granulomatous hepatitis due to combination of amoxicillin and clavulanic acid. Dig Dis Sci 1992;37(1):150–2.

16. Alqahtani SA, Kleiner DE, Ghabril M, et al. Identification and characterization of Cefazolin-induced liver injury. Clin Gastroenterol Hepatol 2015;13(7):1328–36.e2.

17. Bickford CL, Spencer AP. Biliary sludge and hyperbilirubinemia associated with ceftriaxone in an adult: case report and review of the literature. Pharmacotherapy 2005;25(10):1389–95.

18. Bor O, Dinleyici EC, Kebapci M, et al. Ceftriaxone-associated biliary sludge and pseudocholelithiasis during childhood: a prospective study. Pediatr Int 2004; 46(3):322–4.

19. Hopkins S. Clinical toleration and safety of azithromycin. Am J Med 1991; 91(3A):40S–5S.

20. Lockwood AM, Cole S, Rabinovich M. Azithromycin-induced liver injury. Am J Health Syst Pharm 2010;67(10):810–4.

21. Longo G, Valenti C, Gandini G, et al. Azithromycin-induced intrahepatic cholestasis. Am J Med 1997;102(2):217–8.

22. Chandrupatla S, Demetris AJ, Rabinovitz M. Azithromycin-induced intrahepatic cholestasis. Dig Dis Sci 2002;47(10):2186–8.

23. Martinez MA, Vuppalanchi R, Fontana RJ, et al. Clinical and histologic features of azithromycin-induced liver injury. Clin Gastroenterol Hepatol 2015;13(2): 369–76.e3.

24. Van Bambeke F, Tulkens PM. Safety profile of the respiratory fluoroquinolone moxifloxacin: comparison with other fluoroquinolones and other antibacterial classes. Drug Saf 2009;32(5):359–78.

25. Paterson JM, Mamdani MM, Manno M, et al. Fluoroquinolone therapy and idiosyncratic acute liver injury: a population-based study. CMAJ 2012;184(14): 1565–70.

26. Orman ES, Conjeevaram HS, Vuppalanchi R, et al. Clinical and histopathologic features of fluoroquinolone-induced liver injury. Clin Gastroenterol Hepatol 2011; 9(6):517–23.e3.

27. Bataille L, Rahier J, Geubel A. Delayed and prolonged cholestatic hepatitis with ductopenia after long-term ciprofloxacin therapy for Crohn's disease. J Hepatol 2002;37(5):696–9.

28. Bjornsson E, Olsson R, Remotti H. Norfloxacin-induced eosinophilic necrotizing granulomatous hepatitis. Am J Gastroenterol 2000;95(12):3662–4.

29. Surgers L, Lacombe K. Hepatoxicity of new antiretrovirals: a systematic review. Clin Res Hepatol Gastroenterol 2013;37(2):126–33.

30. Nunez M. Clinical syndromes and consequences of antiretroviral-related hepatotoxicity. Hepatology 2010;52(3):1143–55.

31. Cohen CJ, Andrade-Villanueva J, Clotet B, et al. Rilpivirine versus efavirenz with two background nucleoside or nucleotide reverse transcriptase inhibitors in

treatment-naive adults infected with HIV-1 (THRIVE): a phase 3, randomised, non-inferiority trial. Lancet 2011;378(9787):229–37.

32. Molina JM, Cahn P, Grinsztejn B, et al. Rilpivirine versus efavirenz with tenofovir and emtricitabine in treatment-naive adults infected with HIV-1 (ECHO): a phase 3 randomised double-blind active-controlled trial. Lancet 2011;378(9787): 238–46.

33. Katlama C, Haubrich R, Lalezari J, et al. Efficacy and safety of etravirine in treatment-experienced, HIV-1 patients: pooled 48 week analysis of two random-ized, controlled trials. AIDS 2009;23(17):2289–300.

34. Ahmed Y, Siddiqui W, Enoch CB, et al. Rare case of rilpivirine-induced severe allergic hepatitis. J Antimicrob Chemother 2013;68(2):484–6.

35. Mills AM, Nelson M, Jayaweera D, et al. Once-daily darunavir/ritonavir vs. lopi-navir/ritonavir in treatment-naive, HIV-1-infected patients: 96-week analysis. AIDS 2009;23(13):1679–88.

36. Vispo E. Warning on hepatotoxicity of darunavir. AIDS Rev 2008;10(1):63.

37. Gulick RM, Lalezari J, Goodrich J, et al. Maraviroc for previously treated patients with R5 HIV-1 infection. N Engl J Med 2008;359(14):1429–41.

38. Sierra-Madero J, Di Perri G, Wood R, et al. Efficacy and safety of maraviroc versus efavirenz, both with zidovudine/lamivudine: 96-week results from the MERIT study. HIV Clin Trials 2010;11(3):125–32.

39. Mangiafico L, Perja M, Fusco F, et al. Safety and effectiveness of raltegravir in patients with haemophilia and anti-HIV multidrug resistance. Haemophilia 2012;18(1):108–11.

40. Lennox JL, Dejesus E, Berger DS, et al. Raltegravir versus Efavirenz regimens in treatment-naive HIV-1-infected patients: 96-week efficacy, durability, subgroup, safety, and metabolic analyses. J Acquir Immune Defic Syndr 2010;55(1):39–48.

41. Teppler H, Brown DD, Leavitt RY, et al. Long-term safety from the raltegravir clin-ical development program. Curr HIV Res 2011;9(1):40–53.

42. Vispo E, Mena A, Maida I, et al. Hepatic safety profile of raltegravir in HIV-infected patients with chronic hepatitis C. J Antimicrob Chemother 2010; 65(3):543–7.

43. Sax PE, DeJesus E, Mills A, et al. Co-formulated elvitegravir, cobicistat, emtri-citabine, and tenofovir versus co-formulated efavirenz, emtricitabine, and te-nofovir for initial treatment of HIV-1 infection: a randomised, double-blind, phase 3 trial, analysis of results after 48 weeks. Lancet 2012;379(9835): 2439–48.

44. Raffi F, Rachlis A, Stellbrink HJ, et al. Once-daily dolutegravir versus raltegravir in antiretroviral-naive adults with HIV-1 infection: 48 week results from the rand-omised, double-blind, non-inferiority SPRING-2 study. Lancet 2013;381(9868): 735–43.

45. Shah RR, Morganroth J, Shah DR. Hepatotoxicity of tyrosine kinase inhibitors: clinical and regulatory perspectives. Drug Saf 2013;36(7):491–503.

46. Iacovelli R, Palazzo A, Procopio G, et al. Incidence and relative risk of hepatic toxicity in patients treated with anti-angiogenic tyrosine kinase inhibitors for ma-lignancy. Br J Clin Pharmacol 2014;77(6):929–38.

47. O'Brien SG, Guilhot F, Larson RA, et al. Imatinib compared with interferon and low-dose cytarabine for newly diagnosed chronic-phase chronic myeloid leuke-mia. N Engl J Med 2003;348(11):994–1004.

48. Bosutinib. Chronic myeloid leukaemia in treatment failure: major toxicity. Pre-scrire Int 2014;23(151):177.

49. Gambacorti-Passerini C, Cortes JE, Lipton JH, et al. Safety of bosutinib versus imatinib in the phase 3 BELA trial in newly diagnosed chronic phase chronic myeloid leukemia. Am J Hematol 2014;89(10):947–53.
50. Singer JB, Shou Y, Giles F, et al. UGT1A1 promoter polymorphism increases risk of nilotinib-induced hyperbilirubinemia. Leukemia 2007;21(11):2311–5.
51. Bonvin A, Mesnil A, Nicolini FE, et al. Dasatinib-induced acute hepatitis. Leuk Lymphoma 2008;49(8):1630–2.
52. Carlini P, Papaldo P, Fabi A, et al. Liver toxicity after treatment with gefitinib and anastrozole: drug-drug interactions through cytochrome p450? J Clin Oncol 2006;24(35):e60–1.
53. Ho C, Davis J, Anderson F, et al. Side effects related to cancer treatment: CASE 1. Hepatitis following treatment with gefitinib. J Clin Oncol 2005;23(33):8531–3.
54. Shepherd FA, Rodrigues Pereira J, Ciuleanu T, et al. Erlotinib in previously treated non-small-cell lung cancer. N Engl J Med 2005;353(2):123–32.
55. Arora AK. Erlotinib-induced Hepatotoxicity-Clinical presentation and successful management: a case report. J Clin Exp Hepatol 2011;1(1):38–40.
56. Llovet JM, Ricci S, Mazzaferro V, et al. Sorafenib in advanced hepatocellular carcinoma. N Engl J Med 2008;359(4):378–90.
57. Van Hootegem A, Verslype C, Van Steenbergen W. Sorafenib-induced liver failure: a case report and review of the literature. Case Reports Hepatol 2011;2011:941395.
58. Mueller EW, Rockey ML, Rashkin MC. Sunitinib-related fulminant hepatic failure: case report and review of the literature. Pharmacotherapy 2008;28(8):1066–70.
59. Klempner SJ, Choueiri TK, Yee E, et al. Severe pazopanib-induced hepatotoxicity: clinical and histologic course in two patients. J Clin Oncol 2012;30(27):e264–8.
60. Kapadia S, Hapani S, Choueiri TK, et al. Risk of liver toxicity with the angiogenesis inhibitor pazopanib in cancer patients. Acta Oncol 2013;52(6):1202–12.
61. Shamroe CL, Comeau JM. Ponatinib: a new tyrosine kinase inhibitor for the treatment of chronic myeloid leukemia and Philadelphia chromosome-positive acute lymphoblastic leukemia. Ann Pharmacother 2013;47(11):1540–6.
62. Peroukides S, Makatsoris T, Koutras A, et al. Lapatinib-induced hepatitis: a case report. World J Gastroenterol 2011;17(18):2349–52.
63. Spraggs CF, Budde LR, Briley LP, et al. HLA-DQA1*02:01 is a major risk factor for lapatinib-induced hepatotoxicity in women with advanced breast cancer. J Clin Oncol 2011;29(6):667–73.
64. Ribas A, Hodi FS, Callahan M, et al. Hepatotoxicity with combination of vemurafenib and ipilimumab. N Engl J Med 2013;368(14):1365–6.
65. Teo YL, Ho HK, Chan A. Formation of reactive metabolites and management of tyrosine kinase inhibitor-induced hepatotoxicity: a literature review. Expert Opin Drug Metab Toxicol 2015;11(2):231–42.
66. Bunchorntavakul C, Reddy KR. Acetaminophen-related hepatotoxicity. Clin Liver Dis 2013;17(4):587–607, viii.
67. Karczmarek-Borowska B, Salek-Zan A. Hepatotoxicity of molecular targeted therapy. Contemp Oncol (Pozn) 2015;19(2):87–92.
68. Robinson SM, Wilson CH, Burt AD, et al. Chemotherapy-associated liver injury in patients with colorectal liver metastases: a systematic review and meta-analysis. Ann Surg Oncol 2012;19(13):4287–99.
69. Zalinski S, Bigourdan JM, Vauthey JN. Does bevacizumab have a protective effect on hepatotoxicity induced by chemotherapy? J Chir (Paris) 2010;147(Suppl 1):S18–24 [in French].

70. Ishizuna K, Ninomiya J, Ogawa T, et al. Hepatotoxicity induced by trastuzumab used for breast cancer adjuvant therapy: a case report. J Med Case Rep 2014; 8:417.

71. Srinivasan S, Parsa V, Liu CY, et al. Trastuzumab-induced hepatotoxicity. Ann Pharmacother 2008;42(10):1497–501.

72. Cobleigh MA, Vogel CL, Tripathy D, et al. Multinational study of the efficacy and safety of humanized anti-HER2 monoclonal antibody in women who have HER2-overexpressing metastatic breast cancer that has progressed after chemo-therapy for metastatic disease. J Clin Oncol 1999;17(9):2639–48.

73. Verma S, Miles D, Gianni L, et al. Trastuzumab emtansine for HER2-positive advanced breast cancer. N Engl J Med 2012;367(19):1783–91.

74. Ado-trastuzumab emtansine (Kadcyla) for HER2-positive metastatic breast can-cer. Med Lett Drugs Ther 2013;55(1425):75–6.

75. Force J, Saxena R, Schneider BP, et al. Nodular regenerative hyperplasia after treatment with trastuzumab emtansine. J Clin Oncol 2016;34(3):e9–12.

76. Bahirwani R, Reddy KR. Drug-induced liver injury due to cancer chemothera-peutic agents. Semin Liver Dis 2014;34(2):162–71.

77. Wolchok JD, Neyns B, Linette G, et al. Ipilimumab monotherapy in patients with pretreated advanced melanoma: a randomised, double-blind, multicentre, phase 2, dose-ranging study. Lancet Oncol 2010;11(2):155–64.

78. Weber JS, Kahler KC, Hauschild A. Management of immune-related adverse events and kinetics of response with ipilimumab. J Clin Oncol 2012;30(21): 2691–7.

79. Robert C, Thomas L, Bondarenko I, et al. Ipilimumab plus dacarbazine for pre-viously untreated metastatic melanoma. N Engl J Med 2011;364(26):2517–26.

80. Johncilla M, Misdraji J, Pratt DS, et al. Ipilimumab-associated hepatitis: clinico-pathologic characterization in a series of 11 cases. Am J Surg Pathol 2015; 39(8):1075–84.

81. Sarin SK, Kumar M, Lau GK, et al. Asian-Pacific clinical practice guidelines on the management of hepatitis B: a 2015 update. Hepatol Int 2016;10(1):1–98.

82. Reddy KR, Beavers KL, Hammond SP, et al. American Gastroenterological As-sociation Institute guideline on the prevention and treatment of hepatitis B virus reactivation during immunosuppressive drug therapy. Gastroenterology 2015; 148(1):215–9 [quiz: e216–7].

83. Bjornsson ES, Gunnarsson BI, Grondal G, et al. Risk of drug-induced liver injury from tumor necrosis factor antagonists. Clin Gastroenterol Hepatol 2015;13(3): 602–8.

84. Sokolove J, Strand V, Greenberg JD, et al. Risk of elevated liver enzymes asso-ciated with TNF inhibitor utilisation in patients with rheumatoid arthritis. Ann Rheum Dis 2010;69(9):1612–7.

85. Ghabril M, Bonkovsky HL, Kum C, et al. Liver injury from tumor necrosis factor-alpha antagonists: analysis of thirty-four cases. Clin Gastroenterol Hepatol 2013; 11(5):558–64.e3.

86. Carroll MB, Forgione MA. Use of tumor necrosis factor alpha inhibitors in hepa-titis B surface antigen-positive patients: a literature review and potential mech-anisms of action. Clin Rheumatol 2010;29(9):1021–9.

87. Bauer KA. Pros and cons of new oral anticoagulants. Hematology Am Soc Hem-atol Educ Program 2013;2013:464–70.

88. Lee WM, Larrey D, Olsson R, et al. Hepatic findings in long-term clinical trials of ximelagatran. Drug Saf 2005;28(4):351–70.

89. Liakoni E, Ratz Bravo AE, Krahenbuhl S. Hepatotoxicity of New Oral Anticoagulants (NOACs). Drug Saf 2015;38(8):711–20.

90. Caldeira D, Barra M, Santos AT, et al. Risk of drug-induced liver injury with the new oral anticoagulants: systematic review and meta-analysis. Heart 2014; 100(7):550–6.

91. Raschi E, Poluzzi E, Koci A, et al. Liver injury with novel oral anticoagulants: assessing post-marketing reports in the US Food and Drug Administration adverse event reporting system. Br J Clin Pharmacol 2015;80(2):285–93.

92. Russmann S, Niedrig DF, Budmiger M, et al. Rivaroxaban postmarketing risk of liver injury. J Hepatol 2014;61(2):293–300.

93. Liakoni E, Ratz Bravo AE, Terracciano L, et al. Symptomatic hepatocellular liver injury with hyperbilirubinemia in two patients treated with rivaroxaban. JAMA Intern Med 2014;174(10):1683–6.

94. Lambert A, Cordeanu M, Gaertner S, et al. Rivaroxaban-induced liver injury: results from a venous thromboembolism registry. Int J Cardiol 2015;191:265–6.

95. Barrett P, Vuppalanchi R, Masuoka H, et al. Severe drug-induced skin and liver injury from rivaroxaban. Dig Dis Sci 2015;60(6):1856–8.

96. Steinhubl SR, Berger PB, Mann JT 3rd, et al. Early and sustained dual oral antiplatelet therapy following percutaneous coronary intervention: a randomized controlled trial. JAMA 2002;288(19):2411–20.

97. Yusuf S, Zhao F, Mehta SR, et al. Effects of clopidogrel in addition to aspirin in patients with acute coronary syndromes without ST-segment elevation. N Engl J Med 2001;345(7):494–502.

98. Beltran-Robles M, Marquez Saavedra E, Sanchez-Munoz D, et al. Hepatotoxicity induced by clopidogrel. J Hepatol 2004;40(3):560–2.

99. Hollmuller I, Stadlmann S, Graziadei I, et al. Clinico-histopathological characteristics of clopidogrel-induced hepatic injury: case report and review of literature. Eur J Gastroenterol Hepatol 2006;18(8):931–4.

100. Kohli P, Udell JA, Murphy SA, et al. Discharge aspirin dose and clinical outcomes in patients with acute coronary syndromes treated with prasugrel versus clopidogrel: an analysis from the TRITON-TIMI 38 study (trial to assess improvement in therapeutic outcomes by optimizing platelet inhibition with prasugrel-thrombolysis in myocardial infarction 38). J Am Coll Cardiol 2014;63(3):225–32.

101. Serebruany VL, Kipshidze N, Pershukov IV, et al. Fatal sepsis and systemic inflammatory response syndrome after off-label prasugrel: a case report. Am J Ther 2014;21(6):e229–33.

102. Tella SH, Rendell MS. DPP-4 inhibitors: focus on safety. Expert Opin Drug Saf 2015;14(1):127–40.

103. Scheen AJ. Pharmacokinetic and toxicological considerations for the treatment of diabetes in patients with liver disease. Expert Opin Drug Metab Toxicol 2014; 10(6):839–57.

104. Engel SS, Round E, Golm GT, et al. Safety and tolerability of sitagliptin in type 2 diabetes: pooled analysis of 25 clinical studies. Diabetes Ther 2013;4(1): 119–45.

105. Ligueros-Saylan M, Foley JE, Schweizer A, et al. An assessment of adverse effects of vildagliptin versus comparators on the liver, the pancreas, the immune system, the skin and in patients with impaired renal function from a large pooled database of phase II and III clinical trials. Diabetes Obes Metab 2010;12(6): 495–509.

106. Gross BN, Cross LB, Foard J, et al. Elevated hepatic enzymes potentially associated with sitagliptin. Ann Pharmacother 2010;44(2):394–5.

107. Toyoda-Akui M, Yokomori H, Kaneko F, et al. A case of drug-induced hepatic injury associated with sitagliptin. Intern Med 2011;50(9):1015–20.
108. Kurita N, Ito T, Shimizu S, et al. Idiosyncratic liver injury induced by vildagliptin with successful switch to linagliptin in a hemodialyzed diabetic patient. Diabetes Care 2014;37(9):e198–9.
109. Barbehenn E, Almashat S, Carome M, et al. Hepatotoxicity of alogliptin. Clin Pharmacokinet 2014;53(11):1055–6.
110. Kutoh E. Probable linagliptin-induced liver toxicity: a case report. Diabetes Metab 2014;40(1):82–4.
111. Available at: http://www.ema.europa.eu/docs/en_GB/document_library/EPAR_-_Product_Information/human/000771/WC500020327.pdf. Accessed April 14, 2016.
112. Available at: http://www.ema.europa.eu/docs/en_GB/document_library/EPAR_-_Public_assessment_report/human/002182/WC500152273.pdf. Accessed April 14, 2016.
113. Armstrong MJ, Houlihan DD, Rowe IA, et al. Safety and efficacy of liraglutide in patients with type 2 diabetes and elevated liver enzymes: individual patient data meta-analysis of the LEAD program. Aliment Pharmacol Ther 2013;37(2): 234–42.
114. Zhang M, Zhang L, Wu B, et al. Dapagliflozin treatment for type 2 diabetes: a systematic review and meta-analysis of randomized controlled trials. Diabetes Metab Res Rev 2014;30(3):204–21.
115. Devarbhavi H, Andrade RJ. Drug-induced liver injury due to antimicrobials, central nervous system agents, and nonsteroidal anti-inflammatory drugs. Semin Liver Dis 2014;34(2):145–61.
116. Johannessen SI, Landmark CJ. Antiepileptic drug interactions - principles and clinical implications. Curr Neuropharmacol 2010;8(3):254–67.
117. Available at: http://www.accessdata.fda.gov/drugsatfda_docs/label/2009/020189s022lbl.pdf. Accessed September 16, 2016.
118. Amante MF, Filippini AV, Cejas N, et al. Dress syndrome and fulminant hepatic failure induced by lamotrigine. Ann Hepatol 2009;8(1):75–7.
119. Ouellet G, Tremblay L, Marleau D. Fulminant hepatitis induced by lamotrigine. South Med J 2009;102(1):82–4.
120. Tan TC, de Boer BW, Mitchell A, et al. Levetiracetam as a possible cause of fulminant liver failure. Neurology 2008;71(9):685–6.
121. Ragucci MV, Cohen JM. Gabapentin-induced hypersensitivity syndrome. Clin Neuropharmacol 2001;24(2):103–5.
122. Dogan S, Ozberk S, Yurci A. Pregabalin-induced hepatotoxicity. Eur J Gastroenterol Hepatol 2011;23(7):628.
123. Einarsdottir S, Bjornsson E. Pregabalin as a probable cause of acute liver injury. Eur J Gastroenterol Hepatol 2008;20(10):1049.
124. Planjar-Prvan M, Bielen A, Sruk A, et al. Acute oxcarbazepine-induced hepatotoxicity in a patient susceptible to developing drug-induced liver injury. Coll Antropol 2013;37(1):281–4.
125. Sethi NK, Sethi PK, Torgovnick J, et al. Asymptomatic elevation of liver enzymes due to levetiracetam: a case report. Drug Metabol Drug Interact 2013;28(2): 123–4.
126. Voican CS, Corruble E, Naveau S, et al. Antidepressant-induced liver injury: a review for clinicians. Am J Psychiatry 2014;171(4):404–15.
127. Spigset O, Hagg S, Bate A. Hepatic injury and pancreatitis during treatment with serotonin reuptake inhibitors: data from the World Health Organization (WHO)

database of adverse drug reactions. Int Clin Psychopharmacol 2003;18(3): 157–61.

128. Wernicke J, Pangallo B, Wang F, et al. Hepatic effects of duloxetine-I: non-clinical and clinical trial data. Curr Drug Saf 2008;3(2):132–42.

129. Xue F, Strombom I, Turnbull B, et al. Duloxetine for depression and the incidence of hepatic events in adults. J Clin Psychopharmacol 2011;31(4):517–22.

130. McIntyre RS, Panjwani ZD, Nguyen HT, et al. The hepatic safety profile of duloxetine: a review. Expert Opin Drug Metab Toxicol 2008;4(3):281–5.

131. Kim MS, Kim SW, Han TY, et al. Ziprasidone-induced hypersensitivity syndrome confirmed by reintroduction. Int J Dermatol 2014;53(4):e267–8.

132. Parsons B, Allison DB, Loebel A, et al. Weight effects associated with antipsychotics: a comprehensive database analysis. Schizophr Res 2009;110(1–3): 103–10.

Herbal and Dietary Supplement–Induced Liver Injury

Ynto S. de Boer, MD[a,b], Averell H. Sherker, MD, FRCPC[c],*

KEYWORDS

- Herbals • Dietary supplements • Liver • Toxicity • Drug-induced liver injury

KEY POINTS

- The increase in the use of herbal and dietary supplements (HDSs) and a growing awareness of the potential for these agent to cause liver injury has been associated with an increase in reports of HDS-associated hepatotoxicity.
- Limited regulatory oversight, inaccurate product labeling, adulterants, and inconsistent sourcing of constituent ingredients may all contribute to the potential for toxicity.
- The spectrum of HDS-induced liver injury is diverse and the outcome may vary from transient liver test abnormalities to acute hepatic failure requiring liver transplantation, or resulting in death.
- The most commonly implicated products include bodybuilding and weight loss products. There are no validated standardized tools to establish the diagnosis, but some HDS products have a clear clinical signature that can make diagnosis almost certain.

INTRODUCTION
Epidemiology

Herbs and botanicals, as well as their metabolites, constituents, and extracts, are included in the definition of dietary supplements in United States federal law.[1] The term herbal and dietary supplements (HDSs) is redundant but commonly used to categorize these products. Although regulated by the US Food and Drug Administration (FDA), dietary supplements are not subject to the safety monitoring and approval process of pharmaceutical drugs.

Disclosure: The authors have nothing to disclose.
[a] Liver Diseases Branch, National Institute of Diabetes and Digestive and Kidney Diseases, National Institutes of Health, 10 Center Drive, Bethesda, MD 20814, USA; [b] Department of Gastroenterology and Hepatology, VU University Medical Center, De Boelelaan 1117, Amsterdam 1081 HV, The Netherlands; [c] Liver Diseases Research Branch, Division of Digestive Diseases and Nutrition, National Institute of Diabetes and Digestive and Kidney Diseases, National Institutes of Health, 6707 Democracy Boulevard, Room 6003, Bethesda, MD 20892-5450, USA
* Corresponding author.
E-mail address: averell.sherker@nih.gov

Clin Liver Dis 21 (2017) 135–149
http://dx.doi.org/10.1016/j.cld.2016.08.010
1089-3261/17/Published by Elsevier Inc.

Despite these agents generally lacking proof of efficacy and their manufacturers not being permitted to make medical claims, these products have gained extremely wide acceptance and their use has increased over recent decades. During this time, the estimated number of supplements marketed in the United States has increased more than 10-fold, from ~4000 in 1993 to ~55,000 in 2012.[2,3] About half of the adult population in the United States reports having used at least 1 dietary supplement in the past month.[4,5] These products are more commonly used by non-Hispanic white people, at older age, and with higher levels of education.[6–9] Most alternative medicine users think that the use of HDS products is consistent with their attitudes toward health and life, and that these agents contribute to their well-being.[10] The use of HDSs is associated with considerable expense. In 2007, $14.0 billion was spent out of pocket on herbal or complementary nutritional products, equivalent to one-third of the out-of-pocket expenditures associated with prescription drug use in the United States.[11]

Nationally, it is estimated that 23,000 emergency department visits each year can be attributed to adverse effects associated with the use of HDSs.[12] Although there have been well-documented outbreaks of acute liver injury associated with specific dietary supplements, the true incidence of HDS-induced liver injury (HILI) is difficult to estimate. In Spain, 2% of investigated cases of drug-induced liver injury have been attributed to HDS,[13] whereas in Iceland the number is approximately 16%.[14] The National Institutes of Health–funded Drug-Induced Liver Injury Network (DILIN) has recently reported that, of total drug-induced liver injury (DILI) cases adjudicated between 2004 and 2013, attribution to HDSs has increased from 7% to 20% (**Fig. 1**).[15] Among patients presenting with acute liver failure, those whose disease was attributed to

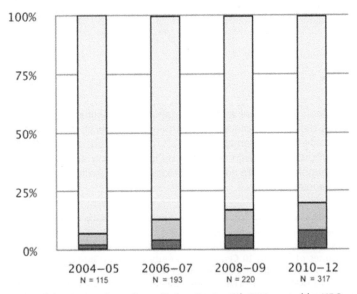

Fig. 1. Increase of the proportion of enrolled patients with DILI caused by HDS products in the DILIN prospective study. Light gray bar represents medications, medium gray bar represents nonbodybuilding HDS, and dark gray bar represents bodybuilding HDS. Trend test for HDS, $P = .0007$; trend test for bodybuilding HDS, $P = .007$; trend test for nonbodybuilding HDS, $P = .05$. (*From* Navarro VJ, Barnhart H, Bonkovsky HL, et al. Liver injury from herbals and dietary supplements in the U.S. Drug-Induced Liver Injury Network. Hepatology 2014;60(4):1403; with permission.)

HDS use are more likely to undergo liver transplant than those associated with prescription medicines (56.1% vs 31.9%; $P<.005$).[16]

REGULATION AND QUALITY CONTROL

In the United States, manufacturers of dietary supplements containing ingredients that were introduced after October 15, 1994, are required to notify the FDA before marketing and to provide a rationale for the safety of the ingredients, such as historical use.[1] Safety testing or FDA approval of dietary supplements is not required before marketing. Only in case of serious adverse events (hospitalization or death) is postmarketing notification of the FDA required.[17] Recent examples of HDS products that were withdrawn from the market include OxyELITE Pro in 2013 (caused acute liver failure)[18] and Hydroxycut (hepatocellular injury with jaundice).[19] In the European Union (EU), herbal and dietary supplements are regulated under the Traditional Herbals Medicine Products Directive 2004/24/EC.[20,21] This directive stipulates that, if a product has been shown to be safely used over an acceptably long period (>30 years, with 15 years' use within the EU), it may be registered through a simplified procedure if the product is not administered parenterally and does not require a medical prescription. In contrast with US regulations, in Europe food supplements such as vitamin and mineral substances are regulated by the European Food Safety Authority according to Directive 2002/46/EC,[22] whereas herbal medical products are overseen by the Committee on Herbal Medicinal Products of the European Medicines Agency. To further complicate the regulatory landscape, many HDS products are acquired online through the Internet, where vendors and manufacturers may not be easily identifiable and enforcement is extremely difficult.

CLINICAL PRESENTATION AND DIAGNOSIS

HILI may manifest virtually the entire spectrum of acute and chronic liver disease. In epidemic outbreaks (eg, OxyELITE Pro) affected individuals may present with a fairly consistent phenotype.[23] A small number of agents (eg, anabolic steroids) have an idiosyncratic clinical presentation that may trigger a high index of suspicion, even in the absence of a disclosed history of exposure. More typically, sporadic cases present with hepatocellular, cholestatic, or mixed pattern of liver injury with varying degrees of severity and hepatic dysfunction. Patients may present with asymptomatic liver enzyme level increases, nonspecific constitutional symptoms, symptoms typical of acute hepatitis (icterus, nausea, fatigue, right upper quadrant abdominal pain), or acute liver failure with hepatic encephalopathy. These cases may have an autoimmune phenotype, because the presence of autoantibodies was reported to be 29% in one series of patients with HILI.[24] Other causes for liver injury, such as biliary obstruction (cholelithiasis and malignancy), viral hepatitis (hepatitis A, B, C, E; cytomegalovirus; and Epstein-Barr virus), alcoholic and nonalcoholic steatohepatitis, autoimmune liver disease (autoimmune hepatitis, primary sclerosing cholangitis and primary biliary cholangitis), hemochromatosis, and Wilson disease, should be considered and excluded. Unlike prescription drugs, HDSs are often perceived as natural (and, by extension, harmless) products by patients and may not be considered relevant to disclose. Individuals who have been using a product for an extended period of time may legitimately discount its role in their acute illness, not recognizing that formulations may change without notice, sourcing of ingredients may vary, and that unregulated quality control processes may lead to significant lot-to-lot variations. Patients may be reluctant or embarrassed to share their use of alternative therapeutics with conventional medical practitioners and, in some cases (eg, anabolic steroids), consumers deny use, knowing that the practice is illegal. Patients with liver disease should be questioned directly about their use of prescription medications, over-the-counter products, and HDSs. If the diagnosis remains uncertain or the index of suspicion is high, the patient should be questioned about HDS use again. It may be helpful to ask the patient or a family member to bring all of the medications and supplements to the clinic or hospital. **Fig. 2** shows a rolling suitcase full of HDS products brought to clinic (and being consumed) by a patient with marked jaundice and advanced subacute liver disease who repeatedly denied HDS use until told of her physician's suspicion after she underwent liver biopsy. **Fig. 3** shows the pharmacopeia of HDSs being used by a patient with liver injury, providing an example of the challenges of ascribing causality to a specific agent. Even when there is a high degree of suspicion for HILI, it may be difficult to establish a diagnosis with a high degree of certainty. To address this issue, Naranjo and colleagues[25] (1981) developed an Adverse Drug Reaction Probability Scale to establish the probability of an adverse drug reaction, primarily in controlled trials and studies. The score is derived from 10 simple questions that can add up to a total score that ranges from −4 to 14.[25] Although widely used, this system was shown to have a limited applicability in estimating liver injury caused by drugs.[26] Instead, they found that the Roussel Uclaf Causality Assessment Method performed better (see article by Amina Ibrahim Shehu and colleagues', "Mechanisms of drug induced hepatotoxicity," in this issue).[26–29]

PATTERN OF INJURY

As with classic DILI, liver injury caused by HDSs can be classified into hepatocellular, mixed, or cholestatic liver injury. This pattern is defined by the R value ([ALT (alanine aminotransferase)/ULN (upper limit of normal)] ÷ [Alk P (alkaline phosphatase)/ULN]), in which a value >5 is interpreted as hepatocellular, less than 2 as cholestatic, and 2 to 5 as mixed hepatic injury. Across the world, HILI seems to be more commonly associated with a hepatocellular pattern of injury than prescription DILI.[14,24,30–34] In

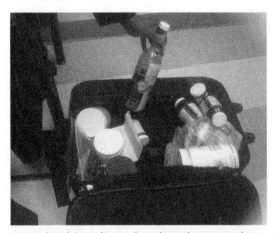

Fig. 2. A patient presented with jaundice and moderately severe subacute hepatitis. She denied any drug or HDS ingestion on repeated questioning over several visits. A liver biopsy was performed because liver tests were slow to improve, and was suspicious for hepatotoxicity. The patient was asked again about ingestions and she admitted that she was taking "1 or 2" HDS products. She wheeled this suitcase in to her next visit and admitted that she was regularly using all the products in the bag.

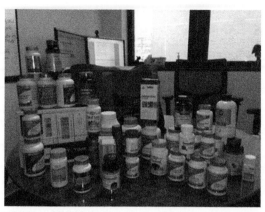

Fig. 3. A patient was referred with abnormal liver tests. He readily admitted to using HDSs and brought in all of the products seen here. This example shows the challenges of ascribing causality to a specific agent. (*Courtesy of* Dr Victor Navarro, Einstein Healthcare Network, Philadelphia, PA, USA.)

DILI, hepatocellular injury with jaundice has been described to have a more severe outcome than is seen in mixed or cholestatic patterns of injury (Hy's law).

UNIQUE ASPECTS OF HERBAL AND DIETARY SUPPLEMENT–INDUCED LIVER INJURY

The mechanisms through which HDS products cause hepatotoxicity are variable and specific to the substance consumed. In HILI, substances may be safe in their natural form but highly concentrated preparations and synthesized chemicals, although marketed as natural, may be associated with toxicities (eg, catechins found in green tea preparations and synthetic aegeline in OxyELITE Pro[35]) (**Tables 1** and **2**). A major challenge in evaluating liver injury caused by HDS products is inaccuracy with respect to product labeling. Contrary to regulations, some products do not display a label listing ingredients. In the DILIN experience, 29 of 73 HDS products (40%) taken for various purposes (eg, bodybuilding, weight loss, immune support) and causing liver injury did not identify green tea extract (GTE) or any of its component catechins on the label despite containing catechins by analytical chemical methods.[36] Note that 3 of 18 (17%) investigated products that did list catechins or GTE on the label did not contain these substances in detectable concentrations. In general, label-reported concentrations of GTE did not accurately reflect the contents.

Adulteration of HDS products has been described. Tablets of the Chinese herbal product Jin Bu Huan Anodyne listed *Polygala chinensis* as its single effective ingredient, but were found to contain levotetrahydropalmatine, which is found in the plant genera *Stephania* and *Corydalis* but not in the genus *Polygala*.[37] This product was responsible for an outbreak of severe hepatotoxicity before it was removed from the market.

Given the lack of regulatory oversight on production and manufacturing, there is a potential for contamination of HDS products. A report on the hepatotoxicity associated with Herbalife products identified bacterial contamination with *Bacillus subtilis* as a potential cause for the products' hepatotoxicity profile.[38]

HEPATOTOXICITY ASSOCIATED WITH SPECIFIC HERBAL AND DIETARY SUPPLEMENTS
Anabolics

Marketed anabolic steroids are generally synthetic chemicals and are not HDSs as strictly defined.[1] However, they are typically included in the discussion of HILI. Liver

Table 1
Use and mechanism of specific HDS products

Herbals	Common Use	Mechanism and Comments	References
Anabolic steroids	Bodybuilding, weight training, or athletics	Unknown	39
Black cohosh (*Cimicifuga/ Actaea racemosa*)	Joint aches, myalgia and menopausal symptoms	Unknown Possibly adulterated with *Actaea pachypoda* Ell. (white cohosh) and *Actaea podocarpa* DC. (yellow cohosh)	45
Chaparral (*Larrea tridentata*)	Antioxidant properties, antiinflammatory, liver disease, skin disorders	Unknown Possibly, interference with cyclooxygenase or CYP450, estrogenlike activity	83
Green tea extracts (*Camellia sinensis*)	Weight loss	EGCG toxicity is possibly heightened in individuals with a genetic predisposition	53
Pyrrolizidine alkaloids/comfrey (*Senecio, Symphytum*)	Natural home remedy	Hepatic sinusoidal cells are damaged, ultimately resulting in sinusoidal obstruction syndrome	54,63
Germander (*Teucrium chamaedrys*)	Dyspepsia, obesity, diabetes, and abdominal colic	CYP3A4-dependent alkylation of microsomal protein leading to autoantibody formation	46–48
Greater celandine (*Chelidonium majus*)	Dyspepsia	Unknown	84
Kava kava (*Piper methysticum*)	Gall bladder disease, biliary colic, cholelithiasis, and jaundice	Immunoallergic and idiosyncratic factors, including CYP2D6 deficiency	64,65
Mistletoe (*Viscum album*)	Asthma, infertility, hypertension	Mistletoe lectins have immunostimulating properties and a strong dose-dependent cytotoxic activity	85
Pennyroyal (*Mentha pulegium, Hedeoma pulegoides*)	Abortifacient	Oxidation of pulegone by cytochrome P450 into menthofuran, depletion of glutathione	86
Skullcap (*Scutellaria baicalensis*)	Arthritic symptoms	CYP3A-dependent apoptosis shown in isolated rat hepatocytes	79–81
Jin Bu Huan	Sedation, analgesic	Adulteration with other plant genera	37
Ma huang	Stimulant, weight loss	Idiosyncratic ephedrine alkaloid toxicity	87

Abbreviations: CYP, cytochrome P; EGCG, epigallocatechin gallate.

Table 2
Use and mechanism of specific HDS proprietary mixes

Proprietary Mixes	Common Use	Mechanism and Comments	References
Herbalife	Weight loss or improvement of well-being	Wide range of different products with listed and unlisted ingredients Hepatotoxicity potentially caused by contamination with *Bacillus subtilis*	38
OxyELITE Pro	Weight loss	Hepatotoxicity emerged after reformulation with synthetic aegeline Product was recalled	18,23
Hydroxycut	Weight loss	Different products, changing formulations Voluntarily recalled in 2009	78
Move Free Advanced	See skullcap, **Table 1**		79–81
SlimQuick	Weight loss, see green tea extracts, **Table 1**		53

injury caused by ingestion of anabolic steroids/bodybuilding compounds has a typical clinical presentation. It mostly involves young men involved in bodybuilding, weight training, or athletics who, despite modest liver enzyme level increases, present with marked jaundice and pruritus.[15,39] It typically has a mild course and completely resolves, albeit often slowly, after the cessation of the product. Pruritus may be debilitating. The use of anabolic steroids or enhancing products is often emphatically denied by the patient, but the diagnosis can be made confidently based on the presentation and clinical course. Frequently, the patient does not return for a scheduled follow-up visit when feeling better (Jay's law [Observation made by Dr Jay H. Hoofnagle in DILIN causality assessment, 2013]). Patients should be warned that the use of these agents may be illegal.

Black Cohosh

Black cohosh (*Cimicifuga/Actaea racemosa*) is an herbal extract that was traditionally used by Native Americans to treat a wide variety of symptoms, including joint aches, myalgia, and gynecologic symptoms. It is now primarily used for the treatment of postmenopausal symptoms. The mechanism of action is unknown, but there have been reports on hepatotoxicity with and without autoimmune features,[40–42] which has led to the publication of a cautionary statement by the US Dietary Supplement Information Expert Committee.[43] However, a more recent meta-analysis of 5 randomized, double-blind, controlled clinical trials found no evidence that isopropanolic extracts of black cohosh have any adverse effect on liver function.[44] Black cohosh has been known to be adulterated with other species of *Actaea* (*Actaea pachypoda* Ell.; white cohosh) and *Actaea podocarpa* DC. (yellow cohosh) from China, which may be responsible for the hepatotoxicity reported.[45]

Germander

The blossoms of wall germander (*Teucrium chamaedrys*) have long been used in folk medicine in the Middle East and Mediterranean region as treatment of dyspepsia, obesity, diabetes, and abdominal colic. Despite its wide use, it was found in the early 1990s that herbal preparations, in the form of tea or capsules, could cause significant liver injury. The injury is characterized by a hepatocellular pattern associated with marked jaundice, in the absence of immunoallergic or autoimmune features.[46] The latency to onset of injury is short, usually within 30 days of starting the preparation. Although fatal cases and liver transplant have been reported, the injury generally resolves after the cessation of the agent.[47] Reexposure to germander leads to rapid recurrence of the injury.[46] The toxicity is thought to arise because of cytochrome P (CYP) 3A4 activation of the component furan ring teucrin A, which can then alkylate intracellular epoxide hydrolase, leading to formation of antimicrosomal epoxide hydrolase autoantibodies.[48] It has been hypothesized that the anorexigenic properties of germander may relate to a mild hepatitis.

Green Tea

Green tea (*Camellia sinensis*) contains polyphenols known as catechins (eg, catechin, gallocatechin, epicatechin, epigallocatechin, epicatechin gallate, and epigallocatechin gallate). An intake of 2 to 3 cups of green tea per day does not generally lead to hepatotoxicity. However, HDS products such as SlimQuick, generally intended for weight loss, may contain higher doses of GTE, which can induce hepatotoxicity.[49–52] Epigallocatechin gallate (EGCG) is the most abundant green tea polyphenol, and is thought to be the most active and potent hepatotoxic component.[49] Genomic investigation in outbred mice identified genes that were associated with EGCG toxicity. There is a suggestion that analogous human genetic variants may be associated with susceptibility to GTE hepatotoxicity.[53]

Pyrrolizidine Alkaloids

Pyrrolizidine alkaloids are found in a large number of plants, including several used as HDSs. Among these are *Senecio*, and *Symphytum* (comfrey) species. Sinusoidal obstruction syndrome (SOS; previously known as hepatic veno-occlusive disease) was first described in 1954 among Jamaicans drinking so-called bush teas brewed from *Senecio*.[54] Reports from South Africa[55] (*Senecio*-contaminated bread), India[56] (*Crotalaria*-contaminated cereal), Afghanistan[57] (*Heliotropium*-contaminated wheat), and the southwestern United States[58–60] (comfrey used as HDS) have implicated pyrrolizidine alkaloids in SOS. Many reports describe the disease in children, suggesting either an increased susceptibility or a dose effect.[61] Note that the pulmonary vascular bed is also sensitive to the effects of pyrrolizidine alkaloids.[62] Sinusoidal obstruction syndrome may present as an acute, subacute, or chronic liver injury characterized by weight gain, ascites, and tender hepatomegaly. Hepatic sinusoidal cells seem to be the primary target of pyrrolizidine alkaloids. These cells are damaged and swell, impeding sinusoidal blood flow, inducing hemorrhage, and ultimately resulting in sinusoidal obstruction.[63]

Kava Kava

Kava kava (*Piper methysticum*) is used to treat anxiety and depressive disorders. However, numerous worldwide reports of fulminant hepatotoxicity, both hepatocellular and cholestatic, have led to the withdrawal of distribution licenses in the United States, Europe, and Australia.[64–66] Both immunoallergic and idiosyncratic factors (including CYP2D6 deficiency) have been implicated.[64,65]

Traditional Chinese Medicine

In the art of traditional Chinese medicine (TCM), specific herbs are selected in different preparations for their supposed properties to treat disease within the human body. TCMs have been used to treat conditions such as viral hepatitis for centuries. In China, currently, approximately 40% of cases of DILI are attributed to the use of TCMs, and have been responsible for cases of acute liver failure with associated coagulopathy.[67,68]

PROPRIETARY MIXES
Herbalife

In 2004, a report by Elinav and colleagues[69] implicated ingestion of Herbalife products in 12 patients who developed DILI, manifest as acute fulminant hepatitis. Herbalife products consist of a wide range of different mixtures, usually being taken for the purpose of weight loss or general well-being. The many identified ingredients include *Solidago gigantea, Ilex paraguariensis, Petroselinum crispum, Garcinia cambogia, Spiraea, Matricaria chamomilla, Liquiritia, Foeniculum amare, Humulus lupulus*, and chromium. In addition, the proprietary formulae of these products contain a wide range of listed and unlisted ingredients, which makes it challenging to identify a single responsible component with any degree of certainty.[70] In the initial cohort of cases implicated, the injury resolved spontaneously in 11 of 12 (92%) patients; 1 patient with preexisting chronic hepatitis B died after undergoing liver transplant. Three patients developed recurrent liver test abnormalities after resuming ingestion of Herbalife products. Since then, several reports have shown similar associations of HILI with Herbalife products, also suggesting contamination with *B subtilis* as a potential cause for its hepatotoxicity profile.[38,71] Employees of Herbalife have aggressively criticized reports of Herbalife-associated hepatotoxicity,[72,73] but their criticisms have been effectively rebutted.[74]

OxyELITE Pro

Between February 2012 and February 2014 the FDA received 55 reports of liver disease in consumers of OxyELITE Pro. The typical clinical course consisted of a severe acute hepatitis pattern of injury with a median time to onset of 60 days. Hospitalization was required in 33 (60%) cases and liver transplant in 3 (5%).[75] In early 2013 the formula of OxyELITE Pro was changed, substituting 1,3-dimethylamylamine, which had been associated with cardiovascular toxicity, with aegeline.[75] Early reports of liver injury were from Hawaii, where an initial cluster of 7 patients was reported to develop liver injury in the period between May and September 2013.[23,76] Following this report, other cases were identified in an outbreak investigation performed by the Hawaii Department of Health, Centers for Disease Control and Prevention (CDC), and FDA.[76] The product was recalled and the manufacturer was required to discontinue the distribution of OxyELITE Pro.[18] Aegeline, derived from the bark of the bael tree in India, has long been used as a traditional remedy but the component implicated in the OxyELITE Pro outbreak was synthetic.[35]

Hydroxycut

Hydroxycut products are generally marketed and used as weight loss supplements. Two published case series implicated the use of some Hydroxycut products in the occurrence of liver injury, presenting predominantly with a hepatocellular pattern of injury and symptoms of jaundice, fatigue, nausea, vomiting, and abdominal pain.[77,78] Several Hydroxycut products were voluntarily recalled in 2009, following a published FDA warning related to the use of Hydroxycut.[19]

Move Free Advanced

Move Free Advanced is a widely distributed dietary supplement, sold over the counter in the United States for treatment of sore joints and to improve flexibility and mobility. The product contains glucosamine, chondroitin, hyaluronic acid, and proprietary

Uniflex consisting of Chinese skullcap (*Scutellaria baicalensis*) and black catechu. In a 2010 report, the ingestion of Move Free was identified as a probable cause for the development of cholestatic hepatitis, which resolved after discontinuation of the supplement.[79] In 1 patient, Move Free was not initially recognized as the agent responsible for the injury and the patient restarted the supplement, after which liver injury recurred. A liver biopsy performed at that time was consistent with acute DILI.[80] In 1 patient, pulmonary infiltrates developed simultaneously with the hepato-toxicity and resolved completely with cessation of the supplement.[81] Diterpenoid compounds in *Scutellaria baicalensis* have previously been shown to cause apoptosis in isolated rat hepatocytes, through reactive metabolites formed by CYP3A.[82]

SUMMARY

The increase in the use of HDSs and a growing awareness of the potential for these agent to cause liver injury has been associated with an increase in reports of HDS-associated hepatotoxicity. Limited regulatory oversight, inaccurate product labeling, adulterants, and inconsistent sourcing of constituent ingredients may all contribute to the potential for toxicity. The spectrum of HILI is diverse and the outcomes vary from transient liver test abnormalities to acute hepatic failure requiring liver transplant, or resulting in death. The most commonly implicated products include bodybuilding and weight loss products. There are no validated standardized tools to establish the diagnosis, but some HDS products have a clear clinical signature that can make diag-nosis almost certain. The keys to diagnosis are a high level of suspicion and a compre-hensive work-up to eliminate competing causes. Management is generally supportive and nonspecific.

REFERENCES

1. US Food and Drug Administration. Dietary Supplement Health and Education Act of 1994. Available at: http://www.fda.gov/RegulatoryInformation/Legislation/Significant AmendmentstotheFDCAct/ucm148003.htm. Accessed September 19, 2016.

2. Commission on Dietary Supplement Labels. Report of the Commission on Dietary Supplement Labels. Washington, DC: Office of Disease Prevention and Health Promotion; 1997.

3. Dietary supplements: FDA may have opportunities to expand its use of reported health problems to oversee products (GAO-13-244). Washington, DC: Govern-ment Accountability Office; 2013.

4. Bailey RL, Gahche JJ, Lentino CV, et al. Dietary supplement use in the United States, 2003-2006. J Nutr 2011;141(2):261–6.

5. Picciano MF, Dwyer JT, Radimer KL, et al. Dietary supplement use among infants, children, and adolescents in the United States, 1999-2002. Arch Pediatr Adolesc Med 2007;161(10):978–85.

6. Radimer K, Bindewald B, Hughes J, et al. Dietary supplement use by US adults: data from the National Health and Nutrition Examination Survey, 1999-2000. Am J Epidemiol 2004;160(4):339–49.

7. Bailey RL, Gahche JJ, Miller PE, et al. Why US adults use dietary supplements. JAMA Intern Med 2013;173(5):355–61.

8. Foote JA, Murphy SP, Wilkens LR, et al. Factors associated with dietary supple-ment use among healthy adults of five ethnicities: the Multiethnic Cohort Study. Am J Epidemiol 2003;157(10):888–97.

9. Block G, Jensen CD, Norkus EP, et al. Usage patterns, health, and nutritional status of long-term multiple dietary supplement users: a cross-sectional study. Nutr J 2007;6:30.

10. Astin JA. Why patients use alternative medicine: results of a national study. JAMA 1998;279(19):1548–53.

11. Nahin RL, Barnes PM, Stussman BJ, et al. Costs of complementary and alternative medicine (CAM) and frequency of visits to CAM practitioners: United States, 2007. Natl Health Stat Report 2009;(18):1–14.

12. Geller AI, Shehab N, Weidle NJ, et al. Emergency department visits for adverse events related to dietary supplements. N Engl J Med 2015;373(16):1531–40.

13. Andrade RJ, Lucena MI, Fernandez MC, et al. Drug-induced liver injury: an analysis of 461 incidences submitted to the Spanish registry over a 10-year period. Gastroenterology 2005;129(2):512–21.

14. Bjornsson ES, Bergmann OM, Bjornsson HK, et al. Incidence, presentation, and outcomes in patients with drug-induced liver injury in the general population of Iceland. Gastroenterology 2013;144(7):1419–25, 1425.e1–3; [quiz: e19–20].

15. Navarro VJ, Barnhart H, Bonkovsky HL, et al. Liver injury from herbals and dietary supplements in the U.S. Drug-Induced Liver Injury Network. Hepatology 2014; 60(4):1399–408.

16. Hillman L, Gottfried M, Whitsett M, et al. Clinical features and outcomes of complementary and alternative medicine induced acute liver failure and injury. Am J Gastroenterol 2016;111(7):958–65.

17. Dietary Supplement and Nonprescription Drug Consumer Protection Act. Public Law 109-462, 120 Stat 4500, Pub. L. No. 109-462 Stat. 4500 (2006).

18. US Food and Drug Administration. FDA Investigation Summary: Acute Hepatitis Illnesses Linked to Certain OxyElite Pro Products. Available at: http://www.fda. gov/Food/RecallsOutbreaksEmergencies/Outbreaks/ucm370849.htm. Accessed September 19, 2016.

19. US Food and Drug Administration. Iovate Health Sciences USA, Inc: Voluntarily Recalls Hydroxycut-Branded Products. Available at: http://www.fda.gov/Safety/Recalls/ArchiveRecalls/2009/ucm145164.htm. Accessed September 19, 2016.

20. Directive 2004/27/EC of the European Parliament and of the Council of 31 March 2004 amending Directive 2001/83/EC on the Community Code relating to medicinal products for human use. Official Journal of the European Union: L136/34; 2004. p. 34–57.

21. Directive 2004/24/EC of the European Parliament and of the Council of 31 March 2004 amending as regards traditional herbal medicinal products, Directive 2001/83/EC on the Community Code relating to medicinal products for human use. Official Journal of the European Union: L183/51; 2004. p. 85–90.

22. Directive 2002/46/EC of the European Parliament and of the Council of 10 June 2002 on the approximation of the laws of the Member States relating to food supplements. Official Journal of the European Union: L183; 2002. p. 51–57.

23. Roytman MM, Porzgen P, Lee CL, et al. Outbreak of severe hepatitis linked to weight-loss supplement OxyELITE Pro. Am J Gastroenterol 2014;109(8):1296–8.

24. Bessone F, Hernandez N, Sanchez A, et al. The Spanish-Latin American DILI Network: preliminary results from a collaborative strategic initiative. J Hepatol 2013;58(Suppl 1):212–3.

25. Naranjo CA, Busto U, Sellers EM, et al. A method for estimating the probability of adverse drug reactions. Clin Pharmacol Ther 1981;30(2):239–45.

26. Garcia-Cortes M, Lucena MI, Pachkoria K, et al. Evaluation of naranjo adverse drug reactions probability scale in causality assessment of drug-induced liver injury. Aliment Pharmacol Ther 2008;27(9):780–9.

27. Benichou C. Criteria of drug-induced liver disorders. Report of an international consensus meeting. J Hepatol 1990;11(2):272–6.

28. Danan G, Benichou C. Causality assessment of adverse reactions to drugs–I. A novel method based on the conclusions of international consensus meetings: application to drug-induced liver injuries. J Clin Epidemiol 1993;46(11):1323–30.

29. Benichou C, Danan G, Flahault A. Causality assessment of adverse reactions to drugs–II. An original model for validation of drug causality assessment methods: case reports with positive rechallenge. J Clin Epidemiol 1003;46(11):1331–6.

30. Chalasani N, Fontana RJ, Bonkovsky HL, et al. Causes, clinical features, and outcomes from a prospective study of drug-induced liver injury in the United States. Gastroenterology 2008;135(6):1924–34, 1934.e1–4.

31. Reuben A, Koch DG, Lee WM. Drug-induced acute liver failure: results of a U.S. multicenter, prospective study. Hepatology 2010;52(6):2065–76.

32. Wai CT, Tan BH, Chan CL, et al. Drug-induced liver injury at an Asian center: a prospective study. Liver Int 2007;27(4):465–74.

33. Suk KT, Kim DJ, Kim CH, et al. A prospective nationwide study of drug-induced liver injury in Korea. Am J Gastroenterol 2012;107(9):1380–7.

34. Medina-Cáliz I, González-Jiménez A, Bessone F, et al. Variations in drug-induced liver injury (DILI) between different prospective DILI registries. Clin Ther 2013; 35(8):e24.

35. US Food and drug Administration. FDA Uses New Authorities To Get OxyElite Pro Off the Market. Available at: http://blogs.fda.gov/fdavoice/index.php/2013/11/fda-uses-new-authorities-to-get-oxyelite-pro-off-the-market/. Accessed September 19, 2016.

36. Navarro VJ, Bonkovsky HL, Hwang SI, et al. Catechins in dietary supplements and hepatotoxicity. Dig Dis Sci 2013;58(9):2682–90.

37. Woolf GM, Petrovic LM, Rojter SE, et al. Acute hepatitis associated with the Chinese herbal product jin bu huan. Ann Intern Med 1994;121(10):729–35.

38. Stickel F, Droz S, Patsenker E, et al. Severe hepatotoxicity following ingestion of Herbalife nutritional supplements contaminated with *Bacillus subtilis*. J Hepatol 2009;50(1):111–7.

39. Robles-Diaz M, Gonzalez-Jimenez A, Medina-Caliz I, et al. Distinct phenotype of hepatotoxicity associated with illicit use of anabolic androgenic steroids. Aliment Pharmacol Ther 2015;41(1):116–25.

40. Lynch CR, Folkers ME, Hutson WR. Fulminant hepatic failure associated with the use of black cohosh: a case report. Liver Transpl 2006;12(6):989–92.

41. van de Meerendonk HW, van Hunsel FP, van der Wiel HE. Auto-immuunhepatitis door zilverkaars. Bijwerking van een kruidenextract. [Autoimmune hepatitis induced by *Actaea racemosa*. Side affects of an herb extract]. Ned Tijdschr Geneeskd 2009;153(6):246–9 [in Dutch].

42. Cohen SM, O'Connor AM, Hart J, et al. Autoimmune hepatitis associated with the use of black cohosh: a case study. Menopause 2004;11(5):575–7.

43. Mahady GB, Low Dog T, Barrett ML, et al. United States Pharmacopeia review of the black cohosh case reports of hepatotoxicity. Menopause 2008;15(4 Pt 1): 628–38.

44. Naser B, Schnitker J, Minkin MJ, et al. Suspected black cohosh hepatotoxicity: no evidence by meta-analysis of randomized controlled clinical trials for isopropanolic black cohosh extract. Menopause 2011;18(4):366–75.

45. Verbitski SM, Gourdin GT, Ikenouye LM, et al. Detection of *Actaea racemosa* adulteration by thin-layer chromatography and combined thin-layer chromatography-bioluminescence. J AOAC Int 2008;91(2):268–75.

46. Larrey D, Vial T, Pauwels A, et al. Hepatitis after germander (*Teucrium chamaedrys*) administration: another instance of herbal medicine hepatotoxicity. Ann Intern Med 1992;117(2):129–32.

47. Dag MS, Aydinli M, Ozturk ZA, et al. Drug- and herb-induced liver injury: a case series from a single center. Turk J Gastroenterol 2014;25(1):41–5.

48. De Berardinis V, Moulis C, Maurice M, et al. Human microsomal epoxide hydrolase is the target of germander-induced autoantibodies on the surface of human hepatocytes. Mol Pharmacol 2000;58(3):542–51.

49. Lambert JD, Kennett MJ, Sang S, et al. Hepatotoxicity of high oral dose (-)-epigallocatechin-3-gallate in mice. Food Chem Toxicol 2010;48(1):409–16.

50. Bonkovsky HL. Hepatotoxicity associated with supplements containing Chinese green tea (*Camellia sinensis*). Ann Intern Med 2006;144(1):68–71.

51. Mazzanti G, Menniti-Ippolito F, Moro PA, et al. Hepatotoxicity from green tea: a review of the literature and two unpublished cases. Eur J Clin Pharmacol 2009;65(4):331–41.

52. Weinstein DH, Twaddell WS, Raufman JP, et al. SlimQuick - associated hepatotoxicity in a woman with alpha-1 antitrypsin heterozygosity. World J Hepatol 2012;4(4):154–7.

53. Church RJ, Gatti DM, Urban TJ, et al. Sensitivity to hepatotoxicity due to epigallocatechin gallate is affected by genetic background in diversity outbred mice. Food Chem Toxicol 2015;76:19–26.

54. Bras G, Jelliffe DB, Stuart KL. Veno-occlusive disease of liver with nonportal type of cirrhosis, occurring in Jamaica. AMA Arch Pathol 1954;57(4):285–300.

55. Wilmot FC, Robertson GW. Senecio disease or cirrhosis of the liver due to Senecio poisoning. The Lancet 1920;196(5069):848–9.

56. Tandon RK, Tandon BN, Tandon HD, et al. Study of an epidemic of venoocclusive disease in India. Gut 1976;17(11):849–55.

57. Mohabbat O, Younos MS, Merzad AA, et al. An outbreak of hepatic veno-occlusive disease in north-western Afghanistan. Lancet 1976;2(7980):269–71.

58. Stillman AS, Huxtable R, Consroe P, et al. Hepatic veno-occlusive disease due to pyrrolizidine (Senecio) poisoning in Arizona. Gastroenterology 1977;73(2):349–52.

59. Bach N, Thung SN, Schaffner F. Comfrey herb tea-induced hepatic veno-occlusive disease. Am J Med 1989;87(1):97–9.

60. Ridker PM, Ohkuma S, McDermott WV, et al. Hepatic venocclusive disease associated with the consumption of pyrrolizidine-containing dietary supplements. Gastroenterology 1985;88(4):1050–4.

61. Steenkamp V, Stewart MJ, Zuckerman M. Clinical and analytical aspects of pyrrolizidine poisoning caused by South African traditional medicines. Ther Drug Monit 2000;22(3):302–6.

62. Shubat PJ, Banner W Jr, Huxtable RJ. Pulmonary vascular responses induced by the pyrrolizidine alkaloid, monocrotaline, in rats. Toxicon 1987;25(9):995–1002.

63. DeLeve LD, Shulman HM, McDonald GB. Toxic injury to hepatic sinusoids: sinusoidal obstruction syndrome (veno-occlusive disease). Semin Liver Dis 2002;22(1):27–42.

64. Russmann S, Lauterburg BH, Helbling A. Kava hepatotoxicity. Ann Intern Med 2001;135(1):68–9.

65. Stickel F, Baumuller HM, Seitz K, et al. Hepatitis induced by Kava (*Piper methysticum rhizoma*). J Hepatol 2003;39(1):62–7.

66. From the Centers for Disease Control and Prevention. Hepatic toxicity possibly associated with kava-containing products–United States, Germany, and Switzerland, 1999-2002. JAMA 2003;289(1):36–7.

67. Zhao P, Wang C, Liu W, et al. Causes and outcomes of acute liver failure in China. PLoS One 2013;8(11):e80991.

68. Zhao P, Wang C, Liu W, et al. Acute liver failure associated with traditional Chinese medicine: report of 30 cases from seven tertiary hospitals in China*. Crit Care Med 2014;42(4):e296–9.

69. Elinav E, Pinsker G, Safadi R, et al. Association between consumption of Herbalife nutritional supplements and acute hepatotoxicity. J Hepatol 2007;47(4): 514–20.

70. Teschke R, Wolff A, Frenzel C, et al. Herbal hepatotoxicity: a tabular compilation of reported cases. Liver Int 2012;32(10):1543–56.

71. Johannsson M, Ormarsdottir S, Olafsson S. Lifrarskadi tengdur notkun a Herbalife. [Hepatotoxicity associated with the use of Herbalife]. Laeknabladid 2010; 96(3):167–72 [in Icelandic].

72. Appelhans K, Frankos V, Shao A. Misconceptions regarding the association between Herbalife products and liver-related case reports in Spain. Pharmacoepidemiol Drug Saf 2012;21(3):333–4 [author reply: 5].

73. Appelhans K, Najeeullah R, Frankos V. Letter: retrospective reviews of liver-related case reports allegedly associated with Herbalife present insufficient and inaccurate data. Aliment Pharmacol Ther 2013;37(7):753–4.

74. Reddy KR, Bunchorntavakul C. Letter: retrospective reviews of liver-related case reports allegedly associated with Herbalife present insufficient and inaccurate data–authors' reply. Aliment Pharmacol Ther 2013;37(7):754–5.

75. Klontz KC, DeBeck HJ, LeBlanc P, et al. The role of adverse event reporting in the FDA response to a multistate outbreak of liver disease associated with a dietary supplement. Public Health Rep 2015;130(5):526–32.

76. Johnston DI, Chang A, Viray M, et al. Hepatotoxicity associated with the dietary supplement OxyELITE Pro - Hawaii, 2013. Drug Test Anal 2016;8(3–4):319–27.

77. Dara L, Hewett J, Lim JK. Hydroxycut hepatotoxicity: a case series and review of liver toxicity from herbal weight loss supplements. World J Gastroenterol 2008; 14(45):6999–7004.

78. Fong TL, Klontz KC, Canas-Coto A, et al. Hepatotoxicity due to Hydroxycut: a case series. Am J Gastroenterol 2010;105(7):1561–6.

79. Linnebur SA, Rapacchietta OC, Vejar M. Hepatotoxicity associated with Chinese skullcap contained in Move Free Advanced dietary supplement: two case reports and review of the literature. Pharmacotherapy 2010;30(7):750, 258e–62e.

80. Yang L, Aronsohn A, Hart J, et al. Herbal hepatoxicity from Chinese skullcap: a case report. World J Hepatol 2012;4(7):231–3.

81. Dhanasekaran R, Owens V, Sanchez W. Chinese skullcap in move free arthritis supplement causes drug induced liver injury and pulmonary infiltrates. Case Reports Hepatol 2013;2013:965092.

82. Haouzi D, Lekehal M, Moreau A, et al. Cytochrome P450-generated reactive metabolites cause mitochondrial permeability transition, caspase activation, and apoptosis in rat hepatocytes. Hepatology 2000;32(2):303–11.

83. Sheikh NM, Philen RM, Love LA. Chaparral-associated hepatotoxicity. Arch Intern Med 1997;157(8):913–9.

84. Benninger J, Schneider HT, Schuppan D, et al. Acute hepatitis induced by greater celandine (*Chelidonium majus*). Gastroenterology 1999;117(5):1234–7.

85. Kienle GS, Grugel R, Kiene H. Safety of higher dosages of *Viscum album* L. in animals and humans–systematic review of immune changes and safety parameters. BMC Complement Altern Med 2011;11:72.

86. Thomassen D, Slattery JT, Nelson SD. Menthofuran-dependent and independent aspects of pulegone hepatotoxicity: roles of glutathione. J Pharmacol Exp Ther 1990;253(2):567–72.

87. Neff GW, Reddy KR, Durazo FA, et al. Severe hepatotoxicity associated with the use of weight loss diet supplements containing ma huang or usnic acid. J Hepatol 2004;41(6):1062–4.

Drug-Induced Acute Liver Failure

Shahid Habib, MD[a], Obaid S. Shaikh, MD, FRCP[b,c],*

KEYWORDS

- Drug hepatotoxicity • Liver failure • Cerebral edema • Encephalopathy
- Liver transplantation

KEY POINTS

- Drug-induced acute liver failure (ALF) disproportionately affects women and nonwhites. It is predominantly caused by antimicrobials, complementary and alternative medications, antimetabolites, antiepileptics, nonsteroidals, and statins.
- It presents as severe hepatic dysfunction characterized by jaundice, encephalopathy, and coagulopathy, in a patient without prior liver disease.
- Cerebral edema and intracranial hypertension are the most serious complications, which require intensive monitoring and therapy.
- Although advances in intensive care have improved survival, ALF has significant mortality without liver transplantation.

INTRODUCTION

Although advancements in intensive care management have considerably improved the outlook of patients with acute liver failure (ALF), it remains a diagnosis that has grave prognostic implications.[1] ALF or fulminant hepatic failure is severe hepatic dysfunction that is characterized by rapid onset, hepatic encephalopathy, and coagulopathy, in the absence of preexisting liver disease.[1,2] Fortunately, it is a rare disease with 2000 to 3000 reported cases in the United States per year.[3] Among 6199 adult liver transplant recipients in the United States in 2014, 239 (3.9%) had ALF.[4] ALF is a syndrome of varied causes, including acetaminophen, idiosyncratic drug-induced liver injury (DILI), viral hepatitis A, B, and E, Epstein-Barr and herpes simplex hepatitis, autoimmune hepatitis, Wilson disease, shock liver, and acute fatty liver of pregnancy.[5]

Disclosures: The authors have nothing to disclose.
[a] Department of Medicine, Southern Arizona Veterans Affairs Healthcare System 3601 S 6th Avenue, Tucson, AZ 85723 USA; [b] Section of Gastroenterology, Department of Medicine, Veterans Affairs Pittsburgh Healthcare System, University Drive C, FU #112, Pittsburgh, PA 15240, USA; [c] Division of Gastroenterology, Hepatology, and Nutrition, University of Pittsburgh School of Medicine, 200 Lothrop Street, Pittsburgh, PA 15213, USA
* Corresponding author. Section of Gastroenterology, Department of Medicine, Veterans Affairs Pittsburgh Healthcare System, University Drive C, FU #112, Pittsburgh, PA 15240.
E-mail address: obaid@pitt.edu

Clin Liver Dis 21 (2017) 151–162
http://dx.doi.org/10.1016/j.cld.2016.08.003
1089-3261/17/Published by Elsevier Inc.

liver.theclinics.com

DILI is a major cause of ALF. In a retrospective population-based study, 62 patients were deemed to have definite or possible ALF, and among them, 32 (52%) had acetaminophen or DILI cause.[6] Acetaminophen was implicated in 18 events (56%), dietary/herbal supplements in 6 events (19%), antimicrobials in 2 events (6%), and miscellaneous medications in 6 events (19%). Acute liver failure study group (ALFSG) is a consortium of major liver centers in the United States that has prospectively collected data from ALF subjects since 1998. Among 1198 patients enrolled at 23 sites over a period of 10 years, acetaminophen toxicity was responsible for 46% of cases, whereas DILI was noted in 11%.[5,7] Sixty-one unique agents were implicated in the causation of DILI, alone or in combination. Antimicrobials were the commonest cause, in particular isoniazid, trimethoprim-sulfamethoxazole, nitrofurantoin, and antifungal agents. Other offending drugs included complementary and alternative medications, antiepileptics, antimetabolites, nonsteroidals, and statins. The implicated DILI ALF agents were taken from 1 to 2 weeks, up to 8 months, and most subjects (65%) did not stop the drug until or after jaundice developed.

CLINICAL FEATURES

Jaundice, hepatic encephalopathy, and coagulopathy are the cardinal manifestations of ALF.[8] However, the syndrome often presents with nonspecific symptoms such as fatigue, malaise, anorexia, nausea, abdominal pain, and fever.[9] These symptoms progress to the development of encephalopathy and coagulopathy, although the rates of progression are somewhat variable. Coagulopathy often precedes the onset of encephalopathy. There are no characteristic features that differentiate DILI ALF from other causes. Nevertheless, DILI can be distinguished from other causes of ALF by the drug history and subacute course. Typical allergic signature drug reactions are less frequently noted in DILI ALF patients than suggested by a survey of common causes of DILI.[7,10]

DILI-associated ALF tends to occur in younger adults and more commonly in women than men. In the ALFSG study, the average age of subjects was 44 years; only 15% were older than 60 years, and the majority was women (71%).[7] In addition, compared with the US general population, nonwhites were overrepresented (43% vs 25%). On admission to the tertiary site, 68% had grade 2 or higher encephalopathy, 25% had clinically detectable ascites, and jaundice was typically noted. Most patients with DILI ALF have hepatocellular pattern of liver injury. In the ALFSG study, 78% had hepatocellular injury, 13% had cholestatic injury, and 10% had mixed pattern. About one-half of patients depicted some degree of renal impairment with serum creatinine greater than or equal to 1.5 mg/dL. Drug injury from herbal medications, traditional therapeutic preparations, and dietary supplements was more commonly associated with hepatocellular liver injury than prescription medications. Skin rash and eosinophilia were noted in a minority (8%), whereas autoantibodies were positive in 63% of the patients tested.

Encephalopathy

Hepatic encephalopathy may vary from subtle changes in affect, insomnia, and difficulties with concentration (grade 1) to deep coma (grade 4).[11] Cerebral edema (CE) is a common neurologic accompaniment of ALF unlike encephalopathy associated with chronic liver disease. It occurs in most patients who progress to grade 4 encephalopathy and is the most commonly identifiable cause of death in autopsy studies. The pathogenesis remains unclear but both vasogenic and cytotoxic mechanisms play a role.[12] CE may be recognized by the development of systemic hypertension, bradycardia (Cushing reflex), decerebrate rigidity, disconjugate eye movements, loss of pupillary reflexes, and papilledema; however, these clinical signs are often unreliable.

Coagulopathy

The liver plays a central role in hemostasis because it synthesizes almost all coagulation factors. In addition, it produces many inhibitors of coagulation and proteins involved in fibrinolysis. Coagulopathy (international normalized ratio [INR] >1.5) is therefore considered a key feature of ALF.[5] There are several factors involved in the bleeding and clotting diatheses seen in ALF, including platelet dysfunction (quantitative and qualitative) and deficiency of several clotting factors both vitamin K dependent (II, VII, IX, and X) and vitamin K independent, such as factor V.[13] There are reduced levels of fibrinolytic proteins, except plasminogen activator inhibitor-1 that is greatly increased, resulting in suppression of fibrinolysis.[14] Anticoagulant factors such as antithrombin III and proteins C and S are also reduced that further helps to rebalance the system.[15] Hemostatic changes in ALF thus incorporate a coagulopathy as well as a tendency to develop thrombotic events, such as disseminated intravascular coagulation.[16] Compared with chronic liver failure, ALF coagulopathy has lower incidence of thrombocytopenia and a more severe reduction in clotting factors.

Other Manifestations

Several systemic and metabolic derangements have been noted to occur in ALF, including acute renal failure, electrolyte abnormalities, hypoglycemia, and acute pancreatitis. Renal failure complicates 40% to 50% of ALF patients and denotes a poor prognosis.[17] It is often multifactorial and may result from prerenal azotemia, acute tubular necrosis, hepatorenal syndrome, or direct nephrotoxicity of a drug such as antibiotics and intravenous contrast. Cardiovascular, hemodynamic, and respiratory complications are notable clinical sequelae of ALF. A major component is systemic vasodilation resulting in diminished systemic vascular resistance, hypotension, and hyperdynamic circulation. Tissue oxygen uptake may be impaired despite adequate oxygen delivery resulting in tissue hypoxia and lactic acidosis ("tissue oxygen debt").[18]

DIAGNOSIS
Definition

Fulminant hepatic failure was originally defined as occurrence of encephalopathy within 8 weeks of the onset of jaundice due to hepatitis in an individual without preexisting liver disease.[2] Over the years, several definitions of ALF have been proposed. A systematic review of 103 published studies noted 41 different definitions of ALF.[19] Such high level of diversity in defining ALF has hindered comparative analysis. Although hepatic encephalopathy remained a cardinal feature, the interval between onset of acute hepatitis (or jaundice) and the occurrence of encephalopathy varied from 2 to 26 weeks.[20] The categorization of ALF as hyperacute, acute, and subacute, based on the interval between onset of symptoms and encephalopathy of up to 7 days, 8 to 28 days, and 5 to 12 weeks, provided prognostic value.[21] Patients with hyperacute ALF, mostly from acetaminophen toxicity, had better spontaneous recovery rate compared with acute or subacute ALF.[9,22] In order to provide uniform definition of ALF, the subcommittee of the International Association for the Study of the Liver developed nomenclature and diagnostic criteria that would allow better comparison of reports from different geographic areas.[23] It is important to differentiate ALF from acute-on-chronic liver failure (ACLF) because patients with ACLF may present without known history of chronic liver disease.[24] Clinical evaluation, biochemical tests, and imaging would help establish the diagnosis.

Establishing Diagnosis

DILI is largely a diagnosis of exclusion because there are no laboratory, imaging, or biopsy findings that are specific for hepatotoxicity from a particular drug.[25] However, there is a growing recognition of the characteristic presentations (signatures) of drug toxicity.[26] Knowledge of such signatures and the incidence rate of DILI with a drug can greatly help establish a diagnosis. Major components of drug signatures include typical latency from the start of treatment to onset of injury, characteristic extrahepatic manifestations, pattern of liver injury (hepatocellular, cholestatic, or mixed), and histologic and serologic features. LiverTox (http://livertox.nih.gov/) is a publicly available online database that provides valuable information regarding hepatotoxicity from more than 600 medications. It calculates the causality score for individual cases using the Roussel Uclaf Causality Assessment Method (RUCAM) and case-specific data entered by the site user.[27] The diagnostic methodology, however, has limitations because DILI signatures are not included in RUCAM. Thus, both causality score and drug signatures have to be subjectively weighed in to reach a diagnosis.[26]

Most DILI ALF cases result from idiosyncratic drug reactions in genetically susceptible individuals.[25] Genetic profiling involving HLA alleles is available, but its significance and clinical utility is uncertain. HLA alleles could help exclude a drug when a patient is exposed to multiple drugs because most alleles have high negative predictive values. Thus, genetic profiling could be an additional causality assessment tool. A recent study used N-acetyltransferase 2 genotyping to determine the appropriate dose of isoniazid in an antituberculosis regimen. It demonstrated that the combination of pharmacogenetic and clinical algorithms could potentially improve drug efficacy and reduce the likelihood of DILI.[28]

MANAGEMENT

Liver has the unique ability to regenerate after acute, self-limiting injury. Because there is no specific therapy for ALF, treatment is limited to supportive measures that anticipate complications, allowing the liver time to regenerate. The management of patients with ALF poses formidable challenges because of the rapidity, unpredictability, and severity of its complications.[29] Very few therapies for ALF have been evaluated in a rigorously controlled fashion. However, in the era of liver transplantation, experience in the management of these critically ill patients has been accrued as a result of channelized referral to the transplant centers. The overall management strategy starts with identification of cause and an initial assessment of prognosis. Especially critical is the decision regarding transplant candidacy. Early transfer to a transplant center should be accomplished where a dedicated multidisciplinary team of experienced hepatologists, critical care intensivists, and transplant surgeons can make the pivotal decisions regarding timing of transplantation and the use of potential "bridges to transplantation."[30]

Identification of the High-Risk Individual

With a mortality in excess of 80% without liver transplantation, it is vital that irreversible ALF be recognized early so that a donor organ is procured before prohibitive complications develop. Equally pivotal is the realization that with the current organ scarcity, short-term risks of surgery, and long-term consequences of immunosuppression, physicians should be able to recognize reversible disease so as to prevent unnecessary transplantations. Several prognostic factors have been studied and validated, including serum alphafetoprotein, bilirubin, and lactic acid levels, INR, arterial pH, histologic features, and mathematical models such as King's College criteria, Clichy criteria, and MELD, Model for End-stage Liver Disease, score.[31] King's College criteria are widely used and appear to have high positive predictive value for an adverse outcome.[9,32]

Treatment of Drug-Induced Liver Injury

In general, the key to the treatment of suspected DILI is to stop using the drug before the development of irreversible hepatic failure. There is limited availability of specific antidotes to acute DILI; one example is carnitine for valproic acid toxicity.[33,34] Cholestyramine may mitigate leflunomide toxicity.[35] N-acetylcysteine (NAC) and corticosteroids have been used in DILI and DILI-ALF.[36,37] Ursodeoxycholic acid, silymarin, and glycyrrhizin have been reported to be effective, but evidence remained largely anecdotal.[38] Primary prevention provides the maximum benefit by avoiding DILI and its consequences.

NAC may be beneficial in some cases of DILI ALF.[36] In a randomized clinical trial comparing NAC with placebo in adults with nonacetaminophen ALF, NAC was associated with an improvement in transplant-free survival in a subgroup of patients with grades 1 to 2 encephalopathy (40% vs 27%).[37] However, there was no difference in the primary outcome of overall survival at 3 weeks after initiation of treatment (70% vs 66%). In a prospective, nonrandomized study conducted in adults with nonacetaminophen ALF at a center without the facility for transplantation, the use of NAC was associated with mortality benefit.[39]

Corticosteroids may be used in DILI if clinical features suggest a prominent immune or hypersensitivity component. However, DILI among patients with classic autoimmune hepatitis is infrequent (9%), with minocycline and nitrofurantoin implicated in 90% of cases.[40] In a case series of 15 severe DILI patients, steroid/ursodeoxycholic acid combination was associated with favorable outcome.[41] Steroids have been reported to be beneficial in ALF from acute sinusoidal obstruction syndrome resulting from myeloablative therapy for hemopoietic stem cell transplantation.[42]

Specific Measures

All patients who present with severe acute liver injury must be monitored for early signs of ALF as described before. Once diagnosis of ALF is established, patients must be monitored and managed for life-threatening complications. A state-of-the-art review of the management of ALF has been published by the authors previously.[29] Key components are discussed here.

Hepatic encephalopathy and cerebral edema

CE and intracranial hypertension (ICH) are among the most serious complications of ALF.[43] CE should be suspected in patients with progressive hepatic encephalopathy. It is rare in patients with grade 1 to 2 encephalopathy but develops in 25% to 35% of those with grade 3 and 65% to 75% of those with grade 4 encephalopathy.[8] Progressive CE can result in fatal cerebral hypoxia and/or uncal herniation. Survivors may suffer from residual neurologic deficits.[44]

Intracranial pressure (ICP) in a healthy, supine adult ranges from 7 to 15 mm Hg.[45] Cerebral blood flow (CBF) autoregulation plays a key role in maintaining cerebral perfusion pressure (CPP), calculated as mean arterial pressure–ICP. ALF is associated with a loss of CBF autoregulation.[46] In the earlier stages, cerebral hyperemia occurs that contributes to the development of CE and ICH; however, as ICP increases, CPP declines, resulting in cerebral ischemia. Monitoring of CBF and ICP may provide useful information in the management of CE.[47] ALFSG has endorsed the use of ICP monitoring among patients at high risk of ICH, including those deemed not to be transplant candidates.[48] ICP is measured by placement of epidural transducers, subdural bolts, or parenchymal catheters. The risk of hemorrhage is lowest with epidural placement and can be further mitigated by the use of recombinant factor VII (rFVIIa).[49–51] Several tools are available to measure CBF and cerebral oxygen consumption, including jugular bulb catheter, transcranial Doppler, and xenon-enhanced computed tomography.[29]

Seizure activity is not uncommon among patients with severe encephalopathy; however, it is often masked by sedatives and paralytics. Seizures may raise ICP, increase cerebral oxygen consumption, and worsen cerebral ischemia.[52] Seizure activity can be monitored by continuous electroencephalography, enabling prompt therapy.

In the management of CE and ICH, the aim is to maintain ICP less than 20 to 25 mm Hg and CPP at 50 to 60 mm Hg.[29] In view of the loss of CBF autoregulation, the head is elevated to 30° and the neck is maintained in a neutral position. A multimodal approach, combining hyperventilation, hemofiltration, hypernatremia, and hypothermia (quadruple-H therapy), is appropriate.[53] Hyperventilation rapidly restores ICP by reducing $Paco_2$ that causes cerebral vasoconstriction.[54] To obviate cerebral hypoxemia, monitoring of cerebral perfusion and oxygen consumption is needed. Hemofiltration corrects volume overload resulting from associated renal dysfunction.[55] Hypernatremia or an increase in serum osmolality can be achieved by intravenous infusion of mannitol or hypertonic saline.[56–58] An increase in serum osmolality causes fluid diffusion from cerebral parenchyma into the circulation, thus reducing ICP. Moderate hypothermia, as defined by a core temperature of 32 to 33°C, restores CBF autoregulation and reactivity to CO_2.[59–61] Possible adverse effects of hypothermia include hypotension, cardiac arrhythmias, coagulopathy, and impaired liver regeneration. Thiopental and phenobarbital are considered second-line therapy for CE and ICH; they act by reducing cerebral oxygen consumption.[62]

Coagulopathy

Coagulopathy is a cardinal feature of ALF and provides important prognostic information.[5] Vitamin K should be administered to all patients with prolonged INR but routine preventive correction of INR with fresh frozen plasma (FFP) infusion is not required. However, in the presence of active bleeding and before invasive procedures, correction of coagulopathy should be attempted with FFP and/or platelet transfusions.[63] An INR less than 1.5 and platelet count greater than 50,000/mL are considered sufficient. Cryoprecipitate is recommended for patients with significant hypofibrinogenemia (blood fibrinogen <100 mg/dL).[48] In patients with ICH, rVIIa may be preferable to FFP infusion to avoid the risk of exacerbating volume overload and CE. It may also be used in patients intolerant or unresponsive to FFP.[64] The effect of rFVIIa lasts for 2 to 6 hours. Because it increases the risk of thrombosis, it should be avoided in patients with prior myocardial infarction, ischemic stroke, or pulmonary embolism.

Sepsis

Infections are commonplace in patients with ALF.[65] Bacterial infections may occur in up to 80% of cases, with pneumonia developing in 50%, bacteremia in about a third, and urosepsis in a quarter.[66] Gram-negative enteric bacilli and gram-positive cocci are commonly implicated. One-third of the patients develop fungal infections, largely

Candida species.[67] Sepsis may progress to systemic inflammatory response syndrome (SIRS), septic shock, and multiorgan failure. Patients with SIRS are more likely to develop progressive encephalopathy and poor outcome.[68] Conversely, patients with worsening encephalopathy are at risk of bacterial infections and may benefit from prophylactic antibiotics.[69] An alternative to prophylaxis is surveillance microbiologic studies that would help in the early detection and treatment of infections.

Metabolic derangements and renal failure

Patients in ALF frequently develop metabolic abnormalities. Hypoglycemia occurs due to glycogen depletion and defective glycolysis and gluconeogenesis.[70] High-concentration dextrose infusion is recommended to avoid exacerbating CE from hypervolemia hyponatremia. Low potassium, magnesium, and phosphate levels develop not too infrequently and require supplementation. One-third of the patients develop adrenal deficiency that requires steroid replacement.[71] Patients in ALF are hypercatabolic; therefore, nutritional support, either enteral or parenteral, should be initiated early.[72]

About 40% to 50% of patients with ALF develop acute kidney injury that may have features of pre-renal failure, hepatorenal syndrome, or acute tubular necrosis.[73] Several factors contribute to the development of renal disease, including direct nephrotoxicity of the DILI agent or of other concomitant medications, sepsis, and volume depletion. Patients with ALF tolerate hemodialysis poorly due to volume shifts causing hemodynamic instability. Continuous renal replacement therapy is therefore recommended in such patients.[74]

Circulatory and respiratory issues

ALF is associated with hyperdynamic circulation that is characterized by increased cardiac output, diminished systemic vascular resistance, and low peripheral blood pressures.[55] Tissue hypoxia may develop due to diminished oxygen delivery and uptake. Intravenous fluid resuscitation is needed and is best achieved with a colloid such as salt poor albumin. In view of the loss of CBF autoregulation, pressors should be used judiciously to avoid exacerbating cerebral hyperemia that may adversely affect ICH.[75,76]

Among patients with ALF, acute lung injury was reported to have increased likelihood of circulatory disturbance, CE, and poor outcome.[77] Hypoxemia occurs commonly, but adult respiratory distress syndrome occurs in about 20% as indicated by a recent study of 200 patients.[78] Such patients require higher positive end expiratory pressure and increased days on ventilator without having an effect on survival.[78]

Liver-Assist Devices

Liver-assist devices could provide vital support to the patients as they await liver transplantation, or during hepatic regeneration leading to spontaneous recovery. Such devices either perform blood detoxification or provide cell-mediated biologic support. Detoxification involves plasma exchange, whole blood exchange, hemoperfusion, standard hemodialysis, or high-permeability dialysis.[79] In clinical studies, those methods showed some increase in the level of consciousness, but there was no persistent improvement.[79] Currently, albumin dialysis methods are preferred because albumin is an effective scavenger of most liver toxins, which are small and hydrophobic.[80] One such device is molecular adsorbent circulatory system (MARS) and another is Prometheus.[81] MARS treatment causes an improvement in mental status; however, larger studies are needed to confirm its utility in ALF.[82] Bioartificial liver (BAL) devices use a cartridge populated with hepatocytes separated from the patient's blood by a semipermeable membrane, which allows passage of small molecules.[83] Hepatocytes provide essential functions and may remain viable for prolonged periods. Further studies are needed to confirm BAL's clinical utility.

Liver Transplantation

Liver transplantation should be considered for all patients determined to have DILI ALF with likely poor prognosis. Such patients should be promptly transferred to a facility providing liver transplant. Patients with ALF receive highest priority for organ allocation (https://optn.transplant.hrsa.gov/governance/policies/). The decision regarding transplantation could be challenging considering the need to transplant before prohibitive complications develop, and concurrently to avoid unnecessary or futile transplants.

SUMMARY

Drug-induced ALF disproportionately affects women and nonwhites. It is most frequently caused by antimicrobials and to a lesser extent by complementary and alternative medications, antiepileptics, antimetabolites, nonsteroidals, and statins. No characteristic features distinguish DILI ALF patients from those caused by other causes. Most DILI ALF patients have hepatocellular injury pattern. CE and ICH are the most serious complications of ALF. Other complications include coagulopathy, sepsis, metabolic derangements, and renal, circulatory, and respiratory dysfunction. Although improvements in intensive care have improved the outlook of patients with DILI ALF, many require liver transplantation. Reliable prognostic assessment is critical in the decision making for transplant. Liver-assist devices may provide a bridge to transplantation or to spontaneous recovery.

REFERENCES

1. Bernal W, Lee WM, Wendon J, et al. Acute liver failure: a curable disease by 2024? J Hepatol 2015;62(1 Suppl):S112–20.
2. Trey C, Lipworth L, Chalmers TC, et al. Fulminant hepatic failure. Presumable contribution to halothane. N Engl J Med 1968;279(15):798–801.
3. Hoofnagle JH, Carithers RL Jr, Shapiro C, et al. Fulminant hepatic failure: summary of a workshop. Hepatology 1995;21(1):240–52.
4. Kim WR, Lake JR, Smith JM, et al. Liver. Am J Transplant 2016;16(S2):69–98.
5. Lee WM, Squires RH Jr, Nyberg SL, et al. Acute liver failure: summary of a workshop. Hepatology 2008;47(4):1401–15.
6. Goldberg DS, Forde KA, Carbonari DM, et al. Population-representative incidence of drug-induced acute liver failure based on an analysis of an integrated health care system. Gastroenterology 2015;148(7):1353–61.e1353.
7. Reuben A, Koch DG, Lee WM, Acute Liver Failure Study Group. Drug-induced acute liver failure: results of a U.S. multicenter, prospective study. Hepatology 2010;52(6):2065–76.
8. Polson J, Lee WM, American Association for the Study of Liver D. AASLD position paper: the management of acute liver failure. Hepatology 2005;41(5):1179–97.
9. Shakil AO, Kramer D, Mazariegos GV, et al. Acute liver failure: clinical features, outcome analysis, and applicability of prognostic criteria. Liver Transpl 2000; 6(2):163–9.
10. BjÖRnsson E, Kalaitzakis E, Olsson R. The impact of eosinophilia and hepatic necrosis on prognosis in patients with drug-induced liver injury. Aliment Pharmacol Ther 2007;25(12):1411–21.
11. Sass DA, Shakil AO. Fulminant hepatic failure. Liver Transpl 2005;11(6):594–605.

12. Rama Rao KV, Jayakumar AR, Norenberg MD. Brain edema in acute liver failure: mechanisms and concepts. Metab Brain Dis 2014;29(4):927–36.
13. Lisman T, Porte RJ. Activation and regulation of hemostasis in acute liver failure and acute pancreatitis. Semin Thromb Hemost 2010;36(4):437–43.
14. Pernambuco JR, Langley PG, Hughes RD, et al. Activation of the fibrinolytic system in patients with fulminant liver failure. Hepatology 1993;18(6):1350–6.
15. Lisman T, Stravitz RT. Rebalanced hemostasis in patients with acute liver failure. Semin Thromb Hemost 2015;41(5):468–73.
16. Lisman T, Caldwell SH, Burroughs AK, et al. Hemostasis and thrombosis in patients with liver disease: the ups and downs. J Hepatol 2010;53(2):362–71.
17. Tujios SR, Hynan LS, Vazquez MA, et al. Risk factors and outcomes of acute kidney injury in patients with acute liver failure. Clin Gastroenterol Hepatol 2015; 13(2):352–9.
18. Bihari DJ, Gimson AE, Williams R. Cardiovascular, pulmonary and renal complications of fulminant hepatic failure. Semin Liver Dis 1986;6(2):119–28.
19. Wlodzimirow KA, Eslami S, Abu-Hanna A, et al. Systematic review: acute liver failure—one disease, more than 40 definitions. Aliment Pharmacol Ther 2012;35(11): 1245–56.
20. Bernuau J, Benhamou JP. Classifying acute liver failure. Lancet 1993;342(8866): 252–3.
21. O'Grady JG, Schalm SW, Williams R. Acute liver failure: redefining the syndromes. Lancet 1993;342(8866):273–5.
22. Larson AM, Polson J, Fontana RJ, et al. Acetaminophen-induced acute liver failure: results of a United States multicenter, prospective study. Hepatology 2005; 42(6):1364–72.
23. Tandon BN, Bernauau J, O'Grady J, et al. Recommendations of the international association for the study of the liver subcommittee on nomenclature of acute and subacute liver failure. J Gastroenterol Hepatol 1999;14(5):403–4.
24. Jalan R, Yurdaydin C, Bajaj JS, et al. Toward an improved definition of acute-on-chronic liver failure. Gastroenterology 2014;147(1):4–10.
25. Chalasani N, Bonkovsky HL, Fontana R, et al. Features and outcomes of 899 patients with drug-induced liver injury: the DILIN prospective study. Gastroenterology 2015;148(7):1340–52.e1347.
26. Watkins PB. How to diagnose and exclude drug-induced liver injury. Dig Dis 2015;33(4):472–6.
27. Danan G, Benichou C. Causality assessment of adverse reactions to drugs–I. A novel method based on the conclusions of international consensus meetings: application to drug-induced liver injuries. J Clin Epidemiol 1993;46(11):1323–30.
28. Aithal GP. Pharmacogenetic testing in idiosyncratic drug-induced liver injury: current role in clinical practice. Liver Int 2015;35(7):1801–8.
29. Sundaram V, Shaikh OS. Acute liver failure: current practice and recent advances. Gastroenterol Clin North Am 2011;40(3):523–39.
30. Struecker B, Raschzok N, Sauer IM. Liver support strategies: cutting-edge technologies. Nat Rev Gastroenterol Hepatol 2014;11(3):166–76.
31. Lee WM. Liver: determining prognosis in acute liver failure. Nat Rev Gastroenterol Hepatol 2012;9(4):192–4.
32. O'Grady JG, Alexander GJ, Hayllar KM, et al. Early indicators of prognosis in fulminant hepatic failure. Gastroenterology 1989;97(2):439–45.
33. Stine JG, Lewis JH. Current and future directions in the treatment and prevention of drug-induced liver injury: a systematic review. Expert Rev Gastroenterol Hepatol 2016;10(4):517–36.

34. Nakamura M, Nagamine T. The effect of carnitine supplementation on hyperammonemia and carnitine deficiency treated with valproic acid in a psychiatric setting. Innov Clin Neurosci 2015;12(9–10):18–24.
35. Sevilla-Mantilla C, Ortega L, Agúndez JAG, et al. Leflunomide-induced acute hepatitis. Dig Liver Dis 2004;36(1):82–4.
36. Chughlay MF, Kramer N, Spearman CW, et al. N-acetylcysteine for non-paracetamol drug-induced liver injury: a systematic review. Br J Clin Pharmacol 2016;81(6):1021–9.
37. Lee WM, Hynan LS, Rossaro L, et al. Intravenous N-acetylcysteine improves transplant-free survival in early stage non-acetaminophen acute liver failure. Gastroenterology 2009;137(3):856–04.
38. Giordano C, Rivas J, Zervos X. An update on treatment of drug-induced liver injury. J Clin Transl Hepatol 2014;2(2):74–9.
39. Mumtaz K, Azam Z, Hamid S, et al. Role of N-acetylcysteine in adults with non-acetaminophen-induced acute liver failure in a center without the facility of liver transplantation. Hepatol Int 2009;3(4):563–70.
40. Czaja AJ. Drug-induced autoimmune-like hepatitis. Dig Dis Sci 2011;56(4):958–76.
41. Wree A, Dechêne A, Herzer K, et al. Steroid and ursodesoxycholic acid combination therapy in severe drug-induced liver injury. Digestion 2011;84(1):54–9.
42. Dignan FL, Wynn RF, Hadzic N, et al. BCSH/BSBMT guideline: diagnosis and management of veno-occlusive disease (sinusoidal obstruction syndrome) following haematopoietic stem cell transplantation. Br J Haematol 2013;163(4):444–57.
43. Blei AT. Brain edema in acute liver failure. Crit Care Clin 2008;24(1):99–114.
44. Jackson EW, Zacks S, Zinn S, et al. Delayed neuropsychologic dysfunction after liver transplantation for acute liver failure: a matched, case-controlled study. Liver Transpl 2002;8(10):932–6.
45. Steiner LA, Andrews PJD. Monitoring the injured brain: ICP and CBF. Br J Anaesth 2006;97(1):26–38.
46. Larsen FS. Cerebral blood flow in hyperammonemia: heterogeneity and starling forces in capillaries. Metab Brain Dis 2002;17(4):229–35.
47. Czosnyka M, Brady K, Reinhard M, et al. Monitoring of cerebrovascular autoregulation: facts, myths, and missing links. Neurocrit Care 2009;10(3):373–86.
48. Stravitz RT, Kramer AH, Davern T, et al. Intensive care of patients with acute liver failure: recommendations of the U.S. acute liver failure study group. Crit Care Med 2007;35(11):2498–508.
49. Blei AT, Olafsson S, Webster S, et al. Complications of intracranial pressure monitoring in fulminant hepatic failure. Lancet 1993;341(8838):157–8.
50. Keays RT, Alexander GJ, Williams R. The safety and value of extradural intracranial pressure monitors in fulminant hepatic failure. J Hepatol 1993;18(2):205–9.
51. Le TV, Rumbak MJ, Liu SS, et al. Insertion of intracranial pressure monitors in fulminant hepatic failure patients: early experience using recombinant factor VII. Neurosurgery 2010;66(3):455–8 [discussion: 458].
52. Gabor AJ, Brooks AG, Scobey RP, et al. Intracranial pressure during epileptic seizures. Electroencephalogr Clin Neurophysiol 1984;57(6):497–506.
53. Warrillow SJ, Bellomo R. Preventing cerebral oedema in acute liver failure: the case for quadruple-H therapy. Anaesth Intensive Care 2014;42(1):78–88.
54. Strauss G, Hansen BA, Knudsen GM, et al. Hyperventilation restores cerebral blood flow autoregulation in patients with acute liver failure. J Hepatol 1998;28(2):199–203.

55. Ellis A, Wendon J. Circulatory, respiratory, cerebral, and renal derangements in acute liver failure: pathophysiology and management. Semin Liver Dis 1996; 16(4):379–88.

56. Canalese J, Gimson AE, Davis C, et al. Controlled trial of dexamethasone and mannitol for the cerebral oedema of fulminant hepatic failure. Gut 1982;23(7): 625–9.

57. Battison C, Andrews PJD, Graham C, et al. Randomized, controlled trial on the effect of a 20% mannitol solution and a 7.5% saline/6% dextran solution on increased intracranial pressure after brain injury. Crit Care Med 2005;33(1): 196–202 [discussion: 257–8].

58. Rockswold GL, Solid CA, Paredes-Andrade E, et al. Hypertonic saline and its effect on intracranial pressure, cerebral perfusion pressure, and brain tissue oxygen. Neurosurgery 2009;65(6):1035–41 [discussion: 1041–2].

59. Jalan R, Olde Damink SW, Deutz NE, et al. Moderate hypothermia in patients with acute liver failure and uncontrolled intracranial hypertension. Gastroenterology 2004;127(5):1338–46.

60. Dmello D, Cruz-Flores S, Matuschak GM. Moderate hypothermia with intracranial pressure monitoring as a therapeutic paradigm for the management of acute liver failure: a systematic review. Intensive Care Med 2010;36(2):210–3.

61. Karvellas CJ, Todd Stravitz R, Battenhouse H, et al. Therapeutic hypothermia in acute liver failure: a multicenter retrospective cohort analysis. Liver Transpl 2015;21(1):4–12.

62. Forbes A, Alexander GJ, O'Grady JG, et al. Thiopental infusion in the treatment of intracranial hypertension complicating fulminant hepatic failure. Hepatology 1989;10(3):306–10.

63. Gazzard BG, Henderson JM, Williams R. Early changes in coagulation following a paracetamol overdose and a controlled trial of fresh frozen plasma therapy. Gut 1975;16(8):617–20.

64. Shami VM, Caldwell SH, Hespenheide EE, et al. Recombinant activated factor VII for coagulopathy in fulminant hepatic failure compared with conventional therapy. Liver Transpl 2003;9(2):138–43.

65. Rolando N, Wade J, Davalos M, et al. The systemic inflammatory response syndrome in acute liver failure. Hepatology 2000;32(4 Pt 1):734–9.

66. Rolando N, Harvey F, Brahm J, et al. Prospective study of bacterial infection in acute liver failure: an analysis of fifty patients. Hepatology 1990;11(1):49–53.

67. Rolando N, Harvey F, Brahm J, et al. Fungal infection: a common, unrecognised complication of acute liver failure. J Hepatol 1991;12(1):1–9.

68. Vaquero J, Polson J, Chung C, et al. Infection and the progression of hepatic encephalopathy in acute liver failure. Gastroenterology 2003;125(3):755–64.

69. Rolando N, Gimson A, Wade J, et al. Prospective controlled trial of selective parenteral and enteral antimicrobial regimen in fulminant liver failure. Hepatology 1993;17(2):196–201.

70. Arai K, Lee K, Berthiaume F, et al. Intrahepatic amino acid and glucose metabolism in a D-galactosamine-induced rat liver failure model. Hepatology 2001; 34(2):360–71.

71. Harry R, Auzinger G, Wendon J. The clinical importance of adrenal insufficiency in acute hepatic dysfunction. Hepatology 2002;36(2):395–402.

72. Schneeweiss B, Pammer J, Ratheiser K, et al. Energy metabolism in acute hepatic failure. Gastroenterology 1993;105(5):1515–21.

73. Ring-Larsen H, Palazzo U. Renal failure in fulminant hepatic failure and terminal cirrhosis: a comparison between incidence, types, and prognosis. Gut 1981; 22(7):585–91.

74. Davenport A, Will EJ, Davidson AM. Improved cardiovascular stability during continuous modes of renal replacement therapy in critically ill patients with acute hepatic and renal failure. Crit Care Med 1993;21(3):328–38.

75. Wendon JA, Harrison PM, Keays R, et al. Effects of vasopressor agents and epoprostenol on systemic hemodynamics and oxygen transport in fulminant hepatic failure. Hepatology 1992;15(6):1067–71.

76. Larsen FS, Strauss G, Knudsen GM, et al. Cerebral perfusion, cardiac output, and arterial pressure in patients with fulminant hepatic failure. Crit Care Med 2000;28(4):996–1000.

77. Baudouin SV, Howdle P, O'Grady JG, et al. Acute lung injury in fulminant hepatic failure following paracetamol poisoning. Thorax 1995;50(4):399–402.

78. Audimoolam VK, McPhail MJW, Wendon JA, et al. Lung injury and its prognostic significance in acute liver failure. Crit Care Med 2014;42(3):592–600.

79. Splendiani G, Tancredi M, Daniele M, et al. Treatment of acute liver failure with hemodetoxification techniques. Int J Artif Organs 1990;13(6):370–4.

80. Mitzner SR, Stange J, Klammt S, et al. Albumin dialysis MARS: knowledge from 10 years of clinical investigation. ASAIO J 2009;55(5):498–502.

81. Kantola T, Koivusalo A-M, Hockerstedt K, et al. The effect of molecular adsorbent recirculating system treatment on survival, native liver recovery, and need for liver transplantation in acute liver failure patients. Transpl Int 2008;21(9):857–66.

82. Khuroo MS, Khuroo MS, Farahat KL. Molecular adsorbent recirculating system for acute and acute-on-chronic liver failure: a meta-analysis. Liver Transpl 2004; 10(9):1099–106.

83. Wang Y, Susando T, Lei X, et al. Current development of bioreactors for extracorporeal bioartificial liver (Review). Biointerphases 2010;5(3):FA116–31.

Management of Acute Hepatotoxicity Including Medical Agents and Liver Support Systems

(®) CrossMark

Humberto C. Gonzalez, MD[a], Syed-Mohammed Jafri, MD[b],
Stuart C. Gordon, MD[b],*

KEYWORDS

- Drug-induced liver injury • Acute liver failure • Liver support systems
- Artificial liver support systems • Bioartificial liver support systems

KEY POINTS

- Drug-induced liver injury (DILI) represents a toxic injury to the liver from prescription drugs, herbals, over-the-counter medications, or dietary supplements.
- Clinical presentation of DILI can vary from asymptomatic liver test elevation to chronic liver injury and acute liver failure (ALF); there is no specific test that confirms DILI and it remains a diagnosis of exclusion.
- The cornerstone of DILI treatment is the discontinuation of the offending drug; only a few medications/toxins, such as acetaminophen, have specific antidotes, otherwise treatment is largely supportive.
- Liver transplantation is the best-proven strategy to improve survival in ALF secondary to DILI; liver support systems artificial (membrane-based) and bioartificial (cell-based) can stabilize liver function.

INTRODUCTION

Drug-induced liver injury (DILI) is a broad term that refers to any injury to the liver by a prescribed medication, over-the-counter medication, herb, or dietary supplement.[1] Manifestations of DILI range from asymptomatic liver test elevations to acute liver failure (ALF). The true incidence of DILI has been difficult to establish given that a

The authors have nothing to disclose.
[a] Department of Transplant Surgery/Center of Advanced Liver Disease, Methodist University Hospital, University of Tennessee Health Science Center, 1211 Union Avenue, Suite 340, Memphis, TN 38104, USA; [b] Division of Gastroenterology and Hepatology, Henry Ford Health System, 2799 West Grand Boulevard, Detroit, MI 48202, USA
* Corresponding author.
E-mail address: sgordon3@hfhs.org

Clin Liver Dis 21 (2017) 163–180
http://dx.doi.org/10.1016/j.cld.2016.08.012
1089-3261/17/© 2016 Elsevier Inc. All rights reserved.

diagnostic test is lacking, the number of persons exposed to individual drugs is unknown, patients can be largely asymptomatic, causality is difficult to establish, and cases are likely underreported. Based on data from France and Iceland, the incidence of DILI has been estimated to be between 13.9 and 19.1 cases per 100,000 persons per year.[2,3]

Most DILI cases resolve with the cessation of the suspected causative agent. Nevertheless, a few cases progress to chronic DILI or ALF requiring liver transplantation. The Drug-Induced Liver Injury Network (DILIN), a cooperative US study, reported that 6 months after having significant DILI, 14% of 300 patients had abnormal liver biochemistries (chronic DILI).[4] Based on 10.5 years of prospective data, The Acute Liver Failure Study Group has reported that 11% of ALF cases are secondary to idiosyncratic DILI.[5] Depending on the causal agent, approximately 2% of patients who experience DILI require liver transplantation, with a 1-year survival rate of 76% to 82%.[4,6] When liver transplantation is contraindicated or there is organ shortage, extracorporeal liver support systems are useful to stabilize liver function.[7]

CHARACTERIZATION OF DRUG-INDUCED LIVER INJURY

DILI is divided into intrinsic and idiosyncratic types. Intrinsic refers to drugs, such as acetaminophen, that reliably result in liver damage on sufficient exposure. Idiosyncratic DILI is unpredictable, has less relationship to the dose, has a variable latency period, and is less common. Examples of drugs that can trigger idiosyncratic DILI include antibiotics, anticonvulsants, nonsteroidal anti-inflammatory drugs, and isoniazid.[1,8]

DILI is also divided into 3 main categories based on biochemical injury patterns: hepatocellular, cholestatic, and mixed. To determine the category, an R ratio or value is established on the basis of the ratio of alanine aminotransferase (ALT) to alkaline phosphate (ALP) to their upper limits of normal (ULN) (R value = [ALT/ULN]/[ALP/ULN]). An R value greater than 5 is defined as hepatocellular injury, less than 2 is cholestatic injury, and between 2 and 5 is a mixed pattern.[8,9] The R value can assist in identifying the causal agent because some drugs produce a typical pattern of injury, although patterns can vary with the same medication.[1]

DILI can be further characterized as immune-mediated versus nonimmune-mediated. Immune-mediated resembles an allergic/hypersensitivity reaction with an early onset and rapid re-injury on reintroduction of the offending agent. It is characterized by fever, rash, eosinophilia, autoantibodies, and includes Stevens-Johnson or toxic epidermal necrolysis syndromes. Nonimmune-mediated DILI has a slow onset, absence of systemic features, and delayed injury on rechallenge.[1]

Workup and Differential Diagnosis

DILI remains a significant diagnostic challenge because many drugs can resemble all known causes of acute or chronic hepatitis.[10] In addition, there is no specific test to rule DILI in or out, and DILI therefore is diagnosed by exclusion. A critical component in evaluating abnormal liver biochemistries is to obtain a detailed history including medications and herbals that have been used in the 6 months before onset. With some drugs (nitrofurantoin and minocycline) latency periods may be longer and the time frame for evaluation should be expanded to 1 year.[8]

The R value can assist in the investigation of DILI. In hepatocellular or mixed patterns, the first line of testing includes viral hepatitis, autoimmune serologies, and liver imaging (usually ultrasound). The second line of testing should be individualized and can include serum ceruloplasmin, and tests for cytomegalovirus, Epstein-Barr virus, and hepatitis E, all potentially followed by a liver biopsy. With a cholestatic pattern of liver injury, imaging is usually the first line of testing. Serologies for primary biliary cholangitis could be performed when the acuity of the onset is in doubt. Cholangiography via endoscopic retrograde pancreatography or magnetic resonance cholangiopancreatography should be performed. A liver biopsy could be the next step if the diagnosis is unclear.[8] LiverTox (http://www.livertox.nih.gov/), an online resource for DILI that contains detailed information on more than 600 agents, should be consulted.

Acute viral infections, such as hepatitis C and hepatitis E, need to be properly ruled out, as they are known masqueraders of DILI. DILIN reports indicate that acute hepatitis C accounts for 1.3% of suspected DILI cases and therefore needs to be ruled out with hepatitis C RNA testing.[4] Moreover, approximately 3% of patients with suspected DILI test positive for hepatitis E.[11] It is recommended that immunoglobulin M antihepatitis E antibodies be investigated, particularly in patients who have traveled to endemic areas.[8]

Autoimmune hepatitis (AIH) should be considered in the differential diagnosis of DILI. In a review of well-established AIH cases at Mayo Clinic, 9% were found to be drug-induced (DIAIH). Common culprits of DIAIH are nitrofurantoin and minocycline. DIAIH and AIH have common histologic findings, but distinguishing between these 2 entities is important because discontinuing immunosuppression is possible in all DIAIH cases but only one-third of AIH cases.[12]

Histopathologic Features of Drug-Induced Liver Injury and the Role of Liver Biopsy

Liver biopsy is a resource for the evaluation process, but it is not mandatory. Among the first 300 patients in the DILIN registry, nearly 50% had a liver biopsy.[4] Kleiner and colleagues[13] described DILI histopathology by pattern of biochemical injury, relationship to laboratory abnormality, and severity. Liver biopsy might be helpful when AIH and DILI diagnosis compete and also when rechallenge with the potentially offending drug is being contemplated.

Differentiation of Drug-Induced Liver Injury from Autoimmune Hepatitis

Histologic features of AIH and DILI commonly overlap, and there is no unique feature that discriminates them. Traditionally, prominent eosinophilic infiltration has been regarded as DILI specific, but recent evidence does not support this observation.[14] The presence of interface hepatitis, focal necrosis, and portal inflammation is common to both conditions, but tends to be severe in AIH. In addition, portal and intra-acinar plasma cells, rosette formation, and emperipolesis favors a diagnosis of AIH. Portal neutrophils and intracellular cholestasis are more prevalent in DILI (cholestatic variety).[14]

Based on predictive modeling,[14] patients are more likely to have hepatocellular DILI than AIH in the presence of prominent intra-acinar lymphocyte infiltrate or canalicular cholestasis without any of the 4 AIH-favorable features (portal inflammation score of >2, rosette formation, prominent portal plasma infiltrates, and prominent intra-acinar eosinophils) or the combination of prominent intra-acinar lymphocyte infiltrate, canalicular cholestasis, and less than 2 of the 4 AIH-favorable features. Fibrosis, portal inflammation, intracellular cholestasis, prominent portal neutrophil infiltrates, and focal necrosis (or portal plasma cell infiltrates) are indicative of cholestatic DILI versus AIH.[14]

Determination of Causality

The Roussel Uclaf Causality Assessment Method (RUCAM) is an instrument to objectively assist clinicians in establishing causality of DILI. Built on expert opinion, it is the most widely used tool for DILI. RUCAM is not free of shortcomings: it is not user-friendly, it requires a high level of expertise to administer (ambiguities on how to score certain sections), does not include histology, and it incorporates rechallenge.[8,9,15–18] To overcome RUCAM pitfalls, the clinical diagnostic scale of Maria and Victorino scale was developed. This tool is simple to administer but is somewhat less predictive in chronic liver injury and in DILI with longer latency periods (see Amina Ibrahim Shehu and colleagues' article, "Mechanisms of drug induced hepatotoxicity," in this issue).[19,20]

MANAGEMENT OF DRUG-INDUCED LIVER INJURY

Most DILI cases are asymptomatic and/or detected incidentally in routine blood screening. When symptomatic, jaundice is the most common presenting symptom.[21] The median duration from diagnosis to resolution of liver biochemical abnormalities is 64 days.[3]

Once the diagnosis of DILI is established, the suspected causal drug must be discontinued, but there is no solid evidence that length of exposure to the drug affects risk of ALF.[8,21] Except in cases in which an antidote is available, therapy for DILI remains largely supportive. In cases in which DILI is severe, liver support systems may be used as a bridge to liver transplantation while awaiting an organ offer or as a long-term therapy (**Fig. 1**).

Drugs That Have Antidotes

Acetaminophen
Acetaminophen (paracetamol) is one of the most common analgesics and antipyretics used worldwide. In the United States, its toxicity is responsible for 56,000 emergency department visits and 26,000 hospitalizations per year, of which 1% develop severe

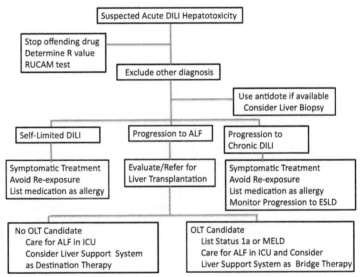

Fig. 1. Algorithm of management in acute hepatotoxicity. ALF, acute liver failure; DILI, drug-induced liver injury; ESLD, end-stage liver disease; ICU, intensive care unit; MELD, Model for End Stage Liver Disease; OLT, orthotopic liver transplantation; RUCAM, Roussel Uclaf Causality Assessment Method.

coagulopathy or encephalopathy. Forty percent to 50% of cases with severe DILI in the United States and Westernized countries are due to acetaminophen.[5,22–25] Acetaminophen toxicity can occur as a consequence of a single overdose (usually with attempt to self-harm) or after repeated excessive doses (usually with therapeutic intent).[26,27]

Acetaminophen is absorbed rapidly in the gastrointestinal tract, and peak concentrations are reached between 30 minutes and 2 hours for therapeutic doses as compared with 4 hours with overdosing.[28–30] Elimination half-lives range between 2 and 4 hours, but this can be delayed with extended formulations.[31] Acetaminophen is mostly metabolized in the liver, 90% by glucuronidation and sulfation,[28,32,33] and the rest by the hepatic cytochrome P450 (CYP2E1, CYP1A2, CYP3A4) into N-Acetyl-p-benzoquinoneimine (NAPQI), which is toxic, reactive, and responsible for liver injury in overdosing.[33–35] NAPQI is rapidly conjugated with hepatic glutathione-forming, nontoxic compounds and then excreted in the urine.[32]

When toxic doses are ingested, the sulfation and glucuronidation pathways are saturated, and more acetaminophen is metabolized by NAPQI via cytochrome P450, leading to glutathione depletion with subsequent liver injury.[32,36] Chronic alcohol ingestion can induce CYP2E1 activity, increasing the rate of NAPQI formation even at recommended doses of acetaminophen, which can lead to DILI.[37]

Therapeutic concentrations of acetaminophen range from 10 to 20 µg/mL (65–130 µmol/L) in serum. An acetaminophen blood level should be drawn at 4 hours after ingestion or immediately any time after 4 hours; levels before 4 hours do not represent peak doses. The level should then be plotted in the Rumack-Matthew nomogram to guide clinical management.[38,39] The ingested dose does not reliably predict serum level concentrations and should be interpreted with caution.[40] In individuals with chronic acetaminophen overdose, serum concentrations tend to be in the therapeutic range; levels do not correlate with toxicity.[27,37] The Rumack-Matthew nomogram has not been validated for extended release preparations.

Gastric decontamination with activated charcoal is advised if toxic acetaminophen ingestion has occurred within 4 hours, and it can be effective up to 16 hours after ingestion.[41] Activated charcoal is more efficacious than gastric lavage or drug-induced emesis and results in decreased hepatotoxicity as well as decreased serum concentration of acetaminophen.[42–44] N-acetylcysteine (NAC) should follow gastric decontamination.

NAC is the universal antidote for acetaminophen intoxication. It is believed that NAC restores glutathione, which subsequently limits or prevents hepatotoxicity. No randomized clinical trials have compared placebo versus NAC, as they would be unethical. NAC can be administered orally or intravenously (ie, 20-hour intravenously [IV], 72-hour orally, 12-hour IV) (**Table 1**).[45–47] A meta-analysis by Green and colleagues[48] comparing oral versus IV administration of NAC indicated that the administration route has no significant effect on hepatotoxicity. Hepatoxicity is 5.7% (95% confidence interval [CI] 4.3%–7.4%) for NAC administered less than 10 hours after ingestion and 26% (95% CI 23.6%–29%) for NAC administered more than 10 hours after ingestion.

The optimal duration of NAC treatment has not been determined. Given that the spectrum of acetaminophen intoxication is broad (acute vs chronic, single vs repeated ingestion, early vs late presentation, known vs unknown exposure time, liver test elevation vs liver failure), a fixed dose or duration seems inadequate. Administration of NAC is usually patient tailored and goal directed. Three criteria commonly guide treatment discontinuation: acetaminophen level should be zero or near zero, ALT level should be markedly improved, and the patient should have clinical improvement or stability.[49]

Table 1
Antidote regimens for drug-mediated acute hepatotoxicity

Drug	Antidote	Route	Regimen
Acetaminophen[45,46,101]	NAC	IV	20-h Load: 150 mg/kg over 15–60 min, then 4 h 12.5 mg/kg/h, then 16 h 6.25 mg/kg/h
		IV	Simplified 20-h 4 h 50 mg/kg/h, then 16 h 6.25 mg/kg/h
		PO	72-h Load: 140 mg/kg, then 70 mg/kg every 4 h for 17 doses
Amanita[54,63]	Benzylpenicillin	IV	0.3–1 million units/kg/d continuous infusion for 2–3 d
	Silymarin	IV	20–50 mg/kg/d in 4 divided doses, continue 48–96 h after ingestion
	NAC	IV	Load: 150 mg/kg over 15 min, then Maint: 50 mg/kg over 4 h, then 100 mg/kg over 16 h
Valproic acid[67]	L-carnitine	IV	Load: 100 mg/kg in 30 min, maximum 3 g, then Maint: 15 mg/kg every 4 h in 1–30 min

Abbreviations: IV, intravenous; Load, loading dose; Maint, maintenance dose, NAC, N-acetylcysteine; PO, oral.

In ALF, NAC should be administered IV and continued until resolution of liver injury or liver transplantation.[50] There is a clear advantage of NAC utilization in liver failure, as it is associated with decreased cerebral edema, hypotension, and mortality.[50]

Acetaminophen is a dialyzable medication, and extracorporeal removal can serve as an adjunctive therapy. The safety and efficacy of this therapy has not been extensively described, and NAC should remain the mainstay treatment. In selected cases, such as concomitant acute renal failure requiring renal replacement, mitochondrial dysfunction, severe metabolic acidosis, and very high concentrations of acetaminophen, extracorporeal removal can be considered.[51,52] Attention is advised on the NAC dosing, as it also can be removed with hemodialysis but not with venovenous hemofiltration.[53]

Amanita phalloides

Mushroom picking and consumption increases the risk of intoxication due to misidentification.[54] In the United States, 6,600 mushroom intoxications were reported in 2012.[55] Most human fatalities are caused by cyclopeptide-containing mushrooms, which have amatoxins. Amatoxins are the main toxic agent of *Amanita* (*Amanita phalloides*, *Amanita virosa*, and *Amanita verna*), *Lepiota* (*Lepiota brunneoincarnata*), and *Galerina* (*Galerina marginata*). Among these, *A phalloides* is responsible for most fatal cases due to mushroom toxicity.[54]

Amatoxins are absorbed in the gastrointestinal tract, and the liver is the first organ to be targeted.[56] The toxins do not undergo any metabolism and are mainly excreted by urine; a small amount is eliminated by bile but might be reabsorbed via the enterohepatic circulation.[54] α-amanitin, the main amatoxin, accumulates in the liver after uptake by an organic anion-transporting octapeptide (OATP1B3) that is located in the sinusoidal membrane.[57] In hepatocytes, α-amanitin binds and inhibits RNA polymerase II. The subsequent decline in messenger RNA leads to decreased protein synthesis and cellular death.[58]

Amanita toxicity is classically divided into 3 phases; gastrointestinal, where acute symptoms such as nausea, vomiting, diarrhea, electrolytes imbalance, and abdominal pain present; latency (asymptomatic); and hepatorenal, in which liver, kidney, and multisystem organ failure may occur.[56]

The first treatment approach should be to decrease absorption of and inactivate toxins; the former includes gastric lavage and/or endoscopic removal and the latter refers to the use of activated charcoal. These interventions start to lose efficacy after 1 hour from ingestion. Although the efficacy of charcoal has not been validated in clinical trials, it is widely used given its potential additional effect in the enterohepatic circulation.[54] Forced diuresis (100–200 mL/h for 4–5 days) can accelerate toxin excretion.[59] In contrast to acetaminophen, *Amanita* does not have a well-established antidote, but benzylpenicillin, NAC, and silymarin are possible options.[60]

Benzylpenicillin (penicillin G) effect is believed to be secondary to a potent inhibition of the OATP13B transporter; blockage of α-amanitin uptake. The use of benzylpenicillin has been described in multiple case reports and small case series. Larger studies have had mixed results. Moroni and colleagues[61] described 47 patients that were treated with benzylpenicillin monotherapy and had a 4% mortality rate. This study is supported by results of a 15-year retrospective analysis in which benzylpenicillin was used with activated charcoal and mortality was 1.8%.[62] On the other hand, a 20-year retrospective study reported a mortality of 7.8% when benzylpenicillin was used in combination with hemoperfusion and hemodialysis as compared with 22% when used with forced diuresis, hemodialysis, and plasmapheresis.[63] Akin and colleagues[64] documented 18.7% mortality when benzylpenicillin was used in combination with gastric lavage, activated charcoal, and hemoperfusion. Despite the varying data, benzylpenicillin alone or in combination with other therapies is the most widely used drug for *Amanita* intoxication.

Amanita intoxication also has been treated with IV NAC. A study from Enjalbert and colleagues,[63] which included 86 patients, reported 7% mortality in those treated with NAC monotherapy. In one analysis, coadministering NAC with benzylpenicillin reduced mortality from 18.7% for benzylpenicillin monotherapy to 4.4% for the combination.[64] Although NAC appears to be safe and effective, both studies of its use are retrospective and should be interpreted cautiously.

Silibinin is an antioxidative and anti-inflammatory acting flavonolignan isolated from milk thistle extracts. Silibinin inhibits hepatocyte uptake of amatoxin by inhibiting OATP1B3 during gastrointestinal and enterohepatic circulation. In addition, silibinin inhibits tumor necrosis factor (TNF)-α and stimulates protein production, both of which contribute to hepatic regeneration. The administration of silibinin with or without forced diuresis, hemoperfusion, and hemodialysis results in a mortality rate of 0% to 4%.[63] In a summary of nearly 1,500 patients treated with silibinin as monotherapy or in combination with benzylpenicillin and NAC, the use of silibinin led to a mortality rate of less than 10%.[65] See **Table 1** for antidote dosing.

Even if done soon after ingestion, *Amanita* toxin removal by hemodialysis, hemoperfusion, or plasmapheresis has limited effectiveness because of the toxin's rapid absorption and excretion.[66]

Valproic acid

Valproic acid is an antiepileptic that is used for both partial and generalized seizures. It has also been approved for stabilization of manic episodes in bipolar disorder.[67] Valproic acid is rapidly absorbed in the gastrointestinal tract, and peak levels occur in 1 to

4 hours. Central nervous system depression and hyperammonemia are common symptoms of toxicity. Valproic acid hepatotoxicity has 4 recognized subtypes: transient elevation of liver tests, hyperammonemia, toxic hepatitis (idiosyncratic reaction that can lead to ALF), and Reye-like syndrome.

Risk factors for valproic acid toxicity include being younger than 2 years, having a coexisting metabolic or neurologic condition, as well as taking concomitant antiepileptics.[68] The exact mechanism of hepatotoxicity is not known, but it has been hypothesized that carnitine deficiency, inhibition of mitochondrial oxidation of long chain fatty acids, and/or inhibition of beta oxidation could explain liver damage. Activated charcoal is used for treating toxicity if overdosing occurred within 1 hour prior.[67] Administering L-carnitine intravenously is proferred in acute and severe hepatotoxicity. A retrospective analysis of patients treated with carnitine versus supportive care revealed that early and IV treatment was associated with improved hepatic survival.[69]

Additional Pharmacologic Therapeutics

Steroids
There is limited available data on treatment options beyond NAC for drug-related hepatotoxicity. Corticosteroids may be effective in managing drug-induced hepatotoxicity associated with systemic hypersensitivity or autoimmune features.[12] Medications including methyldopa, minocycline, and nitrofurantoin may cause injury that mimics the serologic, biochemical, and clinical features of autoimmune hepatitis.[12] Similarly, antiepileptic drugs often have features of hypersensitivity that may respond to corticosteroids. Patients with eosinophilia, rash, and fever may have drug-induced autoimmune disease, which could respond to corticosteroid therapy.[12,70] If DILI is severe, corticosteroid therapy should be considered, although evidence is limited in this setting.[70,71]

Wree and colleagues[72] examined patients with hepatic injury and compared 3-day steroid pulse therapy in 9 patients versus steroid step-down therapy in 15 patients. Therapy was given in combination with ursodeoxycholic acid (UDCA). Patients with no evidence of chronic liver disease had the best outcomes, with bilirubin and liver tests reducing by half within 2 weeks and normalization of laboratory parameters by 8 weeks. However, the study was not designed to demonstrate efficacy of steroid management.

Ursodeoxycholic acid
In patients who have cholestatic features, UDCA may be attempted, although data on its effectiveness is limited. UDCA stabilizes membranes, which enhances function of transporters and replaces bile salts, thereby protecting both cholangiocytes and hepatocytes.[73] Case reports indicate a potential role in vanishing bile duct syndrome and other forms of drug-induced cholestasis.[74]

Cholestyramine
Cholestyramine has been used for bile acid washout in cholestasis and pruritus. Cholestyramine is used for leflunomide toxicity in clinical practice, as drug metabolites undergo extensive enterohepatic circulation with a long half-life that can lead to inflammation even after the causative medication is discontinued.[75] Cholestyramine minimizes liver injury by disrupting the enterohepatic cycle.[75,76]

N-acetylcysteine
The use on NAC in nonacetaminophen ALF was evaluated in a 173-patient, prospective, and double-blinded clinical trial in which subjects received 72 hours of NAC IV infusion versus placebo. DILI was the etiology of ALF in 45 patients (26%). The primary

outcome, a significant increase in overall survival, was not achieved; the NAC group had 70% survival versus 66% for the non-NAC group ($P = .23$).

The percentage of patients with transplant-free survival was 52% in the NAC group versus 30% in the non-NAC group in early (grades I-II) hepatic encephalopathy ($P = .01$). In advanced encephalopathy (grades III-IV), transplant-free survival was 9% with NAC versus 22% without NAC ($P = .91$). The transplantation rate was lower in the NAC group, but the difference did not reach statistical significance (32% vs 45%; $P = .09$).[77] The benefit of NAC for nonacetaminophen ALF does not appear to extend into the pediatric population. Squires and colleagues[78] reported no improvement in 1-year survival and a lower 1-year transplant-free survival in NAC versus non-NAC treatment groups; this study, however, included very few patients with DILI.

Symptom Management

The treatment of DILI remains largely supportive. Most DILI cases do not have specific antidotes, and management revolves around medication discontinuation and symptom control. Pruritus might be particularly bothersome in cases of cholestasis. Treatments for pruritus include emollients, hydroxyzine, diphenhydramine, selective reuptake inhibitors, bile acids resins, and rifampin.[79]

Rechallenging

Rechallenging with the causative agent is discouraged, particularly if the response was severe (Hy law, aminotransferases >5 upper limit of normal and jaundice).[8] Clinicians should consider the possibility of an anamnestic response in the event of reexposure. Rechallenging should be limited to life-threatening situations or where no suitable options are available. If reexposure is considered, liver biopsy to confirm diagnosis is generally recommended as well as seeking advice from a hepatologist.[1,8]

EXTRACORPOREAL LIVER SUPPORT SYSTEMS

In ALF, liver transplantation is the only therapy with well-proven effect on survival.[80] However, transplantation might not be feasible owing to contraindications or organ shortage. Extracorporeal liver support systems can help stabilize the patient's condition in the short or long term.

Extracorporeal liver support systems can be classified into 2 main categories: artificial liver support systems (ALS) and bioartificial liver support systems (BLS). Cell-free and nonbiological, ALS uses membranes and adsorbents to filter circulating toxins. BLS are devices with hepatocytes, which improve synthetic, metabolic, and excretory functions.[7]

Albumin dialysis systems are the best-studied nonbiological liver support systems and are based on the removal of unwanted albumin-bound and water-soluble substances, such as bilirubin, ammonia, nitrotyrosine, and fatty acids. The 3 main albumin dialysis systems are molecular adsorbent reticulating system (MARS), fractionated plasma and adsorption system (Prometheus), and single-pass dialysis (SPAD).

Additional artificial support techniques include hemofiltration, hemodiafiltration, and hemoperfusion. There is limited information about their role in acute hepatotoxicity management. Most recently, high-volume plasma exchange (HVP) has regained attention based on improved survival outcomes as compared with other liver support systems.

Artificial Liver Support Systems

Molecular adsorbent reticulating system
MARS removes protein-bound and water-soluble toxins. It contains 2 dialysis circuits. The first has exogenous human albumin, which establishes contact with the patient's

blood through a semipermeable membrane that clears albumin-bound toxins. The second circuit consists of a hemodialysis unit that cleans water-soluble toxins via a bicarbonate-based dialysate. In addition, the second circuit detoxifies the albumin from the first circuit through charcoal and an anion exchanger and then recirculates the albumin to the semipermeable membrane (first circuit), reestablishing contact with the patient's blood. In Europe, MARS has been approved for acute-on-chronic liver failure (ACLD), severe alcoholic hepatitis, and pruritus secondary to cholestasis. In the United States, MARS has been approved only for acute poisoning intoxication and hepatic encephalopathy.[81]

MARS has been extensively used in noncontrolled clinical trials for acute poisoning acetaminophen toxicity. In this setting, MARS improves biochemical liver parameters, hemodynamic status, intracranial pressure, and hepatic encephalopathy.[66] The beneficial effect could in part result from acceleration of the acetaminophen clearance time from 3.4 to 1.2 hours.[82] In case reports and case series, MARS has been reported to result in biochemical and symptomatic improvement after *Amanita* intoxication.[66] It is hypothesized that the favorable effect of MARS on *Amanita* intoxication is derived from the removal of albumin-bound toxins derived from liver failure rather than *Amanita* toxin removal, because *Amanita* toxin has fast absorption and excretion.

In a clinical trial of 113 patients, in which 55% (62 patients) had a toxic ALF, 22% (32 patients) had acetaminophen toxicity, and 8% (10 patients) had amatoxin toxicity, MARS improved liver recovery in 81% of treated patients as compared with 33% of control patients (*P* = .031). However, the 6-month survival was not statistically different: 84% versus 67% for the MARS and control groups, respectively.[83] The results of this study should be interpreted with caution, as baseline Model for End Stage Liver Disease (MELD) scores were lower among patients treated with MARS, and not quite half of the acetaminophen patients had encephalopathy, whereas all the control patients did.

Saliba and colleagues[84] performed a randomized, prospective, and multicenter clinical trial comparing standard medical therapy (SMT) plus MARS versus SMT in 101 patients with ALF. Thirty-eight percent of patients had acetaminophen intoxication. The study did not find a significant difference in the treatments, with SMT having a 6-month survival rate of 75.5% (95% CI 60.8%–80.2%) and MARS having an 84.9% (95% CI 71.9%–92.8%) rate (*P* = .28). Although this was the first randomized, prospective, and multicenter study in this setting, the short period from enrollment to transplantation precludes evaluating the full potential benefit from MARS (**Table 2**).

Fractionated plasma and adsorption

The Prometheus system eliminates albumin-bound toxins by circulating a patient's blood through a semipermeable membrane. This membrane is capable of filtering albumin and smaller molecules to generate a plasmalike solution that enters a second circuit in which 2 absorbers remove toxins. The purified plasma returns to the patient's blood. A conventional hemodialysis unit is used to remove water-soluble toxins.[85] In a study of acute-on-chronic liver failure, fractionated plasma separation and adsorption led to significant drops in bilirubin levels. The intention-to-treat analysis did not show significant survival advantage at 28 or 90 days when comparing Prometheus versus SMT.[86] Use of Prometheus in ALF remains to be tested in randomized trials.

Single-pass albumin dialysis

In single-pass albumin dialysis, a conventional dialysis circuit is used to circulate an exogenous albumin solution once through a dialysate compartment and later discarded.[81] Most data regarding SPAD is limited to in vitro studies and case reports,

Table 2
Randomized clinical trials of extracorporeal liver support systems

Author	N	Clinical Scenario	Endpoint	Outcome		P	Comments
Saliba et al,[84] 2013	101	ALF 38% APAP	6-mo survival	SMT MARS	75% 84%	.28	16 h from enrollment to transplant precludes efficacy evaluation.
Larsen et al,[90] 2016	182	ALF 59% APAP	In-hospital survival	SMT HVP	48% 59%	.008	13 y to complete enrollment. ALF treatment evolved. Transfusion of FFP could have improved coagulation parameters.
Demetriou et al,[96] 2004	171	ALF/PNF	30-d survival	SMT HepAs	62% 71%	.26	In fulminant/subfulminant ALF there was survival benefit HepAs vs control; risk ratio 0.56, $P = .048$.

Abbreviations: ALF, acute liver failure; APAP, acetaminophen/paracetamol; FFP, fresh frozen plasma; HepAs, HepatAssist; HVP, high volume plasma exchange; MARS, molecular adsorbent recirculating system; PNF, primary nonfunction; SMT, standard medical therapy.

which indicate detoxification capacity. In a small case-control study of SPAD in patients with acetaminophen-induced ALF, there were no reported complications related to SPAD, but neither were there significant changes in clinical, physiologic, or biochemical parameters. There was also no difference in the rates of 1-year survival or liver transplantation referral.[87]

High-volume plasma exchange
HVP involves exchanging 8 to 12 L (or 15% of ideal body weight) of plasma with fresh frozen plasma per day. Exchange usually occurs at a rate of 1 to 2 L per hour. Early noncontrolled studies by Larsen and colleagues[88,89] reported that HVP decreased hepatic encephalopathy and the need for vasopressors in ALF.

More recently, a prospective, multicenter clinical trial randomized patients to HVP plus SMT versus SMT for ALF of any cause. In the treatment group, 54% had acetaminophen intoxication and 23% toxic hepatitis, whereas in the control group 64% had acetaminophen intoxication and 18% had toxic hepatitis. The overall survival was 58.7% for those treated with HVP versus 47.8% who had SMT alone (hazard ratio [HR] with stratification for liver transplantation, 0.56; 95% CI, 0.36–0.86; $P = .0083$). The HVP group had a decrease in international normalized ratio (INR), bilirubin, ammonia, damage-associated molecular patterns, TNF-α, and interleukin 6, with a concordant reduction of systemic inflammatory response syndrome and sequential organ failure assessment scores.[90] Although this is the first randomized controlled study to document transplant-free survival improvement with an extracorporeal liver support system, the results should be interpreted cautiously because it took 13 years to complete enrollment, all patients were treated with NAC, treatment of ALF changed over the years, and the process of plasma exchange can decrease bilirubin and INR.[91]

Bioartificial Liver Support Systems

BLS are devices that incorporate liver cells to improve the detoxification capacity and support the synthetic function of the liver. Most published studies evaluating BLS include a small number of patients.

Extracorporeal liver assist device

The extracorporeal liver assist device (ELAD) incorporates cells derived from human hepatoblastoma, Hep2/C3A. The patient's blood enters an ancillary delivery system where plasma ultrafiltrate is isolated by an ultrafiltrate generator. Next, the plasma ultrafiltrate passes into 4 hollow cartridges containing the human-derived cells. Passage fibers allow 2-way transfer of toxins, metabolites, and nutrients. The fibers, made of a semipermeable membrane, permit passage of macromolecules and other substances from the hepatoblastoma cells to the patient's plasma ultrafiltrate and transfer of toxins (bilirubin), nutrients (glucose), and oxygen from the plasma ultrafiltrate to the cells. The treated plasma ultrafiltrate then returns to the patient.[7] Hep2/C3A cells are viable for 3 to 10 days and have albumin synthetic capacity as well as cytochrome P-450 activity, although at reduced function compared with normal hepatocytes.[92]

The pilot study for ELAD included 24 patients with ALF who were randomly assigned to ELAD versus medical therapy. Patients were divided into 2 groups. In group 1, 50% survival was expected, and in group 2 liver transplant criteria were met. In ELAD-treated individuals, arterial ammonia, bilirubin, and hepatic encephalopathy were improved. There was no survival benefit in any of the groups (78% vs 75% for group 1% and 33% vs 25% in group 2).[93]

Millis and colleagues[94] did a follow-up phase 1 study with the modified ELAD system, in which ultrafiltrate rather than whole blood was used and glucose and O_2 consumption were monitored. The study included 5 patients with ALF (1 related to DILI) who were successfully bridged to transplant with the use of ELAD. This liver support system was well tolerated, and the 30-day survival was 75%. Cardiorespiratory status improved in most patients, who were able to decrease or stop vasopressor support and had improved ventilator parameters.

In 2014, ELAD started enrollment for a phase 2 clinical trial targeting ALF and surgical-induced ALF (VT-212). The study came to an early end as a result of the failure to achieve primary and secondary outcomes in a phase 3 trial (VTI-208) of alcohol-induced liver decompensation. VTI-208 also raised safety concerns for increased risk of adverse effects in patients with coagulopathy and acute kidney injury.[95]

Porcine hepatocyte-based bioartificial liver

HepatAssist comprises porcine hepatocytes contained in a hollow fiber bioreactor. The system contains a perfusion pump, a charcoal column, a combined oxygenator and blood warmer, and custom tubing connecting the components of the machine. Plasma is obtained via plasmapheresis and then passed through the hollow fiber device containing the porcine hepatocytes. The small membrane size prevents hepatocytes and cell debris from reaching the patient.[96]

The most important clinical trial of HepatAssist was a randomized and multicenter clinical trial with 171 patients with ALF or primary nonfunction after liver transplantation.[96] Patients were assigned to a liver support system plus SMT versus SMT. The main outcome was 30-day survival regardless of liver transplantation. There was no significant survival benefit with HepatAssist; 30-day survival was 71% with HepatAssist versus 62% for standard medical care alone ($P = .26$). After adjustment for liver transplantation and exclusion of primary nonfunction, HepatAssist was associated with a 44% reduction in the risk of death in the ALF population (see **Table 2**). Serum bilirubin levels had a statistically significant reduction in patients who received treatment with liver support. There were no changes in encephalopathy, hemodynamics, or other laboratory values. Although HepatAssist had a favorable safety profile, it was in the context of a heterogeneous population. No zoonosis or immune reactions were reported, but these still remain concerns given the origin of the liver cells.[97]

Emerging Therapies

The University College London–Liver Dialysis Device (UCL-LDD) is an artificial ELAD that includes a high cutoff filter extracting albumin and bound toxins by hemofiltration as well as selective endotoxin adsorption cartridges for selective endotoxin extraction by hemoperfusion.[98] Use of the device is combined with human albumin infusions. UCL-LDD was designed to ameliorate innate immune system activation. Pigs with acetaminophen-induced liver failure were randomized to treatment with UCL-LDD versus a control device. The use of UCL-LDD resulted in a 67% reduction of risk of death as compared with the control device (HR = 0.33, P = .043). The survival advantage likely was in part caused by significant reductions in oxidized human non-mercaptalbumin-2, endotoxemia, delayed systemic vasoplegia, decreased acute lung injury, and activation of TLR4 pathway.

The spheroid reservoir bioartificial liver (SRBL) uses porcine hepatocytes contained in an oscillation-based bioreactor.[99] In a trial by Glorioso and colleagues,[100] pigs with induced ALF were randomized to SMT, SMT and no cell device, or SMT and SRBL. The pigs treated with SRBL had a better survival rate (83%) than SMT alone (0%, P = .003) or no cell device (17%, P = .02). Survival correlated with ammonia detoxification and lowering of intracranial pressure, which was function of SRBL duration, hepatocyte dose, and membrane pore size.[100] These novel techniques remain to be tested in humans.

SUMMARY

DILI is rare but nevertheless a common cause of ALF. The mainstays of treatment for DILI include discontinuation of the causal drug, symptomatic treatment, and supportive care. When DILI evolves to ALF, liver transplantation evaluation is granted, as it is the only therapy that has consistently shown survival benefit. Acetaminophen and a few other drugs or toxins causing liver hepatotoxicity have specific antidotes. NAC for nonacetaminophen ALF appears to be useful only in early stages of encephalopathy. The use of UDCA and steroids remains controversial but can be attempted in selected cases.

Determining whether liver support systems are useful in DILI-related ALF is complex because few randomized clinical trials have been done, studies have generally included ALF of any etiology, and the availability of liver transplantation may prevent full understanding of the benefits of support systems. Overall, artificial and bioartificial liver support systems improve liver-related biochemistries, but only a few have shown survival advantage. Liver support systems have not received approval for routine use for the most common causes of ALF. Human data on emerging liver support systems, such as the UCL-LDD and SRBL, are eagerly awaited. Liver support systems will remain an active and evolving field to target the unmet need of high mortality in ALF.

REFERENCES

1. Leise MD, Poterucha JJ, Talwalkar JA. Drug-induced liver injury. Mayo Clin Proc 2014;89(1):95–106.
2. Sgro C, Clinard F, Ouazir K, et al. Incidence of drug-induced hepatic injuries: a French population-based study. Hepatology 2002;36(2):451–5.
3. Bjornsson ES, Bergmann OM, Björnsson HK, et al. Incidence, presentation, and outcomes in patients with drug-induced liver injury in the general population of Iceland. Gastroenterology 2013;144(7):1419–25.e1-3 [quiz: e19–20].

4. Chalasani N, Fontana RJ, Bonkovsky HL, et al. Causes, clinical features, and outcomes from a prospective study of drug-induced liver injury in the United States. Gastroenterology 2008;135(6):1924–34.e1-4.

5. Reuben A, Koch DG, Lee WM, et al. Drug-induced acute liver failure: results of a U.S. multicenter, prospective study. Hepatology 2010;52(6):2065–76.

6. Mindikoglu AL, Magder LS, Regev A. Outcome of liver transplantation for drug-induced acute liver failure in the United States: analysis of the United Network for Organ Sharing database. Liver Transpl 2009;15(7):719–29.

7. Banares R, Catalina MV, Vaquero J. Molecular adsorbent recirculating system and bioartificial devices for liver failure. Clin Liver Dis 2014;18(4):945–56.

8. Chalasani NP, Hayashi PH, Bonkovsky HL, et al. ACG clinical guideline: the diagnosis and management of idiosyncratic drug-induced liver injury. Am J Gastroenterol 2014;109(7):950–66 [quiz: 967].

9. Danan G, Benichou C. Causality assessment of adverse reactions to drugs–I. A novel method based on the conclusions of international consensus meetings: application to drug-induced liver injuries. J Clin Epidemiol 1993;46(11):1323–30.

10. Lewis JH. The art and science of diagnosing and managing drug-induced liver injury in 2015 and beyond. Clin Gastroenterol Hepatol 2015;13(12):2173–89.e8.

11. Davern TJ, Chalasani N, Fontana RJ, et al. Acute hepatitis E infection accounts for some cases of suspected drug-induced liver injury. Gastroenterology 2011; 141(5):1665–72.e1-9.

12. Bjornsson E, Talwalkar J, Treeprasertsuk S, et al. Drug-induced autoimmune hepatitis: clinical characteristics and prognosis. Hepatology 2010;51(6):2040–8.

13. Kleiner DE, Chalasani NP, Lee WM, et al. Hepatic histological findings in suspected drug-induced liver injury: systematic evaluation and clinical associations. Hepatology 2014;59(2):661–70.

14. Suzuki A, Brunt EM, Kleiner DE, et al. The use of liver biopsy evaluation in discrimination of idiopathic autoimmune hepatitis versus drug-induced liver injury. Hepatology 2011;54(3):931–9.

15. Benichou C, Danan G, Flahault A. Causality assessment of adverse reactions to drugs–II. An original model for validation of drug causality assessment methods: case reports with positive rechallenge. J Clin Epidemiol 1993;46(11):1331–6.

16. Rochon J, Protiva P, Seeff LB, et al. Reliability of the Roussel Uclaf causality assessment method for assessing causality in drug-induced liver injury. Hepatology 2008;48(4):1175–83.

17. Shapiro MA, Lewis JH. Causality assessment of drug-induced hepatotoxicity: promises and pitfalls. Clin Liver Dis 2007;11(3):477–505 v.

18. Garcia-Cortes M, Stephens C, Lucena MI, et al. Causality assessment methods in drug induced liver injury: strengths and weaknesses. J Hepatol 2011;55(3):683–91.

19. Maria VA, Victorino RM. Development and validation of a clinical scale for the diagnosis of drug-induced hepatitis. Hepatology 1997;26(3):664–9.

20. Lucena MI, Camargo R, Andrade RJ, et al. Comparison of two clinical scales for causality assessment in hepatotoxicity. Hepatology 2001;33(1):123–30.

21. Giordano C, Rivas J, Zervos X. An update on treatment of drug-induced liver injury. J Clin Transl Hepatol 2014;2(2):74–9.

22. Lee WM. Drug-induced acute liver failure. Clin Liver Dis 2013;17(4):575–86, viii.

23. Gunnell D, Murray V, Hawton K. Use of paracetamol (acetaminophen) for suicide and nonfatal poisoning: worldwide patterns of use and misuse. Suicide Life Threat Behav 2000;30(4):313–26.

24. Nourjah P, Ahmad SR, Karwoski C, et al. Estimates of acetaminophen (Paracetomal)-associated overdoses in the United States. Pharmacoepidemiol Drug Saf 2006;15(6):398–405.
25. Fontana RJ. Acute liver failure including acetaminophen overdose. Med Clin North Am 2008;92(4):761–94, viii.
26. Daly FF, O'Malley GF, Heard K, et al. Prospective evaluation of repeated supratherapeutic acetaminophen (paracetamol) ingestion. Ann Emerg Med 2004; 44(4):393–8.
27. Schiodt FV, Rochling FA, Casey DL, et al. Acetaminophen toxicity in an urban county hospital. N Engl J Med 1997;337(16):1112–7.
28. Forrest JA, Clements JA, Prescott LF. Clinical pharmacokinetics of paracetamol. Clin Pharmacokinet 1982;7(2):93–107.
29. Tighe TV, Walter FG. Delayed toxic acetaminophen level after initial four hour nontoxic level. J Toxicol Clin Toxicol 1994;32(4):431–4.
30. Bizovi KE, Aks SE, Paloucek F, et al. Late increase in acetaminophen concentration after overdose of Tylenol Extended Relief. Ann Emerg Med 1996;28(5): 549–51.
31. Cetaruk EW, Dart RC, Hurlbut KM, et al. Tylenol extended relief overdose. Ann Emerg Med 1997;30(1):104–8.
32. Mitchell JR, Jollow DJ, Potter WZ, et al. Acetaminophen-induced hepatic necrosis. IV. Protective role of glutathione. J Pharmacol Exp Ther 1973;187(1):211–7.
33. Manyike PT, Kharasch ED, Kalhorn TF, et al. Contribution of CYP2E1 and CYP3A to acetaminophen reactive metabolite formation. Clin Pharmacol Ther 2000; 67(3):275–82.
34. Bessems JG, Vermeulen NP. Paracetamol (acetaminophen)-induced toxicity: molecular and biochemical mechanisms, analogues and protective approaches. Crit Rev Toxicol 2001;31(1):55–138.
35. Thummel KE, Lee CA, Kunze KL, et al. Oxidation of acetaminophen to N-acetyl-p-aminobenzoquinone imine by human CYP3A4. Biochem Pharmacol 1993; 45(8):1563–9.
36. Linden CH, Rumack BH. Acetaminophen overdose. Emerg Med Clin North Am 1984;2(1):103–19.
37. Zimmerman HJ, Maddrey WC. Acetaminophen (paracetamol) hepatotoxicity with regular intake of alcohol: analysis of instances of therapeutic misadventure. Hepatology 1995;22(3):767–73.
38. Rumack BH, Matthew H. Acetaminophen poisoning and toxicity. Pediatrics 1975;55(6):871–6.
39. Smilkstein MJ, Douglas DR, Daya MR. Acetaminophen poisoning and liver function. N Engl J Med 1994;331(19):1310–1 [author reply: 1311–2].
40. Ambre J, Alexander M. Liver toxicity after acetaminophen ingestion. Inadequacy of the dose estimate as an index of risk. JAMA 1977;238(6):500–1.
41. Spiller HA, Winter ML, Klein-Schwartz W, et al. Efficacy of activated charcoal administered more than four hours after acetaminophen overdose. J Emerg Med 2006;30(1):1–5.
42. Spiller HA, Krenzelok EP, Grande GA, et al. A prospective evaluation of the effect of activated charcoal before oral N-acetylcysteine in acetaminophen overdose. Ann Emerg Med 1994;23(3):519–23.
43. Underhill TJ, Greene MK, Dove AF. A comparison of the efficacy of gastric lavage, ipecacuanha and activated charcoal in the emergency management of paracetamol overdose. Arch Emerg Med 1990;7(3):148–54.

44. Buckley NA, Whyte IM, O'Connell DL, et al. Activated charcoal reduces the need for N-acetylcysteine treatment after acetaminophen (paracetamol) overdose. J Toxicol Clin Toxicol 1999;37(6):753–7.

45. Smilkstein MJ, Knapp GL, Kulig KW, et al. Efficacy of oral N-acetylcysteine in the treatment of acetaminophen overdose. Analysis of the national multicenter study (1976 to 1985). N Engl J Med 1988;319(24):1557–62.

46. Prescott LF, Park J, Ballantyne A, et al. Treatment of paracetamol (acetaminophen) poisoning with N-acetylcysteine. Lancet 1977;2(8035):432–4.

47. Bateman DN, Dear JW, Thanacoody HK, et al. Reduction of adverse effects from intravenous acetylcysteine treatment for paracetamol poisoning: a randomised controlled trial. Lancet 2014;383(9918).097–704.

48. Green JL, Heard KJ, Reynolds KM, et al. Oral and intravenous acetylcysteine for treatment of acetaminophen toxicity: a systematic review and meta-analysis. West J Emerg Med 2013;14(3):218–26.

49. Dart RC, Rumack BH. Patient-tailored acetylcysteine administration. Ann Emerg Med 2007;50(3):280–1.

50. Keays R, Harrison PM, Wendon JA, et al. Intravenous acetylcysteine in paracetamol induced fulminant hepatic failure: a prospective controlled trial. BMJ 1991; 303(6809):1026–9.

51. Ash SR, Caldwell CA, Singer GG, et al. Treatment of acetaminophen-induced hepatitis and fulminant hepatic failure with extracorporeal sorbent-based devices. Adv Ren Replace Ther 2002;9(1):42–53.

52. Gosselin S, Juurlink DN, Kielstein JT, et al. Extracorporeal treatment for acetaminophen poisoning: recommendations from the EXTRIP workgroup. Clin Toxicol (Phila) 2014;52(8):856–67.

53. Hernandez SH, Howland M, Schiano TD, et al. The pharmacokinetics and extracorporeal removal of N-acetylcysteine during renal replacement therapies. Clin Toxicol (Phila) 2015;53(10):941–9.

54. Garcia J, Costa VM, Carvalho A, et al. Amanita phalloides poisoning: mechanisms of toxicity and treatment. Food Chem Toxicol 2015;86:41–55.

55. Mowry JB, Spyker DA, Cantilena LR Jr, et al. 2012 annual report of the American association of poison control centers' national poison data system (NPDS): 30th annual report. Clin Toxicol (Phila) 2013;51(10):949–1229.

56. Karlson-Stiber C, Persson H. Cytotoxic fungi–an overview. Toxicon 2003;42(4): 339–49.

57. Letschert K, Faulstich H, Keller D, et al. Molecular characterization and inhibition of amanitin uptake into human hepatocytes. Toxicol Sci 2006;91(1):140–9.

58. Wieland T. The toxic peptides from amanita mushrooms. Int J Pept Protein Res 1983;22(3):257–76.

59. Mas A. Mushrooms, amatoxins and the liver. J Hepatol 2005;42(2):166–9.

60. Poucheret P, Fons F, Doré JC, et al. Amatoxin poisoning treatment decision-making: pharmaco-therapeutic clinical strategy assessment using multidimensional multivariate statistic analysis. Toxicon 2010;55(7):1338–45.

61. Moroni F, Fantozzi R, Masini E, et al. A trend in the therapy of Amanita phalloides poisoning. Arch Toxicol 1976;36(2):111–5.

62. Giannini L, Vannacci A, Missanelli A, et al. Amatoxin poisoning: a 15-year retrospective analysis and follow-up evaluation of 105 patients. Clin Toxicol (Phila) 2007;45(5):539–42.

63. Enjalbert F, Rapior S, Nouguier-Soulé J, et al. Treatment of amatoxin poisoning: 20-year retrospective analysis. J Toxicol Clin Toxicol 2002;40(6):715–57.

64. Akın A, Keşkek ŞÖ, Kılıç DA, et al. The effects of N-acetylcysteine in patients with *Amanita phalloides* intoxication. J Drug Metab Toxicol 2013;4:160.
65. Mengs U, Pohl RT, Mitchell T. Legalon(R) SIL: the antidote of choice in patients with acute hepatotoxicity from amatoxin poisoning. Curr Pharm Biotechnol 2012; 13(10):1964–70.
66. Wittebole X, Hantson P. Use of the molecular adsorbent recirculating system (MARS) for the management of acute poisoning with or without liver failure. Clin Toxicol (Phila) 2011;49(9):782–93.
67. Russell S. Carnitine as an antidote for acute valproate toxicity in children. Curr Opin Pediatr 2007;19(2):206–10.
68. Lheureux PE, Penaloza A, Zahir S, et al. Science review: carnitine in the treatment of valproic acid-induced toxicity—what is the evidence? Crit Care 2005; 9(5):431–40.
69. Bohan TP, Helton E, McDonald I, et al. Effect of L-carnitine treatment for valproate-induced hepatotoxicity. Neurology 2001;56(10):1405–9.
70. Czaja AJ. Drug-induced autoimmune-like hepatitis. Dig Dis Sci 2011;56(4): 958–76.
71. Giannattasio A, D'Ambrosi M, Volpicelli M, et al. Steroid therapy for a case of severe drug-induced cholestasis. Ann Pharmacother 2006;40(6):1196–9.
72. Wree A, Dechêne A, Herzer K, et al. Steroid and ursodesoxycholic acid combination therapy in severe drug-induced liver injury. Digestion 2011;84(1):54–9.
73. Stapelbroek JM, van Erpecum KJ, Klomp LW, et al. Liver disease associated with canalicular transport defects: current and future therapies. J Hepatol 2010;52(2):258–71.
74. Smith LA, Ignacio JR, Winesett MP, et al. Vanishing bile duct syndrome: amoxicillin-clavulanic acid associated intra-hepatic cholestasis responsive to ursodeoxycholic acid. J Pediatr Gastroenterol Nutr 2005;41(4):469–73.
75. van Roon EN, Jansen TL, Houtman NM, et al. Leflunomide for the treatment of rheumatoid arthritis in clinical practice: incidence and severity of hepatotoxicity. Drug Saf 2004;27(5):345–52.
76. Stine JG, Lewis JH. Current and future directions in the treatment and prevention of drug-induced liver injury: a systematic review. Expert Rev Gastroenterol Hepatol 2016;10(4):517–36.
77. Lee WM, Hynan LS, Rossaro L, et al. Intravenous N-acetylcysteine improves transplant-free survival in early stage non-acetaminophen acute liver failure. Gastroenterology 2009;137(3):856–64.e1.
78. Squires RH, Dhawan A, Alonso E, et al. Intravenous N-acetylcysteine in pediatric patients with nonacetaminophen acute liver failure: a placebo-controlled clinical trial. Hepatology 2013;57(4):1542–9.
79. Patel T, Yosipovitch G. Therapy of pruritus. Expert Opin Pharmacother 2010; 11(10):1673–82.
80. Jalan R, Gines P, Olson JC, et al. Acute-on chronic liver failure. J Hepatol 2012; 57(6):1336–48.
81. Tsipotis E, Shuja A, Jaber BL. Albumin dialysis for liver failure: a systematic review. Adv Chronic Kidney Dis 2015;22(5):382–90.
82. de Geus H, Mathôt R, van der Hoven B, et al. Enhanced paracetamol clearance with molecular adsorbents recirculating system (MARS(R)) in severe autointoxication. Blood Purif 2010;30(2):118–9.
83. Kantola T, Koivusalo AM, Höckerstedt K, et al. The effect of molecular adsorbent recirculating system treatment on survival, native liver recovery, and need for liver transplantation in acute liver failure patients. Transpl Int 2008;21(9):857–66.

84. Saliba F, Camus C, Durand F, et al. Albumin dialysis with a noncell artificial liver support device in patients with acute liver failure: a randomized, controlled trial. Ann Intern Med 2013;159(8):522–31.

85. Rifai K, Ernst T, Kretschmer U, et al. Prometheus–a new extracorporeal system for the treatment of liver failure. J Hepatol 2003;39(6):984–90.

86. Kribben A, Gerken G, Haag S, et al. Effects of fractionated plasma separation and adsorption on survival in patients with acute-on-chronic liver failure. Gastroenterology 2012;142(4):782–9.e3.

87. Karvellas CJ, Bagshaw SM, McDermid RC, et al. A case-control study of single-pass albumin dialysis for acetaminophen-induced acute liver failure. Blood Purif 2009;28(3):151–8.

88. Larsen FS, Ejlersen E, Hansen BA, et al. Systemic vascular resistance during high-volume plasmapheresis in patients with fulminant hepatic failure: relationship with oxygen consumption. Eur J Gastroenterol Hepatol 1995;7(9):887–92.

89. Larsen FS, Hansen BA, Ejlersen E, et al. Cerebral blood flow, oxygen metabolism and transcranial Doppler sonography during high-volume plasmapheresis in fulminant hepatic failure. Eur J Gastroenterol Hepatol 1996;8(3):261–5.

90. Larsen FS, Schmidt LE, Bernsmeier C, et al. High-volume plasma exchange in patients with acute liver failure: an open randomised controlled trial. J Hepatol 2016;64(1):69–78.

91. Karvellas CJ, Stravitz RT. High volume plasma exchange in acute liver failure: dampening the inflammatory cascade? J Hepatol 2016;64(1):10–2.

92. Lee KC, Stadlbauer V, Jalan R. Extracorporeal liver support devices for listed patients. Liver Transpl 2016;22(6):839–48.

93. Ellis AJ, Hughes RD, Wendon JA, et al. Pilot-controlled trial of the extracorporeal liver assist device in acute liver failure. Hepatology 1996;24(6):1446–51.

94. Millis JM, Cronin DC, Johnson R, et al. Initial experience with the modified extracorporeal liver-assist device for patients with fulminant hepatic failure: system modifications and clinical impact. Transplantation 2002;74(12):1735–46.

95. Vital. Therapies Inc. Vital Therapies® targeting liver disease. Available at: http://vitaltherapies.com/clinical-trials/%5D. Accessed May 1, 2016.

96. Demetriou AA, Brown RS Jr, Busuttil RW, et al. Prospective, randomized, multicenter, controlled trial of a bioartificial liver in treating acute liver failure. Ann Surg 2004;239(5):660–7 [discussion: 667–70].

97. Banares R, Catalina MV, Vaquero J. Liver support systems: will they ever reach prime time? Curr Gastroenterol Rep 2013;15(3):312.

98. Lee KC, Baker LA, Stanzani G, et al. Extracorporeal liver assist device to exchange albumin and remove endotoxin in acute liver failure: results of a pivotal pre-clinical study. J Hepatol 2015;63(3):634–42.

99. Nyberg SL, Hardin J, Amiot B, et al. Rapid, large-scale formation of porcine hepatocyte spheroids in a novel spheroid reservoir bioartificial liver. Liver Transpl 2005;11(8):901–10.

100. Glorioso JM, Mao SA, Rodysill B, et al. Pivotal preclinical trial of the spheroid reservoir bioartificial liver. J Hepatol 2015;63(2):388–98.

101. Wong A, Graudins A. Simplification of the standard three-bag intravenous acetylcysteine regimen for paracetamol poisoning results in a lower incidence of adverse drug reactions. Clin Toxicol (Phila) 2016;54(2):115–9.

Drug Metabolism, Drug Interactions, and Drug-Induced Liver Injury in Living Donor Liver Transplant Patients

CrossMark

Swaytha Ganesh, MD[a],*,
Omar Abdulhameed Almazroo, MSc, CCTS[b], Amit Tevar, MD[a],
Abhinav Humar, MD[a],*, Raman Venkataramanan, PhD[a,c,d]

KEYWORDS

- Living donor liver transplantation • Hepatic regeneration • Drug metabolism
- Cytochrome P450 • Pharmacokinetics • Hepatotoxicity

KEY POINTS

- Living donor liver transplant (LDLT) is increasingly being performed given the shortage of deceased donor livers available for liver transplant.
- Limited pharmacokinetic and metabolism studies have been performed in LDLT patients.
- Given the reduced liver mass, altered blood flow, altered bile production, altered plasma protein production, and increased proinflammatory cytokine levels, the capacity of the liver to metabolize endogenous and exogenous compounds is expected to be decreased in LDLT patients, especially during the hepatic regeneration phase.
- Given these expectations, hepatotoxicity is more likely to be observed in LDLT patients than in deceased donor liver transplant patients.

INTRODUCTION

Liver transplant (LT) has been well established as a therapeutic option for patients with various end-stage liver diseases. Dr Thomas Starzl performed the first successful LT in 1967.[1] Deceased donors have been the primary source of livers for LT. However,

Disclosure: The authors have nothing to disclose.
[a] Thomas Starzl Transplantation Institute, University of Pittsburgh, Pittsburgh, PA 15261, USA;
[b] Department of Pharmaceutical Sciences, School of Pharmacy, University of Pittsburgh, 731 Salk Hall, 3501 Terrace Street, Pittsburgh, PA 15261, USA; [c] Department of Pharmaceutical Sciences, School of Pharmacy, University of Pittsburgh, 718 Salk Hall, 3501 Terrace Street, Pittsburgh, PA 15261, USA; [d] Department of Pathology, School of Medicine, University of Pittsburgh, Pittsburgh, PA, USA
* Corresponding author.
E-mail addresses: ganesx@upmc.edu; humara2@upmc.edu

because of the significant shortage of deceased donor organs and the long waiting time for LT, attempts have been made to expand the donor pool, including the use of livers from extended criteria donors, split livers from deceased donors, and liver segments from living donors.[2] The advantages of living donor LT (LDLT) include shorter waiting time for organs, minimal ischemic time for the grafts, elective surgery time for the patients, the options for the recipients to be medically stabilized before surgery, improved overall transplant outcomes, and improved patient and graft survival compared with those receiving deceased donor LTs (DDLTs).[3–5] LDLT may provide additional advantages depending on the severity of the liver disease, because living donors are typically younger.[6,7] The first successful LDLT was performed in 1989 in a pediatric patient and in 1997 in an adult patient.[8,9] The recipients receive either the left lobe or right lobe of the liver from a living donor. The liver regenerates both in the donor and in the recipient over time to accommodate the needs of the individuals.

DRUG THERAPY IN LIVING DONOR LIVER TRANSPLANT PATIENTS

The donor and recipients of the LDLT receive multiple drug therapy during and after surgery. In the donors, the medications used typically include the following. During surgery, drugs such as lidocaine, metoprolol, midazolam, propofol, rocuronium, succinyl choline, vasopressin, neostigmine, ondansetron, phenylephrine, and labetalol may be used. Following surgery, antibiotics such as ampicillin, sulbactam, amikacin, and vancomycin may be used. Pain medications such as fentanyl, morphine, hydromorphone, oxycodone, or ketorolac may be used intraoperatively or postoperatively. Postoperatively docusate, bisacodyl, pantoprazole, phytonadione, and metoclopramide may be used. In addition to these medications, recipients also receive immunosuppressants such as basiliximab, mycophenolate mofetil (MMF), tacrolimus, methylprednisolone, and prednisone. Postoperative prophylaxis with Bactrim or Dapsone (for sulfa allergy), acyclovir or valganciclovir (cytomegalovirus [CMV] high-risk only), isavuconazole (or voriconazole previously) are also common in recipients. In addition, other drugs, such as docusate, bisacodyl, pantoprazole, entecavir, or tenofovir may also be used in certain patients. Specific information on how these drugs are used in humans is given in **Table 1**. Pharmacokinetics of some selected drugs and hepatotoxicity in LDLT are discussed later.

Immunosuppression

Solid organ transplant recipients normally require lifelong treatment with potent immunosuppressants, which reduce the risk of allograft rejection but increase patient morbidity and mortality after long-term use. Optimal immunosuppressive therapy balances the risk of rejection caused by an inadequately suppressed immune system with potential side effects of immunosuppression. Immunosuppression is personalized to individual patients using several factors, including the underlying cause of original liver disease (eg, hepatitis C virus [HCV], hepatocellular carcinoma), underlying renal function, other comorbidities, and the patient's immunologic state.[10] The most commonly used immunosuppressive regimens in solid organ transplantation include a combination of calcineurin inhibitor (CNIs), antimetabolites (MMF or azathioprine), and corticosteroids. In selected patients, inhibitors of mammalian target of rapamycin (mTORi) such as a sirolimus or everolimus are also used. Some transplant centers use initial induction therapy with biologic T-cell–depleting agents (anti-CD52, OKT3, antithymocyte globulin) or non–T-cell–depleting agents (interleukin [IL]-2 receptor agonists, basiliximab).[11–13]

Calcineurin Inhibitors

Appropriate use of CNIs is critical to transplant recipients' long-term survival. Cyclosporine and tacrolimus are the current CNIs used in LDLT patients. Cyclosporine is a cyclic polypeptide and was introduced clinically in the early 1980s. Tacrolimus is a macrolide that was initially tested in 1989 in LT patients. It was commercially approved in 1994. It is more potent than cyclosporine. Cyclosporine and tacrolimus are chemically distinct molecules that bind to the intracellular immunophilins, cyclophilin and FKBP-12 (FK506 binding protein), respectively.[14] CNIs suppress the immune system by blocking IL-2 production in T cells.

Cyclosporine and tacrolimus have highly variable pharmacokinetics, and narrow therapeutic range. The large variability in drug exposure in patients is attributed to variation in the absorption, distribution, and elimination of these drugs. Both cyclosporine and tacrolimus are highly permeable but poorly soluble drugs. They are well absorbed from the gut, but their oral bioavailability is low because of metabolism by cytochrome P450 (CYP) 3A, a member of the CYP-450 isoenzyme system expressed in the gut and the liver. CYP3A metabolizes many of the drugs used in clinical practice. In addition, efflux in the gut by P-glycoprotein (PGP), which is encoded by the multidrug resistance-1 (MDR1), also known as the ABCB1, also accounts for the low oral bioavailability of CNIs. PGP is a transmembrane transporter capable of transporting numerous endogenous substances from the cytoplasm to the exterior of the cell.[14–16] Prior studies suggest that intraindividual variation in the concentration/dose ratio of tacrolimus is closely related to the variation in the enterocyte messenger ribonucleic acid (mRNA) expression level of multidrug resistance protein (MDR1), but not CYP3A4.

On reaching the vascular system, both cyclosporine and tacrolimus partition into red blood cells (RBCs). The blood to plasma ratio for cyclosporine is around 2 and that for tacrolimus is around 15. Within the body these drugs are also extensively distributed outside the vascular system because of their high lipophilicity. Once in systemic circulation, tacrolimus and cyclosporine are subject to metabolism by CYP enzymes, specifically CYP3A4 and CYP3A5 in the liver. In vivo expression of both CYP3A4/CYP3A5 and PGP vary substantially between individuals. Administration of a drug that is a CYP3A or PGP substrate/inhibitor (ritonavir, ketoconazole) to an LT recipient can lead to high blood levels of the immunosuppressants. At the same time, CYP3A inducers such as rifampin can lead to subtherapeutic levels and graft rejection.

Studies have also shown that the genetic polymorphism in drug metabolizing enzymes such as CYP3A has been linked to differences in the efficacy and toxicity of many medications between different individuals. There is large heterogeneity in the way individuals respond to medications, in terms of both host toxicity and treatment efficacy. This innate nature can provide a scientific basis for optimizing drug therapy using each patient's genetic constitution.[17,18] Patients who express high CYP3A5 levels seem to require a higher dose of tacrolimus and cyclosporine compared with those who poorly express CYP3A5. The dosing of CNIs must be carefully tailored to each transplant recipient because of the differences in sex, race, ethnicity, metabolism, other coadministered drugs, genetic polymorphism, and type of transplant.[19,20] Trough blood concentrations are good surrogate markers of drug exposure (area under the blood concentration vs time curve [AUC]) for cyclosporine and tacrolimus. There is an association between blood levels and outcomes (rejection and toxicity) with these agents. Routine therapeutic monitoring of tacrolimus and cyclosporine (trough blood concentrations) has significantly improved overall outcomes in LT patients.

Table 1
Metabolic pathways and dosing for the drugs used in LDLT recipients

Drug	Primary Route of Elimination	Pathway	Typical Daily Dosing	Dosing with Hepatic Impairment
During Surgery				
Lidocaine	Metabolism	CYP1A2	0.5–1.5 mg/kg	Reduced dose required
Metoprolol	Metabolism	CYP2D6	50–200 mg	Reduced dose required
Midazolam	Metabolism	CYP3A4	0.2–0.6 mg/kg	Reduced dose required
Propofol	Metabolism	UGTs, CYP2B6 and CYP2C9	100–200 µg/kg/min	No dose adjustment necessary
Rocuronium	Hepatic clearance	Bile excretion	Initial dose: 0.6 mg/kg Maintenance dose: 0.6–0.72 mg/kg/h	No dose adjustment necessary
Succinyl choline	Metabolism (hydrolysis)	BCHE	0.5–10 mg/min	No dose adjustment necessary
Vasopressin	Metabolism		0.2–1 unit/min	0.13 unit/min was effective with cirrhotic patients
Surgical Antibiotics				
Ampicillin	Renal	40%–92%	1 g/h	No dose adjustment necessary
Sulbactam	Renal	75%–85%	0.5 g/h	No dose adjustment necessary
Amikacin	Renal	84%–94%	15 mg/kg	No dose adjustment necessary
Vancomycin	Renal	40%–100%	15 mg/kg	No dose adjustment necessary
Pain Medications				
Fentanyl	Metabolism	CYP3A4	20–50 µg/h	50% dose reduction is suggested
Hydromorphone	Metabolism	UGTs	0.1–0.5 mg/h	25%–50% dose reduction is suggested
Oxycodone	Metabolism	CYP3A4; CYP2D6	20–60 mg	30%–50% dose reduction is suggested

Immunosuppressive Drugs

Drug	Process	Pathway	Dose	Adjustment
Basiliximab	Opsonization		20 mg pre-OP; then 20 mg day 4 post-OP	No dose adjustment necessary
Mycophenolic acid	Metabolism	UGTs	1 g BID	No dose adjustment necessary
Tacrolimus	Metabolism	CYP3A	2 mg BID	Reduced dose required
Methylprednisolone	Metabolism	CYP3A	250 mg	No dose adjustment necessary
Prednisone	Metabolism	11β-HSD	5–20 mg	No dose adjustment necessary
Prednisolone	Metabolism	CYP3A4	20 mg	No dose adjustment necessary
Postoperative Antibiotics				
Trimethoprim	Renal	50%	100 mg BID	No dose adjustment necessary
Sulfamethoxazole	Renal	80%–100%	1 g BID	No dose adjustment necessary
Dapsone	Metabolism	CYP3A	100 mg BID	No dose adjustment necessary
Acyclovir	Renal		800 mg QID	No dose adjustment necessary
Valganciclovir	Metabolism	Hydrolysis	900 mg	No dose adjustment necessary
Isavuconazole	Metabolism	CYP3A4/5	Initial dose: 372 mg every 8 h Maintenance dose: 372 mg/d	No dose adjustment necessary
Voriconazole	Metabolism	CYP2C19, CYP2C9, CYP3A4	100–200 mg	Reduced dose required
Others				
Docusate	Hepatic clearance	Bile excretion	100–200 mg	No dose adjustment necessary
Bisacodyl	Metabolism	Esterases	10 mg	No dose adjustment necessary
Pantoprazole	Metabolism	CYP2C19; CYP3A4, CYP2D6, and CYP2C9	40 mg	No dose adjustment necessary
Entecavir	Renal	62%–73%	1 mg	No dose adjustment necessary
Tenofovir	Renal	70%–80%	300 mg	No dose adjustment necessary

Abbreviations: BCHE, butyrylcholinesterase; BID, twice a day; CYP, cytochrome P; HSD, hydroxysteroid dehydrogenase; QID, 4 times a day; UGT, UDP-glucuronosyltransferases.
Data from Refs.[72–75]

Cyclosporine is also a potent inhibitor of uptake (OATP [organic anion-transporting polypeptide]) and efflux transporters (P-glycoprotein) in the hepatocytes.[21] Cyclosporine may alter the pharmacokinetics of certain coadministered drugs as well. Cyclosporine increases statin concentrations by a decrease in hepatic uptake and clearance and an increase in bioavailability. Cyclosporine may also decrease the biliary excretion of certain statins.

Mycophenolic Acid

Mycophenolic acid (MPA) is a noncompetitive inhibitor of inosine monophosphate dehydrogenase (IMPDH), which prevents de novo synthesis of purine nucleotides in proliferating T and B lymphocytes. MPA and its prodrug MMF are often coadministered with CNIs. After oral administration, MMF is rapidly hydrolyzed to the active product, MPA. Subsequently MPA is extensively metabolized by uridine diphosphate glucuronosyltransferase enzymes in the liver, gut, and kidney to its inactive metabolite, phenyl mycophenolic acid glucuronide (MPAG). MPA and MPAG are extensively bound to serum albumin. A second and less abundant metabolite is acyl mycophenolic acid glucuronide (AcMPAG), which is pharmacologically active. Free MPA, rather than total MPA, is the pharmacologically active form of the drug. There is large variability in the pharmacokinetics of MPA in transplant patients. However, routine therapeutic monitoring is not as common for MPA as for CNIs because of the poor correlation between MPA exposure (AUC) and trough MPA concentrations. Partial AUC measurement has been recommended as a method to monitor MPA exposure, but is not routinely used in patients at this time. IMPDH monitoring may offer a better biomarker for optimizing the dose of MMF/MPA.

Mammalian Target of Rapamycin Inhibitors

Sirolimus and everolimus are the two mTORi used in transplantation. Both drugs are available for oral administration and both have low oral bioavailability. Both are highly bound to RBCs and are primarily metabolized by CYP3A enzymes in gut and liver. There is a large variability in the pharmacokinetics of these drugs among patients. The functional status of the liver determines the exposure (AUC) of these drugs in transplant patients. Therapeutic drug monitoring (trough blood concentrations) is routinely used to individualize the dosing of these drugs as well.

PHYSIOLOGIC CHANGES AFFECTING PHARMACOKINETICS AFTER LIVING DONOR LIVER TRANSPLANT

Metabolic and functional changes after hepatic resection are unique, time dependent, and create challenges in patient management. Understanding the hepatic physiology is essential to optimize the care of LDLT donors and recipients.[22] The pathologic changes that occur after liver resection include coagulopathy and fluid and electrolyte imbalances relating to the dysregulation of hepatic metabolism, especially in the donors.[22] The pharmacokinetic parameters of the medications used may be altered by the pathophysiologic changes, including liver regeneration and inflammation during liver regeneration, graft size, altered hepatic blood flow, and concentrations of plasma proteins.[3] The other factors also include abnormal biliary flow rate after LDLT.

Liver Regeneration

The mechanisms of liver regeneration have generated interest from both a biological science and a clinical perspective. Knowledge of the molecular and cellular mechanisms of liver regeneration is both conceptually important and directly relevant to clinical problems. During liver regeneration after hepatectomy, normally quiescent hepatocytes are altered to restore the liver mass by a process of compensatory hyperplasia. Several genes are involved in liver regeneration, and the process can be categorized into 3 networks: cytokine, growth factor, and metabolic.[23,24] Cytokines are important for liver regeneration. Cytokine release is triggered spontaneously after LDLT in both the donors and the recipients. There is limited evidence on the impact of inflammation during liver regeneration on drug metabolism. However, various cytokines involved in hepatic regeneration, including tumor necrosis factor-alpha, IL-1, IL-4, IL-6, and interferons (IFNs), are involved in the changes in CYP gene expressions during inflammation.[25] In addition to cytokines, several other factors contribute to this complex process, including liver graft size, spleen size, portal flow, and hepatic venous flow.[26,27] Prior studies have shown that the liver regeneration process can be divided into 3 phases. The early phase of rapid regeneration occurs during the first 2 postoperative weeks and is associated with vascular engorgement and tissue edema. The second phase is volume decline, attributable to the normalization of developed vascular engorgement or tissue edema at 1 to 2 months after hepatectomy. The third phase is a slow increase in volume, which occurs until the volume reaches a constant level, reaching nearly 90% of the preoperative liver volume by around 6 months to 1 year.[27,28] One study has reported low CYP2C19 protein expression in LDLT recipients and the donors postsurgery.[29]

Graft Size

The vital issue of size matching is determined by the size of the recipient and the degree of portal hypertension in LDLT surgery. Patients with little or no portal hypertension require less graft volume than do patients with more significant portal hypertension, as reflected by ascites, and significant varices. Several formulae have been developed to estimate the volume of the graft. With these equations, it is possible to calculate the expected graft-to-recipient body weight ratio, which should be at least 0.8%.[23,30] During LDLT surgery, the donor undergoes liver resection up to 50%. The right lobe consists of complicated vascular and biliary systems, which may lead to higher risk of surgical complications in the donor, such as impaired blood outflow and bile duct injury, because right lobe graft is now more common for adult LDLT, to avoid small-for-size syndrome (SFSS) in the recipient.[31] In contrast, using a left lobe liver graft improves the donor safety, but shifts the risk of complications to the recipients. The use of a left lobe graft provides only about 30% to 50% of the required liver volume to an adult recipient, which is insufficient to sustain the recipient's metabolic demands, leading to SFSS.[31] The reduced liver size affects drug metabolism because of the decreased metabolic enzyme content and a reduction in the functional capacity of the drug metabolizing enzymes in the liver.[3]

Liver Ischemia/Reperfusion Injury

Metabolic capacity after LT surgery may be affected by the graft size and by hepatic injury during the surgery. It has been shown that the dose of an immunosuppressive drug required to reach a therapeutic target level is significantly correlated with graft weight/standard liver volume, warm ischemia time, and cold ischemic time, indicating limited drug metabolism in LDLT patients.[32] Although the magnitude of the effects of ischemia/reperfusion (I/R) injury on hepatic drug metabolism in LDLT recipients is expected to be lower than in DDLT recipients, injury of the liver following warm I/R still occurs. The warm I/R injury can increase serum levels of proinflammatory cytokines and decrease the activities of enzymes (ie, CYP2C9, CYP2B6).[33]

PHARMACOKINETIC CHANGES IN LIVING DONOR LIVER TRANSPLANT

Liver is essential for bile production. Bile production is expected to be altered after LDLT. This changed in bile production is likely to alter absorption of lipids and lipid-soluble compounds, which should recover to normal over time. The liver is the primary site of plasma protein synthesis. Early after LT patients are hypoalbuminemic, because of decreased hepatic synthesis and malnutrition. Albumin contributes about 80% of the normal oncotic pressure. The altered levels of plasma proteins can affect drug-protein binding, leading to changes in volume of distribution of drugs that are highly bound to these plasma proteins.[34] The major determinant of the extent of drug binding to plasma proteins (albumin and alpha-1 acid glycoprotein) is the concentration of the drug binding protein.[35] Albumin is important for binding acidic drugs, and basic drugs seem to bind preferentially to alpha-1 acid glycoprotein. The concentration of albumin increases with time after transplant, the concentration of alpha-1 acid glycoprotein increases immediately after transplant, and is maintained at high levels over several months after transplant. This finding has been shown in patients after orthotopic LTs, but has not been reported in LDLT. The reduced liver mass in donors and recipients in LDLT are expected lead to altered plasma protein levels until complete hepatic regeneration is reached.[36]

CYP450 enzymes metabolize endogenous substances and a vast variety of drugs. Little is known about the regulation of CYP450s during pathophysiologic conditions in the liver.[37] During hepatic regeneration, cytokine levels are upregulated. Cytokines are known to downregulate various drug-metabolizing enzymes and transporters, which can lead to decreased clearance and prolonged half-life of drugs during the hepatocyte regeneration process. An alteration in hepatic blood flow per unit mass of the liver is also expected to affect drug metabolism in LDLT patients. It has been reported that the first-pass metabolism of the intestines compensates for the metabolism of alcohol in rats in the early postoperative period during liver regeneration.[38]

PHARMACOKINETICS OF CERTAIN MEDICATIONS IN LIVING DONOR LIVER TRANSPLANT PATIENTS

Commonly used medications used both in living donor recipients and donors include narcotic pain medications, proton pump inhibitors, H2 blockers, antibiotics, stool softeners, antiemetics, and antihistamines. However, there have not been any studies describing the clinical pharmacokinetics of several medications that have been commonly used in LDLT recipients. Most of the information in the literature is on immunosuppressive drugs, with limited data on other medications.

The pharmacokinetics and magnitude of drug interactions in recipients of LDLTs are expected to be different from those in the recipients of DDLTs. The dosing requirements of immunosuppressants are significantly different between recipients of living donor and deceased donor liver grafts. There are many potential explanations for this, the most likely of which is that hepatic clearance and metabolism are reduced in patients with partial liver grafts (**Fig. 1**).

Tacrolimus

The impact of reduced size/mass of the hepatic allograft and the process of hepatic regeneration on the pharmacokinetics of drugs used in LDLT patients is crucial for the proper dosing of immunosuppressive drugs such as cyclosporine and tacrolimus. Tacrolimus is the primary immunosuppressive drug currently used in LDLT recipients. Tacrolimus has a narrow therapeutic index. An initial tacrolimus dose reduction of at

A

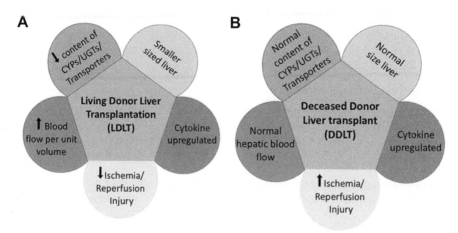

B

Fig. 1. Factors affecting the pharmacokinetics in liver transplant patients. (*A*) Specific for LDLT and (*B*) for DDLT.

least 30% to 40% in the first 14 postoperative days compared with a DDLT recipient has been suggested in LDLT recipients.[35] Because of the marked interpatient variability and reduced clearance of tacrolimus, monitoring of its trough blood levels is necessary to optimize dosing requirements.[24]

Cyclosporine A

For patients unable to tolerate tacrolimus, cyclosporine A (CyA) has been used as a valuable immunosuppressive drug, especially in patients with hepatitis C and primary biliary cirrhosis.[39] LDLT recipients achieve higher trough levels of CyA for a given dose than DDLT recipients. Studies have shown that the overall mean level-dose ratio of cyclosporine in LDLT recipients is significantly (26%) higher than in DDLT recipients. Higher level-dose ratios were seen in LDLT recipients as long as 6 months after transplant, until hepatic regeneration was complete. These observations may be explained by smaller hepatic mass in LDLT recipients compared with DDLT recipients and correspondingly reduced hepatic metabolism.[40] A study has shown that the reduced size of graft liver, prolonged intestinal paralysis because of length of surgery, and posttransplant external bile diversion, which are the features specific for adult LDLT recipients, may contribute to delayed graft functional recovery and poor enteral absorption, which in turn interfere with achieving and maintaining the therapeutic CyA blood concentrations. However, 2 weeks after transplant, when bowel functions returned to normal, less biliary drainage and better CyA exposure were observed after oral administration in LDLT recipients.[39]

Mycophenolic Acid

After oral administration of MMF, glucuronidation of MPA to MPAG and AcMPAG in LDLT patients was less efficient than in DDLT patients. Glucuronide conjugation has been shown to be impaired during hepatic regeneration but recovers after partial hepatectomy in rats. The reduced-size liver clears the drug less readily. The importance of using a lower dosage of its prodrug, MMF, in LDLT recipients has been shown in studies.[37] The MPAG concentrations were higher in DDLT patients than in LDLT recipients, confirming the reduced capacity to conjugate in LDLT patients.[37,41,42] Prior studies have shown that the function of glucuronide conjugation in LDLT patients was decreased compared with that in DDLT patients, and a significantly higher fraction of free MPA in LDLT patients suggested that a lower oral dose of MMF may be administered for LDLT patients.[42]

Sirolimus (Rapamycin)/Everolimus

No information is available on the pharmacokinetics of sirolimus or everolimus in LDLT recipients. Studies in rats suggest that partial hepatectomy does not significantly alter sirolimus exposure. This finding is surprising because there is reduced liver mass and downregulation of the CYP450 system that metabolizes sirolimus during hepatic regeneration.[43]

A comprehensive list of medications used in LT patients with their primary methods of elimination, metabolic pathways, and effects of hepatic impairment is shown in **Table 1**.

IDIOSYNCRATIC DRUG-INDUCED LIVER INJURY IN THE LIVING DONOR LIVER TRANSPLANT SETTING

Drug-induced liver injury (DILI) occurs at an incidence of 10 to 15 in 10,000 to 100,000 in the United States.[44] Evidence has shown that DILI is multifactorial and multifaceted, which suggests that multiple cellular mechanisms may be involved. A common initiating event has been proposed to be the formation of reactive drug metabolites and covalently bound adducts.[45] In transplant patients, drug interactions are of crucial importance because there is a need to keep immunosuppressive drug levels within a therapeutic range and thus alleviate the risk of drug toxicity if levels are too high or acute cellular rejection if levels are too low.[11] Establishing a diagnosis of DILI in the transplant setting is difficult with the variable laboratory features and histopathologic manifestations of hepatotoxicity of different drugs, and the need to exclude competing causes of allograft injury, like rejection. The clinical course of DILI can be categorized as hepatocellular, cholestatic, or mixed based on the presenting laboratory profile and liver histology.[13] Most cases of DILI are idiosyncratic and not associated with the dose or duration of medication administered or obvious clinical risk factors.[46,47]

There is a paucity of data on the frequency, causes, and outcomes of DILI in the LDLT setting. DDLT and LDLT recipients are more susceptible to DILI because of the presence of circulating donor macrophages that may process or present neoantigens to host T cells as well as the frequent use of multiple drugs in LT recipients.[48] In the LDLT setting, it is crucial to exclude biliary, infectious, vascular, and immunologic causes of allograft dysfunction because they are more common causes of liver injury than DILI. LDLT recipients can develop recurrent disease in the allograft, and it is imperative to evaluate for that as well.

Some post-LDLT patients can also develop idiopathic alloimmune hepatitis/de-novo autoimmune hepatitis (AIH) at any time after surgery.[48,49] De novo AIH is a rare condition, occurring late after LT, characterized by histologic and clinical features that are indistinguishable from those of classic AIH. The pathophysiology is still uncertain and whether it represents a specific type of rejection or a genuine form of AIH is under debate.[48] The clinical course of DILI can be divided into hepatocellular, cholestatic, or mixed, based on the presenting laboratory profile and liver histology. Studies have shown the incidence of DILI in LT recipients to be 1.7%, which is substantially higher (ie, 100-fold) than that reported in the general population (0.02%).[48]

HEPATOTOXICITY OF FREQUENTLY USED DRUGS IN LIVING DONOR LIVER TRANSPLANT RECIPIENTS AND DRUG INTERACTIONS

The azole antifungals and non–dihydropyridine calcium channel blockers are commonly used drugs that can increase the blood levels of CNIs and mTORi.

The protease inhibitors telaprevir (TPV) and boceprevir (BOC) have improved outcomes for patients with HCV genotype 1. However, clinically significant drug-drug interactions may limit the use of these drugs and may affect the safety of their use.[50] Telaprevir is both a substrate and an inhibitor of CYP3A4 and can also saturate or inhibit P-glycoprotein in the gut. BOC and TPV are NS3 protease inhibitors. They are potent substrates and inhibitors of CYP3A and have shown significant interactions with the CNIs and mTORi in LT recipients. Studies show that the dose of CNI needs to be markedly reduced during BOC and TPV therapy with highly variable dosing intervals. Also, it is necessary for frequent therapeutic drug monitoring of CNIs in patients on these drugs. A rapid increase in the CNI dosing and frequency is required within 1 to 2 days of discontinuing BOC or TPV to minimize the risk of underimmunosuppression and rejection.[51] Also, the severity of CYP3A interaction is less with cyclosporine compared with tacrolimus, and many centers have opted for conversion to cyclosporine before initiating BOC or TPV therapy in LDLT recipients. Based on the prior studies it is recommended to withhold CNI dosing after the initiation of TPV and then monitor daily CNI blood levels to guide future doses. When using tacrolimus with TPV, it is suggested to use 10% of the initial total daily dose once the morning trough level is less than 3 or 4 ng/mL. The reported dosing interval of tacrolimus ranged from once every 4 days to once every 25 days.[13] The cyclosporine dose is usually 25% of the initial total daily dose and the dosing interval ranged from once every 1 day to once every 7 days. There are limited data available for BOC in LDLT recipients, but one study suggested that cyclosporine could be administered at 50% of the initial total daily dose and given once a day, whereas the tacrolimus dose should be started at approximately 25% of the initial dose and the interval guided by daily assessment of trough levels.[52–54]

A substantial reduction in the clearance of tacrolimus (80%), cyclosporine (50%), and everolimus (53%) was reported in LDLT recipients receiving BOC with peginterferon (PegIFN) and ribavirin (RBV). A significant reduction in the clearance of both cyclosporine and tacrolimus in LT recipients receiving TPV and PegIFN and RBV therapy was reported.[55,56]

Emerging data show that combination of directly acting agents can be more efficacious but drug-drug interactions are still a matter of concern with these regimens.[56] Sofosbuvir, ledipasvir, and daclatasvir do not seem to interact with CNIs. However, simeprevir, a second-generation protease inhibitor, interacts with cyclosporine. With ombitasvir, paritaprevir, ritonavir, dasabuvir, and RBV, dosing modifications for tacrolimus (0.5 mg/wk or 0.2 mg every 3 days) and cyclosporine (one-fifth of the daily pretreatment dose given once daily) resulted in comparable trough concentrations before and during treatment.[56]

In contrast, intake of CYP3A inducers such as carbamazepine, St John's wort, and rifampin can lead to increased metabolism and reduced bioavailability of both CNIs and mTORi.[57,58]

Immunosuppressants

Azathioprine, a prodrug of mercaptopurine that inhibits T-cell maturation, has been used in LDLT recipients. Patients with low levels or deficiency in thiopurine methyltransferase, which affects ∼10% of the population, have a higher rate of myelotoxicity with azathioprine use, but no higher incidence of DILI has been reported with azathioprine use in LT recipients. Nodular regenerative hyperplasia has been reported with prolonged exposure to high-dose azathioprine in LT recipients. The pathophysiology is thought to be endothelial cell damage that leads to sinusoidal dilatation and obliterative pericentral veno-occlusive changes. The acute hepatocellular injury attributed to MMF has been only rarely reported. Hepatotoxicity attributed to cyclosporine and tacrolimus is also uncommon.[59–62] Severe acute hepatocellular injury with jaundice has been reported in transplant patients receiving high doses of cyclosporine with biopsy features of cholestasis and pericholangitis. The mechanism of this intrahepatic cholestasis may be the inhibition of canalicular bile flow and inhibition of bile salt export pump.[62,63] Sirolimus has been reported to cause liver injury in patients with HCV but clinically apparent DILI attributed to everolimus has not been reported.[59–61]

Antibiotics

Amoxicillin-clavulanate is a leading cause of DILI with cholestatic liver injury. This condition is reported both in general and in post-LT and post-LDLT patients. Sulfamethoxazole-trimethoprim can cause a cholestatic liver injury within a few days to weeks of drug initiation, with hypersensitivity features of skin rash, fever, and eosinophilia. Patients may also develop life-threatening DRESS (drug rash and eosinophilia and systemic symptoms) syndrome, whereas others have mild biochemical liver injury and hepatic granulomas on biopsy.[64]

Antifungals

The antifungals (azoles) are frequently used to treat and prevent systemic and superficial fungal infections in LDLT recipients. They are potent inhibitors of CYP3A4 and can also cause mild to moderate increases in serum aminotransferase levels in up to 5% of patients. Fluconazole, as well as the other azole antifungals (itraconazole, voriconazole, ketoconazole), can also rarely lead to severe acute hepatocellular injury.[65,66] Isoniazid is a leading cause of severe acute DILI both in general and post-LT recipients. The optimal time and duration of isoniazid therapy for LT recipients with latent tuberculosis remains unclear, but should generally be deferred until at least 6 months after LT.[67,68]

Antiviral Agents

Ganciclovir and valganciclovir are used to treat and prevent CMV infection in the post-LT setting. None of these agents have been associated with clinically apparent liver injury.[69]

Other Agents

Other drugs associated with DILI in LDLT recipients include sorafenib and amiodarone. It has been reported that weight loss products that contain green tea extract with catechins may cause severe acute hepatocellular injury.[70,71]

SUMMARY

It takes up to 6 months for the liver volume to return to normal after LDLT surgery. In the first 6 months posttransplant in LDLT recipients, drug levels and exposure are generally higher with lower clearance. It is therefore advisable to use lower initial dosages of immunosuppressants in these patients compared with the DDLT recipients. In the absence of data from LDLT, information on the effect of liver disease on the pharmacokinetics of medications can be used as guidance for drug dosing in LDLT patients.

REFERENCES

1. Starzl TE, Groth CG, Brettschneider L, et al. Orthotopic homotransplantation of the human liver. Ann Surg 1968;168(3):392–415.
2. Starzl TE, Fung JJ. Themes of liver transplantation. Hepatology 2010;51(6): 1869–84.
3. Li M, Zhao Y, Humar A, et al. Pharmacokinetics of drugs in adult living donor liver transplant patients: regulatory factors and observations based on studies in animals and humans. Expert Opin Drug Metab Toxicol 2016;12(3):231–43.
4. Saidi RF. Current status of liver transplantation. Arch Iran Med 2012;15(12):772–6.
5. Pomfret EA, Fryer JP, Sima CS, et al. Liver and intestine transplantation in the United States, 1996-2005. Am J Transplant 2007;7(5 Pt 2):1376–89.
6. Terrault NA, Stravitz RT, Lok AS, et al. Hepatitis C disease severity in living versus deceased donor liver transplant recipients: an extended observation study. Hepatology 2014;59(4):1311–9.
7. Berg CL, Gillespie BW, Merion RM, et al. Improvement in survival associated with adult-to-adult living donor liver transplantation. Gastroenterology 2007;133(6): 1806–13.
8. Carlisle EM, Testa G. Adult to adult living related liver transplantation: where do we currently stand? World J Gastroenterol 2012;18(46):6729–36.
9. Strong RW, Lynch SV, Ong TH, et al. Successful liver transplantation from a living donor to her son. N Engl J Med 1990;322(21):1505–7.
10. McCaughan GW, Sze KC, Strasser SI. Is there such a thing as protocol immunosuppression in liver transplantation? Expert Rev Gastroenterol Hepatol 2015; 9(1):1–4.
11. Parikh ND, Levitsky J. Hepatotoxicity and drug interactions in liver transplant candidates and recipients. Clin Liver Dis 2013;17(4):737–47, x–xi.
12. Rostaing L, Saliba F, Calmus Y, et al. Review article: use of induction therapy in liver transplantation. Transplant Rev (Orlando) 2012;26(4):246–60.
13. Tischer S, Fontana RJ. Drug-drug interactions with oral anti-HCV agents and idiosyncratic hepatotoxicity in the liver transplant setting. J Hepatol 2014;60(4): 872–84.
14. Utecht KN, Hiles JJ, Kolesar J. Effects of genetic polymorphisms on the pharmacokinetics of calcineurin inhibitors. Am J Health Syst Pharm 2006;63(23):2340–8.
15. Saeki T, Ueda K, Tanigawara Y, et al. Human P-glycoprotein transports cyclosporin A and FK506. J Biol Chem 1993;268(9):6077–80.
16. Hashida T, Masuda S, Uemoto S, et al. Pharmacokinetic and prognostic significance of intestinal MDR1 expression in recipients of living-donor liver transplantation. Clin Pharmacol Ther 2001;69(5):308–16.
17. Yu S, Wu L, Jin J, et al. Influence of CYP3A5 gene polymorphisms of donor rather than recipient to tacrolimus individual dose requirement in liver transplantation. Transplantation 2006;81(1):46–51.
18. Evans WE, Relling MV. Pharmacogenomics: translating functional genomics into rational therapeutics. Science 1999;286(5439):487–91.
19. Ravaioli M, Neri F, Lazzarotto T, et al. Immunosuppression modifications based on an immune response assay: results of a randomized, controlled trial. Transplantation 2015;99(8):1625–32.

20. He J, Li Y, Zhang H, et al. Immune function assay (ImmuKnow) as a predictor of allograft rejection and infection in kidney transplantation. Clin Transpl 2013;27(4): E351–8.
21. Williams D, Feely J. Pharmacokinetic-pharmacodynamic drug interactions with HMG-CoA reductase inhibitors. Clin Pharmacokinet 2002;41(5):343–70.
22. Wrighton LJ, O'Bosky KR, Namm JP, et al. Postoperative management after hepatic resection. J Gastrointest Oncol 2012;3(1):41–7.
23. Florman S, Miller CM. Live donor liver transplantation. Liver Transpl 2006;12(4): 499–510.
24. Jain A, Venkataramanan R, Sharma R, et al. Pharmacokinetics of tacrolimus in living donor liver transplant and deceased donor liver transplant recipients. Transplantation 2008;85(4):554–60.
25. Morgan ET, Thomas KB, Swanson R, et al. Selective suppression of cytochrome P-450 gene expression by interleukins 1 and 6 in rat liver. Biochim Biophys Acta 1994;1219(2):475–83.
26. Fausto N, Campbell JS, Riehle KJ. Liver regeneration. Hepatology 2006;43(2 Suppl 1):S45–53.
27. Haga J, Shimazu M, Wakabayashi G, et al. Liver regeneration in donors and adult recipients after living donor liver transplantation. Liver Transpl 2008;14(12): 1718–24.
28. Yamanaka N, Okamoto E, Kawamura E, et al. Dynamics of normal and injured human liver regeneration after hepatectomy as assessed on the basis of computed tomography and liver function. Hepatology 1993;18(1):79–85.
29. Chiu KW, Nakano T, Chen KD, et al. Cytochrome P450 in living donor liver transplantation. J Biomed Sci 2015;22:32.
30. Urata K, Kawasaki S, Matsunami H, et al. Calculation of child and adult standard liver volume for liver transplantation. Hepatology 1995;21(5):1317–21.
31. Raut V, Alikhanov R, Belghiti J, et al. Review of the surgical approach to prevent small-for-size syndrome in recipients after left lobe adult LDLT. Surg Today 2014; 44(7):1189–96.
32. Al-Jahdari WS, Kunimoto F, Saito S, et al. Total body propofol clearance (TBPC) after living-donor liver transplantation (LDLT) surgery is decreased in patients with a long warm ischemic time. J Anesth 2006;20(4):323–6.
33. Friedman BH, Wolf JH, Wang L, et al. Serum cytokine profiles associated with early allograft dysfunction in patients undergoing liver transplantation. Liver Transpl 2012;18(2):166–76.
34. Mukhtar A, EL Masry A, Moniem AA, et al. The impact of maintaining normal serum albumin level following living related liver transplantation: does serum albumin level affect the course? A pilot study. Transplant Proc 2007;39(10):3214–8.
35. Troisi R, Militerno G, Hoste E, et al. Are reduced tacrolimus dosages needed in the early postoperative period following living donor liver transplantation in adults? Transplant Proc 2002;34(5):1531–2.
36. Huang ML, Venkataramanan R, Burckart GJ, et al. Drug-binding proteins in liver transplant patients. J Clin Pharmacol 1988;28(6):505–6.
37. Jain A, Venkataramanan R, Sharma R, et al. Pharmacokinetics of mycophenolic acid in live donor liver transplant patients vs deceased donor liver transplant patients. J Clin Pharmacol 2008;48(5):547–52.
38. Morales-Gonzalez JA, Gutierrez-Salinas J, Hernandez-Munoz R. Pharmacokinetics of the ethanol bioavailability in the regenerating rat liver induced by partial hepatectomy. Alcohol Clin Exp Res 1998;22(7):1557–63.

39. Hibi T, Tanabe M, Hoshino K, et al. Cyclosporine A-based immunotherapy in adult living donor liver transplantation: accurate and improved therapeutic drug monitoring by 4-hr intravenous infusion. Transplantation 2011;92(1):100–5.

40. Trotter JF, Stolpman N, Wachs M, et al. Living donor liver transplant recipients achieve relatively higher immunosuppressant blood levels than cadaveric recipients. Liver Transpl 2002;8(3):212–8.

41. Shen B, Chen B, Zhang W, et al. Comparison of pharmacokinetics of mycophenolic acid and its metabolites between living donor liver transplant recipients and deceased donor liver transplant recipients. Liver Transpl 2009;15(11):1473–80.

42. Jain A, Venkataramanan R, Hamad IS, et al. Pharmacokinetics of mycophenolic acid after mycophenolate mofetil administration in liver transplant patients treated with tacrolimus. J Clin Pharmacol 2001;41(3):268–76.

43. Lodewijk L, Mall A, Spearman CW, et al. Effect of liver regeneration on the pharmacokinetics of immunosuppressive drugs. Transplant Proc 2009;41(1):379–81.

44. Yuan L, Kaplowitz N. Mechanisms of drug-induced liver injury. Clin Liver Dis 2013;17(4):507–18, vii.

45. Tailor A, Faulkner L, Naisbitt DJ, et al. The chemical, genetic and immunological basis of idiosyncratic drug-induced liver injury. Hum Exp Toxicol 2015;34(12):1310–7.

46. Aithal PG, Day CP. The natural history of histologically proved drug induced liver disease. Gut 1999;44(5):731–5.

47. Bjornsson E, Davidsdottir L. The long-term follow-up after idiosyncratic drug-induced liver injury with jaundice. J Hepatol 2009;50(3):511–7.

48. Guido M, Burra P. De novo autoimmune hepatitis after liver transplantation. Semin Liver Dis 2011;31(1):71–81.

49. Heneghan MA, Portmann BC, Norris SM, et al. Graft dysfunction mimicking autoimmune hepatitis following liver transplantation in adults. Hepatology 2001;34(3):464–70.

50. Garg V, Chandorkar G, Farmer HF, et al. Effect of telaprevir on the pharmacokinetics of midazolam and digoxin. J Clin Pharmacol 2012;52(10):1566–73.

51. Oo YH, Mutimer DJ. Rapid recovery of cytochrome P450 3A4 after protease inhibitor withdrawal in post-liver transplant patients. Liver Transpl 2012;18(10):1264–5.

52. Coilly A, Roche B, Dumortier J, et al. Safety and efficacy of protease inhibitors to treat hepatitis C after liver transplantation: a multicenter experience. J Hepatol 2014;60(1):78–86.

53. Pungpapong S, Aqel BA, Koning L, et al. Multicenter experience using telaprevir or boceprevir with peginterferon and ribavirin to treat hepatitis C genotype 1 after liver transplantation. Liver Transpl 2013;19(7):690–700.

54. Werner CR, Egetemeyr DP, Lauer UM, et al. Telaprevir-based triple therapy in liver transplant patients with hepatitis C virus: a 12-week pilot study providing safety and efficacy data. Liver Transpl 2012;18(12):1464–70.

55. Coilly A, Furlan V, Roche B, et al. Practical management of boceprevir and immunosuppressive therapy in liver transplant recipients with hepatitis C virus recurrence. Antimicrob Agents Chemother 2012;56(11):5728–34.

56. Audrey C, Raffaele B. Liver transplantation for hepatitis C virus in the era of direct-acting antiviral agents. Curr Opin HIV AIDS 2015;10(5):361–8.

57. Hebert MF, Park JM, Chen YL, et al. Effects of St. John's wort (*Hypericum perforatum*) on tacrolimus pharmacokinetics in healthy volunteers. J Clin Pharmacol 2004;44(1):89–94.

58. Burton JR Jr, Everson GT. Management of the transplant recipient with chronic hepatitis C. Clin Liver Dis 2013;17(1):73–91.
59. Jacques J, Dickson Z, Carrier P, et al. Severe sirolimus-induced acute hepatitis in a renal transplant recipient. Transpl Int 2010;23(9):967–70.
60. Neff GW, Ruiz P, Madariaga JR, et al. Sirolimus-associated hepatotoxicity in liver transplantation. Ann Pharmacother 2004;38(10):1593–6.
61. Chang GJ, Mahanty HD, Quan D, et al. Experience with the use of sirolimus in liver transplantation–use in patients for whom calcineurin inhibitors are contraindicated. Liver Transpl 2000;6(6):734–40.
62. Lorber MI, Van Buren CT, Flechner SM, et al. Hepatobiliary and pancreatic complications of cyclosporine therapy in 466 renal transplant recipients. Transplantation 1987;43(1):35–40.
63. Oto T, Okazaki M, Takata K, et al. Calcineurin inhibitor-related cholestasis complicating lung transplantation. Ann Thorac Surg 2010;89(5):1664–5.
64. Neuman MG, McKinney KK, Nanau RM, et al. Drug-induced severe adverse reaction enhanced by human herpes virus-6 reactivation. Transl Res 2013;161(5):430–40.
65. Bronstein JA, Gros P, Hernandez E, et al. Fatal acute hepatic necrosis due to dose-dependent fluconazole hepatotoxicity. Clin Infect Dis 1997;25(5):1266–7.
66. Cruciani M, Mengoli C, Malena M, et al. Antifungal prophylaxis in liver transplant patients: a systematic review and meta-analysis. Liver Transpl 2006;12(5):850–8.
67. Jafri SM, Singal AG, Kaul D, et al. Detection and management of latent tuberculosis in liver transplant patients. Liver Transpl 2011;17(3):306–14.
68. Rubin RH. Management of tuberculosis in the transplant recipient. Am J Transplant 2005;5(11):2599–600.
69. Cvetković RS, Wellington K. Valganciclovir: a review of its use in the management of CMV infection and disease in immunocompromised patients. Drugs 2005;65(6):859–78.
70. Herden U, Fischer L, Schafer H, et al. Sorafenib-induced severe acute hepatitis in a stable liver transplant recipient. Transplantation 2010;90(1):98–9.
71. von Vital JM, Karachristos A, Singhal A, et al. Acute amiodarone hepatotoxicity after liver transplantation. Transplantation 2011;91(8):e62–64.
72. Circeo LE, Reeves ST. Multicenter trial of prolonged infusions of rocuronium bromide in critically ill patients: effects of multiple organ failure. South Med J 2001;94(1):36–42.
73. Suh SJ, Yim HJ, Yoon EL, et al. Is propofol safe when administered to cirrhotic patients during sedative endoscopy? Korean J Intern Med 2014;29(1):57–65.
74. Verbeeck RK. Pharmacokinetics and dosage adjustment in patients with hepatic dysfunction. Eur J Clin Pharmacol 2008;64(12):1147–61.
75. Zhou SF, Zhou ZW, Yang LP, et al. Substrates, inducers, inhibitors and structure-activity relationships of human cytochrome P450 2C9 and implications in drug development. Curr Med Chem 2009;16(27):3480–675.

Evolution of Experimental Models of the Liver to Predict Human Drug Hepatotoxicity and Efficacy

 CrossMark

Lawrence A. Vernetti, PhD[a],*, Andreas Vogt, PhD[a],
Albert Gough, PhD[a], D. Lansing Taylor, PhD[a,b]

KEYWORDS

- Human liver models • Liver toxicology • Drug discovery • In vitro hepatotoxicity
- Quantitative system pharmacology • Microphysiology liver
- Drug-induced liver injury

KEY POINTS

- Quantitative Systems Pharmacology is a multiscale, iterative, and integrated computational and experimental approach for optimizing the development of therapeutic strategies.
- Limited efficacy and drug safety methods continue to limit the efficiency of the discovery and development of therapeutics.
- Mammalian in vivo models have low concordance to clinical hepatotoxicity.
- The predictive concordance between the existing in vitro experimental models coupled with computational modeling and clinical hepatotoxicity has reached a limit.
- Three-dimensional, multicellular, microfluidic, human tissue and organ experimental models are a promising alternative to whole animal and cultured cell methods for efficacy and safety testing.

Research reported in *Clinics in Liver Disease* was supported by the NIH National Center for Advancing translational Sciences (NCATS) of the National Institutes of Health under award number UH2TR000503.

The authors have nothing to disclose.

[a] Department of Computational and Systems Biology, University of Pittsburgh Drug Discovery Institute, Biomedical Science Tower 200 Lothrop Street, University of Pittsburgh, Pittsburgh, PA 15260, USA; [b] University of Pittsburgh Cancer Institute, 5150 Centre Avenue, Pittsburgh, PA 15232, USA

* Corresponding author.

E-mail address: vernetti@pitt.edu

In this article, we review the past applications of in vitro models in identifying human hepatotoxins and then focus on the use of multiscale experimental models in drug development, including the use of zebrafish and human cell-based, 3-dimensional (3D), microfluidic systems of liver functions as key components in applying Quantitative Systems Pharmacology (QSP). We have implemented QSP as a platform to improve the rate of success in the process of drug discovery and development of therapeutics.[1,2] Our working definition of QSP is "Determining the mechanism(s) of disease progression and mechanism(s) of action of drugs on multiscale systems through iterative and integrated computational and experimental methods to optimize the development of therapeutic strategies" (**Fig. 1**).

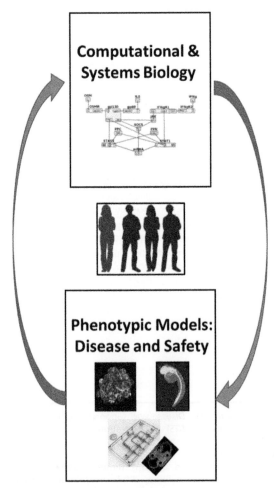

Fig. 1. QSP is an approach to drug discovery and development that applies iterative and integrated computational and experimental methods to determine the mechanism(s) of disease progression and mechanism(s) of action of drugs on multiscale systems. QSP starts with patients and patient samples, applies computational and experimental models, and ends with fundamental knowledge that optimizes therapeutic treatments for patients. This article focuses on the use of multiscale experimental models for liver toxicity and efficacy testing, especially phenotypic models.

The stakeholders involved in drug development from academia, industry, and government agencies have long understood the need to improve drug candidate selection by optimizing efficacy while screening out potential toxins so as to concentrate efforts on candidates with favorable chances for market approval. A survey of the number of new drugs released between 2000 and 2009 demonstrated a 25-year low in drug approvals despite increases in research and development (R&D) investment.[3] Laverty and colleagues[4] reported that 66% of failed clinical trials were due to a lack of efficacy and 21% for unacceptable drug toxicity. However, Sacks and colleagues[5] evaluated clinical drug trials between 2000 and 2012 using additional criteria to further refine the analysis and reported that lack of efficacy alone accounted for only 41% of failures, while the combination of poor efficacy and safety accounted for 35%, and safety alone accounted for 19% of drug failures. Together, cardiovascular and liver toxicity accounted for nearly 75% of all postmarket drug withdrawals in the United States between 1975 and 2007.[6] Although cardiotoxicity has recently surpassed hepatotoxicity as the main organ toxicity ending clinical trials or causing postmarket drug withdrawal, hepatotoxicity has been the most frequent cause of drug product recalls between 1953 and 2014.[7]

CURRENT STATUS OF DRUG HEPATOTOXICITY PREDICTION USING MAMMALIAN IN VIVO MODELS

The liver is responsible for a wide range of functions, including xenobiotic detoxification, protein synthesis, synthesis and storage of glucose, production of the bile necessary for digestion, and regulation of blood cholesterol and triglycerides. The organ is positioned downstream of the gastrointestinal tract to enable "first-pass" clearance of orally ingested drugs and toxins. The structural organization of the liver sinusoidal space facilitates close contact between circulating compounds and the transporter-rich hepatocyte membrane proteins that allow for rapid and efficient transport of drugs from the portal blood. The high capacity for biotransformation in the hepatocyte also facilitates the generation of reactive metabolites that can cause liver damage.[8]

The key data for assessing hepatotoxicity derives from drug safety study protocols approved by regulatory agencies. Although evidence suggests that preclinical animal studies can predict up to approximately 70% of human toxicity, several problems are apparent from this approach.[6] First, the traditional animal studies clearly fail to identify all possible adverse liver effects, because many compounds pass safely through animal testing only to be found hepatotoxic in the clinical trials or in the postmarketing. Second, the traditional drug safety protocols were designed only to ask broad questions with a simple yes or no answer; for example, is the compound hepatotoxic? Is the compound a reproductive toxin? Traditional preclinical drug safety assessments essentially ignored the why and the how of toxicity.[9] Historically, few efforts were made to link the observational results from drug safety studies to molecular and cell level events, mechanisms of toxicity (MOTs), or to interactions between tissues and organs.

Adherence to the regulatory agencies' drug safety protocols also failed to account for the poor concordance between animal and human organ toxicity (**Table 1**). The concordance can be as low as 40% for the liver to better than 90% for drugs with hematological liability.[10] A good demonstration of how animal testing failed to identify clinical hepatotoxic drugs is exemplified by a series of structurally similar and marketed drug pairs for the same therapeutic indication (**Table 2**). In each case, one of the drugs in the pair exhibited no hepatotoxicity during preclinical and clinical trials or in postmarket surveillance, but the other was "silent" during the animal studies,

Table 1
Concordance of animal and human organ toxicity

Target Organ	Concordance, %
Liver	40–54[10,52]
Cutaneous/Ophthalmic	36
Endocrine	60
Urinary tract	64
Neurologic	70
Cardiovascular	80
Gastrointestinal	85
Hematologic	91

Data from Olson H, Betton G, Robinson D, et al. Concordance of the toxicity of pharmaceuticals in humans and in animals. Regul Toxicol Pharmacol 2000;32(1):56–67.

yet induced hepatotoxicity in clinical trials or in the postmarket release. This discordance in the liver findings has been attributed to differences in the metabolism and metabolic clearance pathways between man and animal test species.[11]

After expensive postmarket drug recalls for Troglitazone and Bromfenac and the restrictive labeling for Trovafloxacin and Tolcapone, the pharmaceutical industry

Table 2
Clinical liver effects of structurally similar drugs found safe in animals

Human Liver Toxic Drug	Structure	Human Liver Safe Drug	Structure
Nefazodone		Trazodone	
Bromfenac		Diclofenac	
Alpidem		Zolpidem	
Trovafloxacin		Moxifloxacin	
Ibufenac		Ibuprofen	
Tolcapone		Entacapone	

initiated strategies to prescreen compounds for liver toxicity. In one example, the industry successfully implemented in vitro and specialized in vivo pharmacokinetic (PK) screening early in the lead optimization process. Although in 1993 nearly 39% of compounds failed in clinical trials due to poor PK, this fell dramatically to 7% by 2003 following implementation of early drug discovery PK profiling.[12] However, during the same period of time, the rate of compounds failing in the clinic due to toxicity rose from 10% to 16%.[12] Based on the success in PK profiling, it was projected that a strategy similar to early PK screening also would be successful in identifying and eliminating potential hepatotoxins before proceeding into preclinical testing.

IN VITRO MODELS FOR PREDICTING DRUG-INDUCED HEPATOTOXICITY

Many commonly used in vitro hepatotoxicity assays rely on subcellular liver fractions, established hepatoma cell lines, primary animal and human hepatocytes, liver slices, and whole perfused livers. The use of in vitro data from microsomes, primary hepatocytes and S9 subcellular fractions to predict in vivo drug clearance is generally a well-accepted procedure.[13,14] Whole perfused livers and liver slices on the other hand are low throughput, require continual usage of animals, are costly, and still suffer the lack of concordance with human toxic liabilities. These models have been reviewed elsewhere.[11]

Rodent and human primary hepatocytes have become a mainstay of hepatotoxicity testing in the in vitro laboratory.[11] Large numbers of healthy hepatocytes can be isolated from a single rat or from a human liver resection or autopsy. This has allowed moderate to high-throughput screening to identify potential hepatotoxins, while at the same time reducing animal use, amount of test agent, cost per compound tested, and the time required to make a toxic liability decision. The primary hepatocyte has been a convenient model for investigating MOT, pharmacokinetics, identification of metabolites, and dose response toxicity. However, an important limitation in the use of isolated primary hepatocytes is a reduction in function and differentiation after 24 to 48 hours in culture.[15] To avoid this issue, many in vitro hepatotoxicity tests have been conducted using established human hepatoma cell lines such as HepG2 and HepaRG or with immortalized primary hepatocytes such the Corning HepatoCell (Corning, NY).[16-18] The limitation to these cell types, however, is low or absent biotransformation for many of the important cytochrome P450 enzymes and phase II conjugation reactions involved in drug clearance.[11,19] The advantages and disadvantages of the more commonly used single-cell and cell fraction in vitro models are compared in **Table 3**.

The primary hepatocyte and immortalized hepatocytes have been used in 2D monolayers, 2D co-cultures, 3D single-cell type, and 3D co-cultures depending on the questions posed. Two-dimensional monolayer assays have been applied to collect simple cell death end points to triage large numbers of compounds.[11] In recent years, high-throughput screening (HTS) assays have been used to measure MOTs known to be relevant to mechanisms of clinical hepatotoxicity. The latter assay type, which is often referred to as "fit-for-purpose," tests compounds in a model designed solely to identify a specific mechanism of toxicity. Examples of "fit-for-purpose" hepatocyte assays include mitochondrial dysfunction, oxidative stress, bile salt exporter protein inhibition, covalent binding, and pregnane X receptor nuclear receptor modulation. These 5 mechanisms have a demonstrable association to increased risk for clinical hepatotoxicity.[20-24]

Although preclinical animal testing remains critical for Investigational New Drug and New Drug Application approval, a significant shift to alternative approaches using quantitative structure-activity relationships (QSAR) computational models, simple

Table 3
Commonly used cell and cellular fraction in vitro models for absorption, distribution, metabolism, excretion, and toxicity (ADMET)

Model	Application	Advantage	Disadvantage	Reference
Hepatocyte cell fractions microsomes	Liver clearance, metabolite ID	Fast, inexpensive, individual variation can be studied	Overestimates in vivo metabolism; only CYP and UGT enzymes	14,53
S9	Liver clearance, metabolite ID	Phase I and phase II activity	Lower enzyme activity in the S9 fraction, may miss low level metabolites	14
1° hepatocyte suspensions	Liver clearance, metabolite ID	In vivo levels of drug metabolism and transport proteins, cryopreservation	4-h time limit	19
Transgenic cell lines for PK	Metabolite ID	Single enzyme reactions generate high levels of metabolites for structural ID	Overestimate involvement of one enzyme species	14
Established liver cells lines HepG2	Toxicity testing, MOT, induction	Established cell line, inexpensive	Absence or low expression of most phase I and phase II enzymes	14,19
HepaRG	Toxicity testing, MOT, induction, metabolite ID	CYP1A2 and 3A4 inducible, established cell line	High CYP3A4, Cyp 7A1 expression, but low in all other CYP levels compared with primary hepatocytes	19,54
Primary Heps	PK, toxicity testing, metabolite ID	Well characterized, intact metabolism, intact transporters, cryopreservation	Decline in differentiated functions; no immune or fibrosis cells; single donor variation	14
Spheroids: established cell lines HepG2, HepaRG	PK, toxicity testing, metabolite ID	Extend differentiated cell functions from days to weeks, 3D, improved metabolism	Cell functions lower than primary hepatocytes, low urea, albumin production	55–57

Abbreviations: CYP, cytochrome p450; Heps, hepatocytes; MOT, mechanisms of toxicity; PK, pharmacokinetic; UGT, udp-glucuronosyltransferase.

in vitro cytotoxicity and "fit-for-purpose" HTS assays have been promoted by governmental agencies such as the Environmental Protection Agency, the National Center for the Advancement of Translational Sciences (NCATS), and the National Toxicology Program. These initiatives have resulted in the development of a number of databases (eg, Tox21, ToxCast) and models for prioritizing compounds based on HTS assay hepatotoxicity, as well as other organ toxicities.[25] In addition to the government initiatives, most R&D organizations in academia and the pharmaceutical industry have a slate of in vitro toxicity assays and computational approaches designed to eliminate unfavorable compounds early in the drug discovery process.[26]

PAST EXPERIENCES WITH IN VITRO LIVER ABSORPTION, DISTRIBUTION, METABOLISM, EXCRETION, AND TOXICITY MODELS PREDICTING HUMAN CLINICAL TOXICITY

The concordance of in vitro toxicity testing with clinical hepatotoxicity varies from only 25% for the simple in vitro assays to nearly 80% for the more complex assays and analyses.[17,27] **Table 4** presents a subset of computational approaches: in vitro 2D human cell-based HTS assays; a human cell co-culture model; and one in vitro covalent binding assay selected from a joint Food and Drug Administration (FDA) National Center for Toxicology Research, California Institute of Technology, and Hannover Medical School report which cross-validated the concordance of these methods to human drug-induced liver injury (DILI).[27] Three interesting findings are noteworthy from the results: (1) multiparametric cell-based models performed better than the computational or cell-free covalent binding assays; (2) the predictive result for DILI-negative drugs (assay specificity) was always higher than the predictive result for DILI-positive drugs (assay sensitivity); and (3) an apparent upper limit to the predicted DILI nearing 75% to 80% was reached with the existing in vitro cell-based systems.[27] A likely explanation for the plateau of predictive concordance of 80% with existing in vitro cell models is the reductionist strategy used to simplify the organized, multicellular complexity of the liver microenvironment to single-cell or even 2-cell type testing assays.

ZEBRAFISH LARVAE AS A LOW-COST, MEDIUM-THROUGHPUT, WHOLE-ORGANISM PLATFORM TO PREDICT DRUG HEPATOTOXICITY

The use of animals for experimentation, especially warm-blooded species, presents ethical concerns, and governing bodies now strive to implement the reduction, refinement, and replacement ("3R") of animals strategy in research.[28] The European Union Directive 2010/63/EU on the protection of animals used for scientific purposes requires the use of species with the lowest capacity to experience pain, suffering, and distress, and mandates that the smallest number of animals be used to obtain scientifically valid results. Studies in rodents are further limited by the high costs for acquisition and maintenance.

In recent years, there has been an increased recognition that in vitro phenotypic experimental cell models, as well as small multicellular organisms, can be used in the multiscale approach described as part of QSP.[1] Zebrafish in particular have attracted attention not only as a model for drug discovery, but also as a preclinical model for toxicity assessments.[29–32] Their prospective position in drug discovery and toxicity assessment is envisioned to be a bridge between simple cell-based and the still mandated mammalian testing.[33]

Zebrafish are uniquely positioned for large-scale experimentation. Zebrafish are vertebrate animals with high similarity to mammals, both organotypically and physiologically. They have a tractable, diploid genome that is 70% to 80% similar to humans and that is amenable to both forward and reverse genetics. Because of their small size, zebrafish, at the larval stage, are compatible with multiwell plate formats used in HTS, requiring only small amounts of compounds/drugs. Their high fecundity makes it possible to obtain large numbers of specimens for experimentation, dramatically reducing cost compared with rodent models. The zebrafish embryo therefore provides a cost-effective opportunity to discover potential drug liabilities using functional assays in a living animal as a complement to the emerging human tissue models.

The zebrafish embryonic liver is completely developed and functional by 72 hours post fertilization (hpf), as judged by organ appearance and functional markers, such

Table 4
Concordance of large-scale in vitro screening to human hepatotoxicity[a]

Model	Name/Type	# Compounds	Overall[b] Concordance, %	True Positives, %	True Negatives, %	Reference
In silico models						
Structural alert	DEREK[c]	623	56	46	73	58
QSAR/Molecular descriptors	4 commercial programs[d]	~1600	63	39	87	59
	2D molecular descriptor	382	76	76	75	60
	PaDel molecular descriptor[e]	1087	69	67	70	27,61
	ECF 6 molecular descriptors[f]	295	59	53	65	62
2D in vitro cell models						
HepG2	6 endpoint[g]	102	70	40	100	63
HepG2	11 endpoint[h]	136	76	N/A[i]	N/A	17
1° Human hepatocytes	4 endpoint[j]	344	75–80	50–60	95–100	64
Co-cultured 1° human hepatocytes, stromal cells	Micropattern surface 4 endpoint[k]	45	78	66	90	65
In vitro cell-free assays	Covalent binding assay-glutathione adduct formation	223	68	45	90	66

Abbreviations: QSAR, quantitative structure-activity relationship; 2D, 2-dimensional.

[a] Cross-validated results.
[b] Concordance = True positives (sensitivity) + true negatives (specificity)/2.
[c] DEREK - toxicity prediction software (Lhasa, Leeds, UK)
[d] MC4PC, MDL-QSAR, BioEpisteme, Predictive Data Miner.
[e] PaDel open source software for calculating molecular descriptors.
[f] ECF (extended connectivity functional fingerprints).
[g] Cell counts, nuclear area, plasma membrane integrity, lysosomal activity, mitochondrial membrane potential and mitochondrial area.
[h] Cell count, DNA degradation, nuclear size, cytoskeletal disruption, DNA damage response, oxidative stress, mitosis, stress kinase, mitochondrial membrane potential and area, cell cycle arrest. Results not cross validated.
[i] Not available.
[j] Cell count, mitochondrial damage, oxidative stress, and intracellular glutathione.
[k] Glutathione levels, ATP levels, albumin, and urea secretion.
Data from Chen M, Bisgin H, Tong L, et al. Toward predictive models for drug-induced liver injury in humans: are we there yet? Biomark Med 2014;8(2):201–13.

as phase I and phase 2 biotransformation capabilities, serum protein secretion, glycogen storage, and lipogenesis.[34–36] Importantly, transgenic zebrafish larvae expressing human Cyp3A4 have been developed and will find use in PK and toxicity testing.[37]

Assays for zebrafish hepatotoxicity have thus far mainly been observational. In zebrafish larvae, necrotic cells can be visually identified by a change in appearance from translucency to opaque black.[31] A major shortcoming of macroscopic cell death assays is that they are not sensitive enough to detect early toxicity.[38] Nonetheless, a variant of this methodology using liver degeneration, changes in size, and yolk sac retention as endpoints has recently been published and shown to predict 8 of 8 known hepatotoxicants.[39] Changes in liver appearance, for example, cellular organization, interactions, and shape, also can be detected by histopathology from tissue slices, although this method is time-consuming, requires a trained pathologist, and therefore is usually reserved to validate observations by other measurements. Last, hepatotoxicity can be assessed in the adult zebrafish using canonical liver enzyme assays (eg, alanine aminotransferase), although the use of adults eliminates the convenience, ethical impact, and high-throughput compatibility that embryos offer.[40] Our own data suggest that even gross organism toxicity, assessed by visual inspection of morphologic changes in 72 hpf larvae (ie, bent tails, distended peritoneum and edema, pericardial congestion) can distinguish hepatotoxic from nontoxic agents (**Table 5**).

Zebrafish toxicity research is now shifting from observational to mechanism-based toxicity assays. Mesens and colleagues[41] explored a molecular endpoint that captures effects on lipid metabolism because liver injury is frequently associated with perturbations in lipid metabolism. Hence, the group looked at expression of liver-specific fatty acid binding protein 10a (L-FABP 10a) as a molecular biomarker for hepatotoxicity and found that changes in expression were predictive of specific mechanisms. A corollary example was recently published by Verstraelen and colleagues,[42] in which they evaluated the expression of 5 liver-specific genes (including 2 apoptosis, and 2

Table 5
Gross morphologic observations in zebrafish larvae identify known toxicants including hepatotoxic amiodarone

Compound/ Dose Range	Gross Morphology	Concentration, μM						
Dose range		200	66	20	6.6	2	0.66	DMSO
Menadione	Live/dead[a]	0/4	0/4	0/4	4/0	4/0	4/0	4/0
	Visual toxicity[b]				1/4	2/4	0/4	0/4
Amiodarone	Live/dead	0/4	0/4	4/0	4/0	4/0	4/0	4/0
	Visual toxicity			2/4	3/4	0/4	1/4	0/4
Dose range		1000	300	100	30	10	3	DMSO
Caffeine	Live/dead	4/0	4/0	4/0	4/0	4/0	4/0	4/0
	Visual toxicity	3/4	4/4	0/4	0/4	0/4	0/4	0/4
Dose range		20	6.6	?	0.66	0.2	0.07	DMSO
CCCP	Live/dead	1/4	4/0	4/0	4/0	4/0	4/0	4/0
	Visual toxicity	0/1	2/4	3/4	3/4	4/4	2/4	0/4
Rotenone	Live/dead	1/4	3/4	4/0	4/0	4/0	4/0	4/0
	Visual toxicity	1/1	0/3	1/4	2/4	3/4	2/4	0/4

Abbreviations: CCCP, Carbonyl cyandide m-chorophenyl hydrazone; DMSO, dimethyl sulfoxide.
[a] Translucent (live), Opaque (dead).
[b] Bent tail, distended peritoneum, edema, pericardial congestion.

metabolism-related) following exposure with 5 known toxicants. Their results confirmed those of Mesens and colleagues[41] with L-FABP 10a and further documented that biomarker responses are compound-dependent, mechanism-dependent, and concentration-dependent. At the present time, the utility of biomarkers for prediction of toxicity appears to have potential in "fit-for-purpose" studies. If highly predictive biomarkers can be found, the zebrafish offers the opportunity to generate transgenic reporter lines that would greatly increase throughput.

Our own work has embraced adaptation of in vitro, human mechanism-based toxicity models and screening in zebrafish. In addition to morphologic observations (see **Table 5**), this suite of assays includes measurements of reactive oxygen species (ROS) and mitochondrial membrane perturbations because they are very good predictors of clinical toxicity.[24] **Fig. 2** illustrates the utility of ROS measurements in zebrafish larvae using menadione. Menadione is a naphthoquinone that generates ROS in cells through redox cycling. Menadione caused time-dependent and dose-dependent generation of ROS in zebrafish that correlated with embryonal toxicity and ROS induction and death in cultured hepatocytes, although there were quantitative differences between these types of models, likely due to differences in drug uptake, glutathione levels, and possibly metabolism. Additional development of these methods is required.

CASE STUDY: USING "FIT-FOR-PURPOSE" ASSAY EVALUATIONS TO RANK-ORDER COMPOUNDS

Given the limits to predicting human hepatotoxicity from current in vitro and in vivo methods, additional improvements to the test systems and analytical methods are needed to select better compounds for preclinical testing. A case study is presented

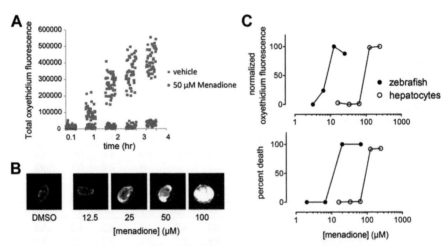

Fig. 2. ROS generation correlates with death in zebrafish larvae and rat hepatocytes. (A) Zebrafish larvae at 72 hpf were arrayed in 96-well microplates, loaded with dihydroethidium (DHE) for 30 minutes, and treated with menadione (50 μM). At the indicated time points, plates were scanned and analyzed for red oxyethidium fluorescence on an ArrayScan VTi high-content reader (ThermoFisher, Waltham, MA, USA). (B) Fluorescence micrographs of dose-dependent menadione-induced oxyethidium generation at 48 hpf. (C) Zebrafish larvae at 72 hpf (*closed circles*) or cultured rat hepatocytes (*open circles*) were treated in 96-well plates with various concentrations of menadione and oxyethidium fluorescence quantified. Toxicity correlated with production of ROS in both zebrafish embryos and hepatocytes.

to Illustrate one strategy used at the University of Pittsburgh Drug Discovery Institute to rank-order compounds for hepatotoxicity risk. Compounds are screened through zebrafish embryos and a set of in vitro "fit-for-purpose" cytotoxicity and mechanism of toxicity assays are then applied (**Fig. 3**). Rank ordering does not rely on any one single assay, but as a profile of risk factors calculated from the safety margin (the ratio of toxic level to therapeutic level) categorically binned into high, moderate, or low risk. The development of this approach was an extension of the time-dependent and concentration-dependent multiplexed MOT endpoint assays for mitochondrial function, oxidative stress, and cytotoxicity analyses developed and validated in the Cell-Ciphr HepG2 and primary hepatocyte toxicity panels. Our use of the safety margin to classify risk, taken together with a Pfizer study that reported an increase in concordance between in vitro assays and clinical hepatotoxicity with drugs that induced 2 or more MOTs, suggested that some improvements are possible.[17,23,43] In the case study described here, the chance of clinical hepatotoxicity increases in compounds with more high and moderate risk factors.

EMERGENCE OF HUMAN TISSUE AND ORGAN MODELS

For the reasons presented previously, new strategies are required to better identify hepatotoxic compounds, especially chronic toxicity, as well as to develop better

SAR Compound Seriess Rank Ordered by Hepatotoxicity Risk

Compound	ZebraFish Embryo μM ALD[a]	HepG2 1h mito function μM IC50	HepG2 72h cytotoxicity μM IC50	Primary Hepatocytes 1h mito function μM IC50	Primary Hepatocytes 4h ROS μM IC50	Primary Hepatocytes 5-d Cytotoxicity μM IC50	cLogP	pKa
Cmpd 1							4.16	2.41
Cmpd 2							2.75	2.22
Cmpd 3			34				2.54	2.21
Cmpd 4			73				1.59	3.38
Cmpd 5		48	169	284			2.37	3.39
Cmpd 6			49			155	4.03	2.21
Cmpd 7		169	28			280	4.03	2.21
Cmpd 8		70	202				4.61	3.77
Cmpd 9			16				2.92	3.4
Cmpd 10	86		183		197	210	3.74	5.28
Cmpd 11		11	160				3.48	2.41
Cmpd 12	21	35	75				4.24	2.22
Cmpd 13	21	20	24			140	4.61	4.61
Cmpd 14	5	8	18	80	143	147	4.16	2.42
Cmpd 15	6.2	25	15				5.05	4.91
Cmpd 16	<9[b]	4	6	2	180	230	5.86	2.42
Cmpd 17	0.3	2	31	10	6	62	4.46	2.42
Cmpd 18	5	8	7	33	17	63	4.82	2.43
Cmpd 19	14	6	11	13	15	45	4.92	2.42

Less Risk ↑ **More Risk**

Color Coded Safety Margin

<10 X Cmax | 10–30 X Cmax | >30 Cmax

Fig. 3. Case use of multiple "fit-for-purpose" assays to determine hepatotoxicity risk. The concentration of inhibitor in which the response is reduced by half (IC_{50}) results from 6 different assays in zebrafish, HepG2 and primary hepatocytes are used to calculate the safety margin, defined as the toxic IC_{50} response/Cmax blood concentration. The lower the safety window the higher the risk for hepatotoxicity. To rank-order compounds, the safety margin is categorized into high (*red*), moderate (*yellow*), or low (*green*) risk to generate the heat map. The overall rank order is determined by the number of high and moderate risks. [a] Acute lethal dose at which one-half of zebrafish embryos are dead by 24-hour exposure. [b] Drug quantity not sufficient (QNS) to repeat study to calculate safety margin.

human efficacy and disease models. The development of biomimetic, multicellular, 3D, microfluidic microphysiology models of the human liver and other organs are in development.[44,45]

Cellular responses to drugs in the intact human organ are more accurately represented by 3D human cell cultures than the traditional static 2D cell cultures, with additional advantages provided by the inclusion of media perfusion to provide nutrients, oxygen, chemicals, and remove waste products.[46–48] Researchers are now capitalizing on the increased availability of human primary, immortalized, or induced pluripotent stem cell (iPSC)-derived hepatocytes, new bioengineering materials, microfabrication techniques, and microfluidic devices to construct reasonable representations of the adult human liver acinus in 3D multicellular microphysiological systems (MPS).[48,49] These MPS can be maintained for a month or longer, allowing chronic, as well as acute, responses to drug challenges. In our recent study, we demonstrated acute and chronic drug effects, including the induction of fibrosis by methotrexate and the induction of immune-mediated hepatotoxicity.[48] A comparison of some current static and perfused 3D, multicell models are presented in **Table 6**.

Of particular interest to those who study hepatotoxicity is the creation of a "liver on a chip" with iPSC-derived adult hepatocytes from patients who have susceptibility to DILI events or other defined genetic and disease backgrounds. This would place liver MPS platforms at the center of personalized medicine and in the continuum of the QSP approach to drug discovery and evaluation of disease progression.[1,2] The potential ramifications and promises of this new paradigm for drug discovery, disease progression, and toxicity assessments are discussed in more detail in the Prospectus.

PROSPECTUS: MOVING TO THE FUTURE: INTEGRATING THE HUMAN LIVER ON A CHIP, COMPUTATIONAL MODELS, AND QUANTITATIVE SYSTEMS PHARMACOLOGY

Collectively, the limited concordance of laboratory animal drug safety testing with human safety, the apparent 80% limit of success of human-based 2D in vitro models and the 65% to 75% rate of success with computational models to predict drug-induced clinical hepatotoxicity has shifted the focus to the creation of human, 3D, microfluidic systems, referred to as MPS. One such platform has been developed at the University of Pittsburgh Drug Discovery Institute and integrates an MPS liver model using 4 human liver cell types organized into a microfluidic, 3D, sinusoidal complex, with the capacity for live cell monitoring of MOT using fluorescence-based biosensors over a period of several weeks. Secreted proteins, cytokines, and metabolites collected from the efflux are analyzed by biochemical assays and mass spectrometry along with the results from imaging biosensors for parameters such as apoptosis, ROS production, and free calcium levels. All of the data are linked in a database designed to collect, manage, and model the data (**Fig. 4**). Integrated human MPS platforms that are biomimetics of normal organ structure and function have the potential to improve on the current predictive limit (approximately 80%) and diminish the odds of "silent" human hepatotoxins from being introduced into clinical trials or the market.

Continued improvements to the MPS liver models will include the application of renewable cells (eg, human iPSC-derived adult hepatocytes, as well as the nonparenchymal cells) to permit the investigation of the heterogeneous human genetic backgrounds, as well as specific diseases (eg, nonalcoholic fatty liver disease, hepatocarcinoma, and rare childhood liver diseases). Further advances also will

Table 6
Examples of multicellular static and microfluidic liver models for absorption, distribution, metabolism, excretion, and toxicity (ADMET) testing

Model	Application	Advantage	Disadvantage	References
Static models				
Co-culture spheroids	Stellate cell activation	Long term 3D culturing with improved drug metabolism and output of albumin, urea	Specialized plates to from spheroids, specialized culturing techniques	67
Co-culture micropatterned primary hepatocytes with fibroblasts	Hepatotoxicity Metabolite ID Disease models	Hepatocytes maintain differentiated function 2–3 wk	2D cultures, specialized plates	65,68
Four-cell spheroids primary hepatocytes, primary liver NPC	Hepatotoxicity Metabolite ID	Hepatocytes maintain differentiated function >3 wk, 3D, immune-mediated toxicity	Specialized culturing techniques	69
3D microfluidic, multicellular liver models				
Primary hepatocytes, endothelial cells	Hepatotoxicity	Hepatocytes maintain differentiated function >3 wk, microfluidic improves function	Specialized culturing techniques, perfusion system	70
Hepatocytes, endothelial cells, stellate cells, Kupffer-like immune cells	PK, toxicity, therapeutic intervention, liver disease model	Hepatocytes maintain differentiated function >3 wk, immune-mediated toxicity, fibrosis activation microfluidic improves function	Specialized culturing techniques, perfusion system	48,51,71

Abbreviations: 2D, 2 dimensional; 3D, 3 dimensional; NPC, non parenchymal cells; PK, pharmacokinetic.

include liver metabolic zonation and higher throughput arrays of MPS. The microphysiology database also will continue to evolve as a tool to manage, mine, and model the experimental data, as well as public sources of preclinical and clinical findings, expert-based drug knowledge, physical properties, pharmacology targets, adverse event reporting, and large datasets from "omics," including toxicogenomics, metabolomics, proteomics, reactive metabolite proteomics, and transcriptomics.[50] Furthermore, QSP is expected to increase our understanding of the integrated and interacting cellular, tissue, and organ networks; genes; proteins; and metabolic processes that give rise to liver disease progression, therapeutic efficacy, and drug-induced hepatotoxicity.[1,50]

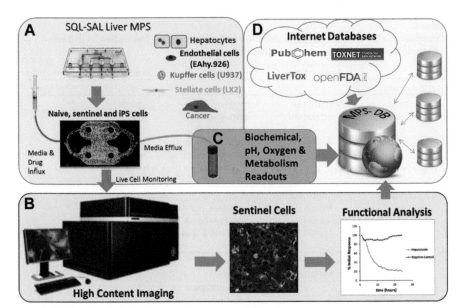

Fig. 4. Overview of the Human Liver Microphysiology Platform for studying human liver physiology, disease models and drug safety testing. The platform is composed of the following: (*A*) the Sequentially Layered, *Self-Assembly Liver* model (SQL-SAL) constructed from a microfluidic device and 4 human cell types, a fraction of which are "sentinel" cells expressing fluorescence-based biosensors, and that can include disease-specific cells, such as cancer cells. Data are collected from the model via (*B*) high-content imaging readouts of transmitted light contrast and fluorescence; and (*C*) biochemical and mass spectrometry readouts.[48,51] (*D*) The multiplexed data are uploaded into the *Microphysiology Systems Database* (MPS-Db) to manage data, associate external data sources, and build predictive models of human efficacy and toxicity.[50]

REFERENCES

1. Stern AM, Schurdak ME, Bahar I, et al. A perspective on implementing a quantitative systems pharmacology platform for drug discovery and the advancement of personalized medicine. J Biomol Screen 2016;21(6):521–34.
2. Sorger PK, Allerheiligen SBR, Abernathy DR, et al. Quantitative and systems pharmacology in the post-genomic era: new approaches to discovering drugs and understanding therapeutic mechanisms. In an NIH white paper by the QSP workshop group – October, 2011. Bethesda (MD): NIH; 2011. Ward R, Editor.
3. Kaitin KI, DiMasi JA. Pharmaceutical innovation in the 21st century: new drug approvals in the first decade, 2000-2009. Clin Pharmacol Ther 2011;89(2):183–8.
4. Laverty H, Benson C, Cartwright E, et al. How can we improve our understanding of cardiovascular safety liabilities to develop safer medicines? Br J Pharmacol 2011;163(4):675–93.
5. Sacks LV, Shamsuddin HH, Yasinskaya YI, et al. Scientific and regulatory reasons for delay and denial of FDA approval of initial applications for new drugs, 2000-2012. JAMA 2014;311(4):378–84.
6. Stevens JL, Baker TK. The future of drug safety testing: expanding the view and narrowing the focus. Drug Discov Today 2009;14(3–4):162–7.

7. Onakpoya IJ, Heneghan CJ, Aronson JK. Post-marketing withdrawal of 462 medicinal products because of adverse drug reactions: a systematic review of the world literature. BMC Med 2016;14:10.

8. Yuan L, Kaplowitz N. Mechanisms of drug-induced liver injury. Clin Liver Dis 2013;17(4):507–18, vii.

9. Doull J, Bruce M. General principles of toicology. In: Klaassen CD, editor. Cassertt and Doull's toxicology: the basic science of poisons. New York: Macmillan Publishing Company; 1986. p. 11–32.

10. Olson H, Betton G, Robinson D, et al. Concordance of the toxicity of pharmaceuticals in humans and in animals. Regul Toxicol Pharmacol 2000;32(1):56–67.

11. Godoy P, Hewitt NJ, Albrecht U, et al. Recent advances in 2D and 3D in vitro systems using primary hepatocytes, alternative hepatocyte sources and non-parenchymal liver cells and their use in investigating mechanisms of hepatotoxicity, cell signaling and ADME. Arch Toxicol 2013;87(8):1315–530.

12. Kubinyi H. Drug research: myths, hype and reality. Nat Rev Drug Discov 2003; 2(8):665–8.

13. Ito K, Houston JB. Comparison of the use of liver models for predicting drug clearance using in vitro kinetic data from hepatic microsomes and isolated hepatocytes. Pharm Res 2004;21(5):785–92.

14. Brandon EF, Raap CD, Meijerman I, et al. An update on in vitro test methods in human hepatic drug biotransformation research: pros and cons. Toxicol Appl Pharmacol 2003;189(3):233–46.

15. Soldatow VY, Lecluyse EL, Griffith LG, et al. In vitro models for liver toxicity testing. Toxicol Res (Camb) 2013;2(1):23–39.

16. Mennecozzi M, et al. Hepatotoxicity screening taking a mode-of-action approach using HepaRG cells and HCA. Altex Proceedings 2012;1:193–204.

17. Vernetti L, et al. Cellular systems biology applied to preclinical safety testing: a case study of CellCiphr™ profiling. In: Ekins S, Xu JJ, editors. Drug efficacy, safety, and biologics discovery: Emerging technologies and tools. Hoboken (NJ): John Wiley & Sons; 2009. p. 53–73.

18. Faris RA, Hong YL, Liu J, et al. Corning (R) hepatocell-cells closely model the behavior of parental cells for predicting hepatotoxicity. In drug metabolism reviews. Abingdon (United Kingdom): Taylor & Francis Ltd; 2015.

19. Bi YA, Kazolias D, Duignan DB. Use of cryopreserved human hepatocytes in sandwich culture to measure hepatobiliary transport. Drug Metab Dispos 2006; 34(9):1658–65.

20. Wang YM, Chai SC, Brewer CT, et al. Pregnane X receptor and drug-induced liver injury. Expert Opin Drug Metab Toxicol 2014;10(11):1521–32.

21. Usui T, Mise M, Hashizume T, et al. Evaluation of the potential for drug-induced liver injury based on in vitro covalent binding to human liver proteins. Drug Metab Dispos 2009;37(12):2383–92.

22. Will Y, Dykens J. Mitochondrial toxicity assessment in industry–a decade of technology development and insight. Expert Opin Drug Metab Toxicol 2014;10(8): 1061–7.

23. Aleo MD, Luo Y, Swiss R, et al. Human drug-induced liver injury severity is highly associated with dual inhibition of liver mitochondrial function and bile salt export pump. Hepatology 2014;60(3):1015–22.

24. Pereira CV, Nadanaciva S, Oliveira PJ, et al. The contribution of oxidative stress to drug-induced organ toxicity and its detection in vitro and in vivo. Expert Opin Drug Metab Toxicol 2012;8(2):219–37.

25. Collins FS, Gray GM, Bucher JR. Toxicology. Transforming environmental health protection. Science 2008;319(5865):906–7.
26. Blomme EA, Will Y. Toxicology strategies for drug discovery: present and future. Chem Res Toxicol 2016;29(4):473–504.
27. Chen M, Bisgin H, Tong L, et al. Toward predictive models for drug-induced liver injury in humans: are we there yet? Biomark Med 2014;8(2):201–13.
28. Russell WMS, Burch RL. The principles of humane experimental technique. London: Methuen; 1959. p. 238.
29. Rubinstein AL. Zebrafish assays for drug toxicity screening. Expert Opin Drug Metab Toxicol 2006;2(2):231–40.
30. McGrath P, Li CQ. Zebrafish: a predictive model for assessing drug-induced toxicity. Drug Discov Today 2008;13(9–10):394–401.
31. Hill A, Mesens N, Steemans M, et al. Comparisons between in vitro whole cell imaging and in vivo zebrafish-based approaches for identifying potential human hepatotoxicants earlier in pharmaceutical development. Drug Metab Rev 2012; 44(1):127–40.
32. Zon LI, Peterson RT. In vivo drug discovery in the zebrafish. Nat Rev Drug Discov 2005;4(1):35–44.
33. Parng C. In vivo zebrafish assays for toxicity testing. Curr Opin Drug Discov Devel 2005;8(1):100–6.
34. Chu J, Sadler KC. New school in liver development: lessons from zebrafish. Hepatology 2009;50(5):1656–63.
35. Behra M, Etard C, Cousin X, et al. The use of zebrafish mutants to identify secondary target effects of acetylcholine esterase inhibitors. Toxicol Sci 2004; 77(2):325–33.
36. Jones HS, Panter GH, Hutchinson TH, et al. Oxidative and conjugative xenobiotic metabolism in zebrafish larvae in vivo. Zebrafish 2010;7(1):23–30.
37. Poon KL, Wang X, Ng AS, et al. Humanizing the zebrafish liver shifts drug metabolic profiles and improves pharmacokinetics of CYP3A4 substrates. Arch Toxicol 2016. [Epub ahead of print].
38. Wolf JC, Wolfe MJ. A brief overview of nonneoplastic hepatic toxicity in fish. Toxicol Pathol 2005;33(1):75–85.
39. He JH, Guo SY, Zhu F, et al. A zebrafish phenotypic assay for assessing drug-induced hepatotoxicity. J Pharmacol Toxicol Methods 2013;67(1):25–32.
40. Murtha JM, Qi W, Keller ET. Hematologic and serum biochemical values for zebrafish (Danio rerio). Comp Med 2003;53(1):37–41.
41. Mesens N, Crawford AD, Menke A, et al. Are zebrafish larvae suitable for assessing the hepatotoxicity potential of drug candidates? J Appl Toxicol 2015;35(9): 1017–29.
42. Verstraelen S, Peers B, Maho W, et al. Phenotypic and biomarker evaluation of zebrafish larvae as an alternative model to predict mammalian hepatotoxicity. J Appl Toxicol 2016;36:1194–206.
43. Abraham VC, Towne DL, Waring JF, et al. Application of a high-content multiparameter cytotoxicity assay to prioritize compounds based on toxicity potential in humans. J Biomol Screen 2008;13(6):527–37.
44. Bhatia SN, Ingber DE. Microfluidic organs-on-chips. Nature 2014;201:4.
45. Wikswo J. Annual thematic issue: the biology and medicine of microphysiological systems [special issue]. Exp Biol Med 2014;239(9):1061–3.
46. Nam KH, Smith AS, Lone S, et al. Biomimetic 3D tissue models for advanced high-throughput drug screening. J Lab Autom 2015;20(3):201–15.

47. Ouattara DA, Choi SH, Sakai Y, et al. Kinetic modelling of in vitro cell-based assays to characterize non-specific bindings and ADME processes in a static and a perfused fluidic system. Toxicol Lett 2011;205(3):310–9.

48. Vernetti LA, Senutovitch N, Boltz R, et al. A human liver microphysiology platform for investigating physiology, drug safety, and disease models. Exp Biol Med (Maywood) 2016;241(1):101–14.

49. Sarkar U, Rivera-Burgos D, Large EM, et al. Metabolite profiling and pharmacokinetic evaluation of hydrocortisone in a perfused three-dimensional human liver bioreactor. Drug Metab Dispos 2015;43(7):1091–9.

50. Gough A, Vernetti L, Bergenthal L, et al. The microphysiology systems database for analyzing and modeling compound interactions with human and animal organ models. Applied In Vitro Toxicology 2016;2(2):103–17.

51. Senutovitch N, Vernetti L, Boltz R, et al. Fluorescent protein biosensors applied to microphysiological systems. Exp Biol Med (Maywood) 2015;240(6):795–808.

52. Cross H, Tower B. Pre-market evaluation of hepatotoxicity in health products, Health Canada Guidance document # 12-104742-88, 2012.

53. Jia L, Liu X. The conduct of drug metabolism studies considered good practice (II): in vitro experiments. Curr Drug Metab 2007;8(8):822–9.

54. Kanebratt KP, Andersson TB. Evaluation of HepaRG cells as an in vitro model for human drug metabolism studies. Drug Metab Dispos 2008;36(7):1444–52.

55. Ramaiahgari SC, den Braver MW, Herpers B, et al. A 3D in vitro model of differentiated HepG2 cell spheroids with improved liver-like properties for repeated dose high-throughput toxicity studies. Arch Toxicol 2014;88(5):1083–95.

56. Wang Z, Luo X, Anene-Nzelu C, et al. HepaRG culture in tethered spheroids as an in vitro three-dimensional model for drug safety screening. J Appl Toxicol 2015;35(8):909–17.

57. Lubberstedt M, Müller-Vieira U, Mayer M, et al. HepaRG human hepatic cell line utility as a surrogate for primary human hepatocytes in drug metabolism assessment in vitro. J Pharmacol Toxicol Methods 2011;63(1):59–68.

58. Greene N, Fisk L, Naven RT, et al. Developing structure-activity relationships for the prediction of hepatotoxicity. Chem Res Toxicol 2010;23(7):1215–22.

59. Matthews EJ, Ursem CJ, Kruhlak NL, et al. Identification of structure-activity relationships for adverse effects of pharmaceuticals in humans: part B. Use of (Q) SAR systems for early detection of drug-induced hepatobiliary and urinary tract toxicities. Regul Toxicol Pharmacol 2009;54(1):23–42.

60. Cheng A, Dixon SL. In silico models for the prediction of dose-dependent human hepatotoxicity. J Comput Aided Mol Des 2003;17(12):811–23.

61. Liew CY, Lim YC, Yap CW. Mixed learning algorithms and features ensemble in hepatotoxicity prediction. J Comput Aided Mol Des 2011;25(9):855–71.

62. Ekins S, Williams AJ, Xu JJ. A predictive ligand-based Bayesian model for human drug-induced liver injury. Drug Metab Dispos 2010;38(12):2302–8.

63. Persson M, Løye AF, Mow T, et al. A high content screening assay to predict human drug-induced liver injury during drug discovery. J Pharmacol Toxicol Methods 2013;68(3):302–13.

64. Xu JJ, Henstock PV, Dunn MC, et al. Cellular imaging predictions of clinical drug-induced liver injury. Toxicol Sci 2008;105(1):97–105.

65. Khetani SR, Kanchagar C, Ukairo O, et al. Use of micropatterned cocultures to detect compounds that cause drug-induced liver injury in humans. Toxicol Sci 2013;132(1):107–17.

66. Sakatis MZ, Reese MJ, Harrell AW, et al. Preclinical strategy to reduce clinical hepatotoxicity using in vitro bioactivation data for >200 compounds. Chem Res Toxicol 2012;25(10):2067–82.
67. Basu A, Saito K, Meyer K, et al. Stellate cell apoptosis by a soluble mediator from immortalized human hepatocytes. Apoptosis 2006;11(8):1391–400.
68. Khetani SR, Bhatia SN. Microscale culture of human liver cells for drug development. Nat Biotechnol 2008;26(1):120–6.
69. Messner S, Agarkova I, Moritz W, et al. Multi-cell type human liver microtissues for hepatotoxicity testing. Arch Toxicol 2013;87(1):209–13.
70. Schutte J, Hagmeyer B, Holzner F, et al. Artificial micro organs–a microfluidic device for dielectrophoretic assembly of liver sinusoids. Biomed Microdevices 2011;13(3):493–501.
71. Prodanov L, Jindal R, Bale SS, et al. Long-term maintenance of a microfluidic 3D human liver sinusoid. Biotechnol Bioeng 2016;113(1):241–6.

Moving?

Make sure your subscription moves with you!

To notify us of your new address, find your **Clinics Account Number** (located on your mailing label above your name), and contact customer service at:

Email: journalscustomerservice-usa@elsevier.com

800-654-2452 (subscribers in the U.S. & Canada)
314-447-8871 (subscribers outside of the U.S. & Canada)

Fax number: 314-447-8029

Elsevier Health Sciences Division
Subscription Customer Service
3251 Riverport Lane
Maryland Heights, MO 63043

ELSEVIER

Printed and bound by CPI Group (UK) Ltd, Croydon, CR0 4YY

03/10/2024

01040392-0006